T0402079

Hematologic Malignancies

Tiziano Barbui • Ayalew Tefferi
Editors

Myeloproliferative Neoplasms

Critical Concepts and Management

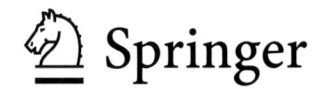 Springer

Editors
Prof. Dr. Tiziano Barbui
Research Foundation
Ospedale Maggiore (FROM)
and Hematology Department
Ospedali Riuniti
Bergamo
Italy
tbarbui@ospedaliriuniti.bergamo.it

Ayalew Tefferi, MD
Division of Hematology
Department of Medicine
Mayo Clinic
Rochester, MN
USA
tefferi.ayalew@mayo.edu

ISBN 978-3-642-24988-4   e-ISBN 978-3-642-24989-1
DOI 10.1007/978-3-642-24989-1
Springer Heidelberg Dordrecht London New York

British Library Cataloguing in Publication Data
A catalogue record for this book is available from the British Library

Library of Congress Control Number: 2012930007

Springer is part of Springer Science+Business Media (www.springer.com)

On behalf of all contributing authors who have sacrificed their valuable time, we dedicate this book to all patients with myeloproliferative neoplasms and acknowledge their tremendous courage and tenacity.

Barbui
Tefferi

Contents

Part I
Biology

Update on the Biology of Myeloproliferative Neoplasms

1

Robert Kralovics

Contents

R. Kralovics
Center for Molecular Medicine (CeMM)
of the Austrian Academy of Sciences, Vienna, Austria

Division of Hematology and Blood Coagulation,
Department of Internal Medicine I,
Medical University of Vienna, Vienna, Austria
e-mail: robert.kralovics@cemm.oeaw.ac.at

1.1 Introduction

Single cell origin of hematopoiesis is considered to be a hallmark of all myeloid malignancies. In hematological malignancies, the mutations initiating stem cell clonality can have various forms such as translocated chromosomes, chromosomes with deleted or amplified regions, or point mutations in single genes. Once a stem cell clone has been established, it expands and its progeny competes with healthy cells for "habitat" in the bone marrow microenvironment. As the clone expands, more mutagenesis occurs in the next generation of cells. Although vast majority of these newly acquired genomic mutations do not provide any benefit to the clone, some lesions may prove to be useful and provide a selective advantage. Therefore, selection is the main driving force that shapes the cancer genome in the given environment. Different tissues have different selective forces that evolve the cancer genome. In hematological malignancies, the stem cell clone of each patient takes on a unique evolutionary path even though the accompanying genetic defects are often recurrently detected when many myeloid cancer genomes are compared. The mutations acquired in the evolution of the myeloid cancer genome and their combined effects may have different influence on the differentiation dynamics of the hematopoietic progenitors. Some mutations reduce and others may increase the output of the terminally differentiated cells. Each clonal evolution has a certain phenotypic outcome often detectable by differential blood count and histopathologic evaluation of the

T. Barbui and A. Tefferi (eds.), *Myeloproliferative Neoplasms*, Hematologic Malignancies,
DOI 10.1007/978-3-642-24989-1_1, © Springer-Verlag Berlin Heidelberg 2012

bone marrow. The clinical classification of these different phenotypic outcomes provided the foundations for diagnosis in the past. Inclusion of the genetic defects that associate with certain clinical entity into the diagnosis has brought significant improvements in the diagnostic process. The developments in the field of myeloproliferative neoplasms (MPN) in the past decade are an excellent example of this process.

MPN represent a phenotypically diverse group of hematological malignancies. MPN are characterized by a single or multilineage overproduction of terminally differentiated blood elements and pronounced predisposition to thrombosis, bleeding, and leukemic transformation. There are three major MPN phenotypes characterized by distinct clinical features: polycythemia vera (PV), essential thrombocythemia (ET), and primary myelofibrosis (PMF). The vast majority of patients have a stable disease often lasting many years. However, the chronic phase phenotype may progress to a stage characterized by secondary (post-PV or post-ET) myelofibrosis, variable degrees of pancytopenia, and accumulation of blasts in the bone marrow and peripheral blood. Further evolution of this stage results in acute leukemia. Although there were certain exceptions described, the majority of myeloid cells in MPN have single cell origin and are derived from a stem cell clone dominating the productive myelopoiesis. MPN is a phenotypic outcomes of clonal stem cell evolution driven by a certain set of somatic mutations. Mutations of the JAK2 kinase gene are found in approximately two thirds of patients with MPN (Baxter et al. 2005; James et al. 2005; Kralovics et al. 2005; Levine et al. 2005). Almost all patients with PV carry JAK2 kinase mutations, whereas only about half of PMF and ET cases test positive for JAK2 mutations. Only a minority of PMF and ET cases carry mutations of the thrombopoietin receptor gene MPL (Beer et al. 2008; Pardanani et al. 2006; Pikman et al. 2006). JAK2 and MPL oncogenic mutations are often preceded or followed by cytogenetic lesions such as deletions or chromosomal gains (Kralovics 2008). Cytogenetic lesions in MPN contribute to clonal outgrowth and have a potential to contribute to the overall clinical phenotype. Despite recent efforts to define the mutation profile of MPN patients, about one third of MPN cases do not carry a detectable cytogenetic lesion or mutations in JAK2 or MPL. Many studies are ongoing that focus on this "gap" in MPN biology. New genetic lesions with diagnostic value will likely emerge in the near future.

1.2 Diversity of Gene Defects in the Pathogenesis of MPN

Despite a number of newly discovered somatic defects in the MPN pathogenesis, JAK2 and MPL mutations remain the most prominent and show highest specificity for MPN. High-resolution mapping of deletions on chromosome 4 led to the identification of TET2 – an important tumor suppressor gene in most myeloid malignancies including MPN (Delhommeau et al. 2009). In addition to deletions of TET2, loss-of-function point mutations occur even more frequently than deletions. TET2 mutations are detectable in about 13% of MPN patients depending on the studied cohort and MPN entity with highest frequencies observed in PV and PMF (up to 20%) (Delhommeau et al. 2009; Tefferi et al. 2009a, b). TET2 deletions occur in about 3% of MPN patients (Klampfl et al. 2011). Interestingly, most patients carry only heterozygous mutations or hemizygous deletions. Thus, only slight decrease of active gene dosage of TET2 is sufficient to grant clonal advantage to hematopoietic stem cells (Delhommeau et al. 2009). As TET2 encodes an enzyme that converts 5-methylcytosine to 5-hydroxymethylcytosine, loss of TET2 function might alter epigenetic gene regulation. Regulation of gene expression seems to be frequently altered in myeloid malignancies by mutations or deletions of genes involved in transcription. Examples of these lesions include losses/mutations of IKZF1, CUX1, and EZH2, all located on chromosome 7 and found in all myeloid malignancies including MPN (Ernst et al. 2010; Jager et al. 2010; Klampfl et al. 2011). It might explain why monosomy 7 is one of the most severe cytogenetic lesions in myeloid malignancies as at least three tumor suppressor genes are affected at the same time. Another example is mutations in the ASXL1 gene, a gene encoding a polycomb transcription factor involved in negative regulation of HOX genes (Abdel-Wahab et al. 2010). Cytogenetic studies using high-resolution microarrays implicated additional transcription factors such as ETV6, FOXP1, RUNX1, and CUX2 that are frequently deleted in MPN (Klampfl et al. 2011). It remains unclear what function of hematopoietic stem cells is impaired by decreased functional dosage of transcription factor genes. As most of these proteins are involved in transcriptional repression, their loss might be associated with increased frequency of cell cycle entry and/or alterations of differentiation dynamics within the progenitor compartment.

Another large group of defects in MPN is directly involved in cytokine signaling. In addition to JAK2 and MPL mutations, frequent mutations are found in the E3 ubiquitin ligase CBL (Dunbar et al. 2008; Grand et al. 2009; Sanada et al. 2009). It regulates the stability of proteins involved in cytokine signaling by ubiquitination that leads to proteasome-dependent degradation (Schmidt and Dikic 2005). CBL ubiquitinates cytokine receptors (Epo-R, c-Kit), tyrosine kinases (JAK2, Tyk2, Abl), as well as signaling adaptors (Grb2) (Schmidt and Dikic 2005). CBL mutations act as dominant negative and are found in the RING finger motif of the protein encoded by exons 8 and 9 (Grand et al. 2009; Ogawa et al. 2010a, b; Sanada et al. 2009). Activation of cytokine signaling induces STAT-dependent transcription. Among the genes induced by cytokines are the SOCS proteins that negatively regulate the signaling cascade by binding to the receptors or JAK2 (Nicola et al. 1999). SOCS genes can be impaired in MPN either due to hypermethylation (Jost et al. 2007; Teofili et al. 2008) or due to deletions (Klampfl et al. 2011). In addition to the JAK-STAT signaling, two members of the MAP-kinase pathway NRAS and NF1 have been shown to be targeted by mutagenesis in MPN (Beer et al. 2009; Stegelmann et al. 2010). Activating NRAS mutations have been found in MPN patients that transformed to leukemia, whereas NF1 deletions and mutations are often detected in chronic phase ET and PMF. Mutations in the signaling adaptor LNK (SH2B3) have been recently identified in MPN although they are rare and predominantly present in patients with advanced disease (Gery et al. 2009; Oh et al. 2010; Pardanani et al. 2010a). LNK negatively regulates JAK2 and c-KIT (Simon et al. 2008; Tong and Lodish 2004; Tong et al. 2005), and mice deficient for LNK develop myeloproliferative phenotype (Velazquez et al. 2002). In a different SH2B family member (SH2B2), a single somatic mutation found in a case of post-MPN AML (Klampfl et al. 2011).

The V617F and exon 12 mutations of JAK2 as well as MPL mutations have clearly been shown to have high selectivity for MPN and also induce a myeloproliferative phenotype in mice. Mutations in the rest of the above mentioned genes do not show specificity for MPN and are distributed at variable frequencies across all myeloid malignancies. It remains to be seen if murine models might clarify their potential to induce a myeloproliferative phenotype. Furthermore, more than a third of MPN patients are negative for JAK2 or MPL mutations, and none of the other genes explain MPN phenotype in these patients. Functional studies of individual mutations may not be sufficient as patients often carry several mutations and cytogenetic lesions. As the acquisition order of mutations turned out to be insignificant, the combination of different mutations might be important. It is possible that certain combinations of somatic lesions of weaker phenotypic effect will result in MPN in the absence of dominant lesions such as JAK2-V617F. If this is the case, JAK2-and MPL-negative patients will represent a very heterogeneous population with many types of somatic lesions and their combinations. Whole-genome sequencing will provide some answers, but it is already clear that MPN is a remarkably complex disease both genetically as well as phenotypically.

1.3 Mutations Associated with Disease Progression

At least three disease stages can be defined in MPN. The chronic phase is characterized by a stable disease with minimal evidence for progression. In ET and PV, disease progression is evident when patients develop secondary myelofibrosis. Another stage that is clinically recognizable is often referred to as "accelerated" phase characterized by variable degree of cytopenia (most often anemia) and gradual increase of blasts in bone marrow and peripheral blood. The last stage is the leukemic stage where the frequency of blasts increases over 20% in the bone marrow.

To date, MPN is associated with somatic lesions in over 20 different genes; however, their role in the pathogenesis remains unclear. It is important to classify the MPN-associated molecular lesions based on their impact on the severity of phenotype they induce. These studies are often difficult to achieve as large patient cohorts are needed, and many genes due to their shear size are laborious to screen for mutations. For example, TET2, ASXL1, and NF1 combined have a over 19,000 base pairs of coding sequence in over 80 exons, and as their mutation frequencies are relatively low, large patient numbers are needed to test association with clinical features. In certain cases, mutation frequencies are reported only in patients that show disease progression, whereas no data are available on the frequency in the chronic phase of the disease. Thus, rigorous statistical evidence is often missing when a certain lesion is implicated in disease progression.

The first lesion studied in terms of implications for disease progression was the JAK2-V617F mutation. Patients exhibit difference in V617F mutational burden due to variable populations' sizes of myeloid cells with wild-type, heterozygous, and homozygous genotypes for JAK2-V617F. A number of studies addressed the clinical impact of high V617F burden, and a clear association was found with secondary myelofibrosis (Vannucchi et al. 2007). This means that PV and ET patients with high JAK2-V617F burden are more likely to develop secondary myelofibrosis. Similarly, progression to secondary myelofibrosis in PV and ET was confirmed for uniparental disomy 9p associated with high JAK2-V617F burden (Klampfl et al. 2011).

Mutations of the p53 tumor suppressor (encoded by the TP53 gene) have previously been reported in few post-MPN AML cases (Beer et al. 2009). The TP53 mutation frequency in the chronic phase of MPN was unknown, and therefore the significance of TP53 mutations the transformation process was unclear. In recent studies, the TP53 mutation frequency was determined both in chronic phase as well as in post-MPN AML cases (Harutyunyan et al. 2011b; Klampfl et al. 2011). TP53 mutations were found common in the leukemic phase (20%), whereas only few patients in the chronic phase carried a mutation (1.6%). Interestingly, TP53 mutation positive chronic phase patients carried only monoallelic mutations while post-MPN AML patients carried mostly biallelic TP53 mutations. Another p53 pathway related lesion associated with post-MPN AML is gain of chromosome 1q as the MDM4 gene was found within the 1q amplicon (Harutyunyan et al. 2011b). Since MDM4 is a potent inhibitor of p53, 1q gains may increase the MDM4 gene dosage and result in a similar effect as TP53 mutations. Gains of 1q and TP53 mutations never found together in the same patient – an observation made also in solid tumors (Veerakumarasivam et al. 2008). If the frequencies of TP53 mutations and MDM4 gains are combined, they might explain about 40% of transformation event in MPN. As TP53 mutation rate in de novo AML is low (Wattel et al. 1994), the question arises to what degree pharmacologic management of MPN and/or MPN biology influence acquisition of p53 pathway lesions. Long-term treatment of MPN patients with DNA damage-inducing agents might target the p53 pathway for mutagenesis to facilitate clonal progression. However, such link has not been established as yet (Bjorkholm et al. 2011).

The transformation of MPN to post-MPN AML tuned out to share common defects with de novo AML. However, mutations in genes previously implicated in de novo AML are found mutated at somewhat lower frequencies in post-MPN AML. These genes include IDH1/2 (Andrulis et al. 2010; Green and Beer 2010; Klampfl et al. 2011; Kosmider et al. 2010; Pardanani et al. 2010b), RUNX1 (Ding et al. 2009; Klampfl et al. 2011; Taketani et al. 2002), FLT3 (Klampfl et al. 2011; Lin et al. 2006), NPM1 (Klampfl et al. 2011; Oki et al. 2006; Schnittger et al. 2011), and DNMT3A (Abdel-Wahab et al. 2011; Stegelmann et al. 2011).

Mutations of TET2 have been linked to more aggressive disease; however, their leukemic potential remains questionable as TET2 mutation frequencies in chronic phase and in post-MPN AML do not differ dramatically (Tefferi 2010). Moreover, TET2 is often acquired before JAK2-V617F, and thus, TET2 mutations likely play a role in initiation of clonal hematopoiesis. Mutations of CBL and EZH2 seem to have stronger association with leukemic transformation; however, strong evidence is still missing.

The cytogenetic lesions have been extensively investigated using single-nucleotide polymorphism (SNP) array technologies. These microarrays allow the measurement of copy number and provide simultaneous assessment of SNP heterozygosity across the whole genome (Klampfl et al. 2011; Stegelmann et al. 2010; Thoennissen et al. 2010). Marker densities used depended on the microarray platform ranging from 50,000 to 1.8 million. In the most recent study using SNP arrays with 1.8 million marker/genome resolution, over 400 MPN patients were evaluated in various disease stages (Klampfl et al. 2011). Cytogenetic complexity of MPN patients did not differ among the three MPN entities, and JAK2 mutations status and disease duration did not associate with increased number of cytogenetic lesions. The cytogenetic complexity considerably increased with disease progression. Among the 25 recurrent aberrations, only 8 showed association with leukemic transformation including gains of 1q (MDM4) and 3q, deletions of chromosomes 7q (CUX1), 7p (IKZF1), 5q, and 6p, as well as uniparental disomies on 19q and 22q. Post-MPN AML patients carrying these chromosomal aberrations also had other mutations in TP53, RUNX1, or IDH1/2; however, one third of patients had not detectable somatic lesion and had a normal karyotype (Klampfl et al. 2011).

As more data are available on the leukemic association of individual lesions, we might have come closer to assemble a set of molecular markers with prognostic value. Those lesions that are strongly inducing leukemic transformation are of less prognostic value as they are almost never observed in the chronic phase of MPN, and the time between acquisition of the lesion and transformation is short. Mutations in TP53, CBL, and perhaps EZH2 and LNK might be of some value, but their usefulness needs to be examined in prospective studies.

1.4 Hereditary Factors Influence MPN Pathogenesis

Existence of familial clustering of MPNs is considered to be the strongest evidence that germline mutations may cause an MPN like phenotype. This concept was further strengthened when a clear molecular distinction of true familial MPN from other familial syndromes such as familial erythrocytosis and hereditary thrombocythemia has become possible using clonality markers, cellular studies, and JAK2 mutation analysis. Familial MPN remains clinically indistinguishable from sporadic MPN, and this applies also for the presence of somatically occurring JAK2, MPL, TET2 mutations. Only MPL mutations were found germline in some pedigrees with an ET-like phenotype. Germline TET2 mutations/variants were reported, but they were not segregating in familial MPN cases, and thus their role remains elusive.

Another example of germline genetic factors influencing MPN pathogenesis was the discovery of the GGCC (also known as 46/1) haplotype of the JAK2 gene (Jones et al. 2009; Kilpivaara et al. 2009; Olcaydu et al. 2009a, b). Somatic mutations of JAK2 in MPN do not distribute equally between the two most common JAK2 gene haplotypes in Caucasian populations. The GGCC haplotype acquires over 80% of all V617F mutations as well as exon 12 mutations. The molecular reason why this deviation from random mutagenesis exists remains unclear. The GGCC haplotype predisposes carries for JAK2 mutation positive MPN, and thus its major role is in the disease initiation. The hypothesis that the GGCC haplotype might account for familial clustering of MPN has recently been disproved in a study showing equal haplotype frequency in sporadic and familial MPN cases (Olcaydu et al. 2011). The reason why the GGCC haplotype has negligible role in familial MPN is its weak ability (low penetrance) to initiate the disease phenotype. An as yet unknown, germline mutation(s) in familial MPN has an estimated three orders of magnitude higher penetrance than the GGCC haplotype (Olcaydu et al. 2011).

Another interesting way how germline mutations or polymorphisms may influence disease course in cancer has recently been described (Harutyunyan et al. 2011a). Harutyunyan et al. studied a polycythemia vera patient who was a germline carrier of a rare Fanconi anemia nonsense mutation (FANCM) on chromosome 14. The patient acquired uniparental disomy on chromosome 14 that switched the FANCM mutation from heterozygosity to homozygosity and caused the shift from polycythemia to anemia. Rare recessive mutations each patient carries have no phenotypic effect in heterozygous state (when the wild-type gene copy is present). However, loss of heterozygosity (LOH) often occurs in the cancer tissue that may expose recessive mutations. This way cancer cells may tap into a resource of germline recessive mutations from which some may prove advantageous for cancer growth; others may have unpredictable phenotypic effects.

1.5 Future Directions

With the advances of whole-genome analysis, more somatic lesions are expected to be discovered in MPN. Thus, genetic complexity of MPN will increase. To sort out the role of these, molecular lesions in the disease pathogenesis and their clinical significance will require coordinated multicenter studies that ensure large cohort size and access to high-throughput genome analysis. Genotypic stratification of patients may also be the key to successful treatment as well as to proper clinical management of patients.

References

Abdel-Wahab O, Manshouri T, Patel J, Harris K, Yao J, Hedvat C, Heguy A, Bueso-Ramos C, Kantarjian H, Levine RL et al (2010) Genetic analysis of transforming events that convert chronic myeloproliferative neoplasms to leukemias. Cancer Res 70:447–452

Abdel-Wahab O, Pardanani A, Rampal R, Lasho TL, Levine RL, Tefferi A (2011) DNMT3A mutational analysis in primary myelofibrosis, chronic myelomonocytic leukemia and advanced phases of myeloproliferative neoplasms. Leukemia 25(7):1219–1220

Andrulis M, Capper D, Meyer J, Penzel R, Hartmann C, Zentgraf H, von Deimling A (2010) IDH1 R132H mutation is a rare event in myeloproliferative neoplasms as determined by a mutation specific antibody. Haematologica 95:1797–1798

Baxter EJ, Scott LM, Campbell PJ, East C, Fourouclas N, Swanton S, Vassiliou GS, Bench AJ, Boyd EM, Curtin N et al (2005) Acquired mutation of the tyrosine kinase JAK2 in human myeloproliferative disorders. Lancet 365:1054–1061

Beer PA, Campbell PJ, Scott LM, Bench AJ, Erber WN, Bareford D, Wilkins BS, Reilly JT, Hasselbalch HC, Bowman R et al (2008) MPL mutations in myeloproliferative disorders: analysis of the PT-1 cohort. Blood 112(1):141–149

Beer PA, Delhommeau F, LeCouedic JP, Dawson MA, Chen E, Bareford D, Kusec R, McMullin MF, Harrison CN, Vannucchi AM et al (2009) Two routes to leukemic transformation after a JAK2 mutation-positive myeloproliferative neoplasm. Blood 115:2891–2900

Bjorkholm M, Derolf AR, Hultcrantz M, Kristinsson SY, Ekstrand C, Goldin LR, Andreasson B, Birgegard G, Linder O, Malm C et al (2011) Treatment-related risk factors for transformation to acute myeloid leukemia and myelodysplastic syndromes in myeloproliferative neoplasms. J Clin Oncol 29:2410–2415

Delhommeau F, Dupont S, Della Valle V, James C, Trannoy S, Masse A, Kosmider O, Le Couedic JP, Robert F, Alberdi A et al (2009) Mutation in TET2 in myeloid cancers. N Engl J Med 360:2289–2301

Ding Y, Harada Y, Imagawa J, Kimura A, Harada H (2009) AML1/RUNX1 point mutation possibly promotes leukemic transformation in myeloproliferative neoplasms. Blood 114:5201–5205

Dunbar AJ, Gondek LP, O'Keefe CL, Makishima H, Rataul MS, Szpurka H, Sekeres MA, Wang XF, McDevitt MA, Maciejewski JP (2008) 250 K single nucleotide polymorphism array karyotyping identifies acquired uniparental disomy and homozygous mutations, including novel missense substitutions of c-Cbl, in myeloid malignancies. Cancer Res 68:10349–10357

Ernst T, Chase AJ, Score J, Hidalgo-Curtis CE, Bryant C, Jones AV, Waghorn K, Zoi K, Ross FM, Reiter A et al (2010) Inactivating mutations of the histone methyltransferase gene EZH2 in myeloid disorders. Nat Genet 42:722–726

Gery S, Cao Q, Gueller S, Xing H, Tefferi A, Koeffler HP (2009) Lnk inhibits myeloproliferative disorder-associated JAK2 mutant, JAK2V617F. J Leukoc Biol 85:957–965

Grand FH, Hidalgo-Curtis CE, Ernst T, Zoi K, Zoi C, McGuire C, Kreil S, Jones A, Score J, Metzgeroth G et al (2009) Frequent CBL mutations associated with 11q acquired uniparental disomy in myeloproliferative neoplasms. Blood 113:6182–6192

Green A, Beer P (2010) Somatic mutations of IDH1 and IDH2 in the leukemic transformation of myeloproliferative neoplasms. N Engl J Med 362:369–370

Harutyunyan A, Gisslinger B, Klampfl T, Berg T, Bagienski K, Gisslinger H, Kralovics R (2011a) Rare germline variants in regions of loss of heterozygosity may influence clinical course of hematological malignancies. Leukemia 12:1782–1784

Harutyunyan A, Klampfl T, Cazzola M, Kralovics R (2011b) p53 lesions in leukemic transformation. N Engl J Med 364:488–490

Jager R, Gisslinger H, Passamonti F, Rumi E, Berg T, Gisslinger B, Pietra D, Harutyunyan A, Klampfl T, Olcaydu D et al (2010) Deletions of the transcription factor Ikaros in myeloproliferative neoplasms. Leukemia 24:1290–1298

James C, Ugo V, Le Couedic JP, Staerk J, Delhommeau F, Lacout C, Garcon L, Raslova H, Berger R, Bennaceur-Griscelli A et al (2005) A unique clonal JAK2 mutation leading to constitutive signalling causes polycythaemia vera. Nature 434:1144–1148

Jones AV, Chase A, Silver RT, Oscier D, Zoi K, Wang YL, Cario H, Pahl HL, Collins A, Reiter A et al (2009) JAK2 haplotype is a major risk factor for the development of myeloproliferative neoplasms. Nat Genet 41:446–449

Jost E, do ON, Dahl E, Maintz CE, Jousten P, Habets L, Wilop S, Herman JG, Osieka R, Galm O (2007) Epigenetic alterations complement mutation of JAK2 tyrosine kinase in patients with BCR/ABL-negative myeloproliferative disorders. Leukemia 21:505–510

Kilpivaara O, Mukherjee S, Schram AM, Wadleigh M, Mullally A, Ebert BL, Bass A, Marubayashi S, Heguy A, Garcia-Manero G et al (2009) A germline JAK2 SNP is associated with predisposition to the development of JAK2(V617F)-positive myeloproliferative neoplasms. Nat Genet 41:455–459

Klampfl T, Harutyunyan A, Berg T, Gisslinger B, Schalling M, Bagienski K, Olcaydu D, Passamonti F, Rumi E, Pietra D et al (2011) Genome integrity of myeloproliferative neoplasms in chronic phase and during disease progression. Blood 118:167–176

Kosmider O, Gelsi-Boyer V, Slama L, Dreyfus F, Beyne-Rauzy O, Quesnel B, Hunault-Berger M, Slama B, Vey N, Lacombe C et al (2010) Mutations of IDH1 and IDH2 genes in early and accelerated phases of myelodysplastic syndromes and MDS/myeloproliferative neoplasms. Leukemia 24:1094–1096

Kralovics R (2008) Genetic complexity of myeloproliferative neoplasms. Leukemia 22:1841–1848

Kralovics R, Passamonti F, Buser AS, Teo SS, Tiedt R, Passweg JR, Tichelli A, Cazzola M, Skoda RC (2005) A gain-of-function mutation of JAK2 in myeloproliferative disorders. N Engl J Med 352:1779–1790

Levine RL, Wadleigh M, Cools J, Ebert BL, Wernig G, Huntly BJ, Boggon TJ, Wlodarska I, Clark JJ, Moore S

et al (2005) Activating mutation in the tyrosine kinase JAK2 in polycythemia vera, essential thrombocythemia, and myeloid metaplasia with myelofibrosis. Cancer Cell 7:387–397

Lin P, Jones D, Medeiros LJ, Chen W, Vega-Vazquez F, Luthra R (2006) Activating FLT3 mutations are detectable in chronic and blast phase of chronic myeloproliferative disorders other than chronic myeloid leukemia. Am J Clin Pathol 126:530–533

Nicola NA, Nicholson SE, Metcalf D, Zhang JG, Baca M, Farley A, Willson TA, Starr R, Alexander W, Hilton DJ (1999) Negative regulation of cytokine signaling by the SOCS proteins. Cold Spring Harb Symp Quant Biol 64:397–404

Ogawa S, Sanada M, Shih LY, Suzuki T, Otsu M, Nakauchi H, Koeffler HP (2010a) Gain-of-function c-CBL mutations associated with uniparental disomy of 11q in myeloid neoplasms. Cell Cycle 9:1051–1056

Ogawa S, Shih LY, Suzuki T, Otsu M, Nakauchi H, Koeffler HP, Sanada M (2010b) Deregulated intracellular signaling by mutated c-CBL in myeloid neoplasms. Clin Cancer Res 16:3825–3831

Oh ST, Simonds EF, Jones C, Hale MB, Goltsev Y, Gibbs KD Jr, Merker JD, Zehnder JL, Nolan GP, Gotlib J (2010) Novel mutations in the inhibitory adaptor protein LNK drive JAK-STAT signaling in patients with myeloproliferative neoplasms. Blood 116:988–992

Oki Y, Jelinek J, Beran M, Verstovsek S, Kantarjian HM, Issa JP (2006) Mutations and promoter methylation status of NPM1 in myeloproliferative disorders. Haematologica 91:1147–1148

Olcaydu D, Harutyunyan A, Jager R, Berg T, Gisslinger B, Pabinger I, Gisslinger H, Kralovics R (2009a) A common JAK2 haplotype confers susceptibility to myeloproliferative neoplasms. Nat Genet 41:450–454

Olcaydu D, Skoda RC, Looser R, Li S, Cazzola M, Pietra D, Passamonti F, Lippert E, Carillo S, Girodon F et al (2009b) The 'GGCC' haplotype of JAK2 confers susceptibility to JAK2 exon 12 mutation-positive polycythemia vera. Leukemia 23(10):1924–1926

Olcaydu D, Rumi E, Harutyunyan A, Passamonti F, Pietra D, Pascutto C, Berg T, Jager R, Hammond E, Cazzola M et al (2011) The role of the JAK2 GGCC haplotype and the TET2 gene in familial myeloproliferative neoplasms. Haematologica 96:367–374

Pardanani AD, Levine RL, Lasho T, Pikman Y, Mesa RA, Wadleigh M, Steensma DP, Elliott MA, Wolanskyj AP, Hogan WJ et al (2006) MPL515 mutations in myeloproliferative and other myeloid disorders: a study of 1182 patients. Blood 108:3472–3476

Pardanani A, Lasho T, Finke C, Oh ST, Gotlib J, Tefferi A (2010a) LNK mutation studies in blast-phase myeloproliferative neoplasms, and in chronic-phase disease with TET2, IDH, JAK2 or MPL mutations. Leukemia 24:1713–1718

Pardanani A, Lasho TL, Finke CM, Mai M, McClure RF, Tefferi A (2010b) IDH1 and IDH2 mutation analysis in chronic- and blast-phase myeloproliferative neoplasms. Leukemia 24:1146–1151

Pikman Y, Lee BH, Mercher T, McDowell E, Ebert BL, Gozo M, Cuker A, Wernig G, Moore S, Galinsky I et al (2006) MPLW515L is a novel somatic activating mutation in myelofibrosis with myeloid metaplasia. PLoS Med 3:e270

Sanada M, Suzuki T, Shih LY, Otsu M, Kato M, Yamazaki S, Tamura A, Honda H, Sakata-Yanagimoto M, Kumano K et al (2009) Gain-of-function of mutated C-CBL tumour suppressor in myeloid neoplasms. Nature 460:904–908

Schmidt MH, Dikic I (2005) The Cbl interactome and its functions. Nat Rev Mol Cell Biol 6:907–918

Schnittger S, Bacher U, Haferlach C, Alpermann T, Dicker F, Sundermann J, Kern W, Haferlach T (2011) Characterization of NPM1-mutated AML with a history of myelodysplastic syndromes or myeloproliferative neoplasms. Leukemia 25:615–621

Simon C, Dondi E, Chaix A, de Sepulveda P, Kubiseski TJ, Varin-Blank N, Velazquez L (2008) Lnk adaptor protein down-regulates specific Kit-induced signaling pathways in primary mast cells. Blood 112:4039–4047

Stegelmann F, Bullinger L, Griesshammer M, Holzmann K, Habdank M, Kuhn S, Maile C, Schauer S, Dohner H, Dohner K (2010) High-resolution single-nucleotide polymorphism array-profiling in myeloproliferative neoplasms identifies novel genomic aberrations. Haematologica 95:666–669

Stegelmann F, Bullinger L, Schlenk RF, Paschka P, Griesshammer M, Blersch C, Kuhn S, Schauer S, Dohner H, Dohner K (2011) DNMT3A mutations in myeloproliferative neoplasms. Leukemia 25(7):1217–1219

Taketani T, Taki T, Takita J, Ono R, Horikoshi Y, Kaneko Y, Sako M, Hanada R, Hongo T, Hayashi Y (2002) Mutation of the AML1/RUNX1 gene in a transient myeloproliferative disorder patient with Down syndrome. Leukemia 16:1866–1867

Tefferi A (2010) Novel mutations and their functional and clinical relevance in myeloproliferative neoplasms: JAK2, MPL, TET2, ASXL1, CBL, IDH and IKZF1. Leukemia 24:1128–1138

Tefferi A, Lim KH, Abdel-Wahab O, Lasho TL, Patel J, Patnaik MM, Hanson CA, Pardanani A, Gilliland DG, Levine RL (2009a) Detection of mutant TET2 in myeloid malignancies other than myeloproliferative neoplasms: CMML, MDS, MDS/MPN and AML. Leukemia 23:1343–1345

Tefferi A, Pardanani A, Lim KH, Abdel-Wahab O, Lasho TL, Patel J, Gangat N, Finke CM, Schwager S, Mullally A et al (2009b) TET2 mutations and their clinical correlates in polycythemia vera, essential thrombocythemia and myelofibrosis. Leukemia 23(5):905–911

Teofili L, Martini M, Cenci T, Guidi F, Torti L, Giona F, Foa R, Leone G, Larocca LM (2008) Epigenetic alteration of SOCS family members is a possible pathogenetic mechanism in JAK2 wild type myeloproliferative diseases. Int J Cancer 123:1586–1592

Thoennissen NH, Krug UO, Lee DH, Kawamata N, Iwanski GB, Lasho T, Weiss T, Nowak D, Koren-Michowitz M, Kato M et al (2010) Prevalence and prognostic impact of allelic imbalances associated with leukemic transformation of Philadelphia chromosome-negative myeloproliferative neoplasms. Blood 115:2882–2890

Tong W, Lodish HF (2004) Lnk inhibits Tpo-mpl signaling and Tpo-mediated megakaryocytopoiesis. J Exp Med 200:569–580

Tong W, Zhang J, Lodish HF (2005) Lnk inhibits erythropoiesis and Epo-dependent JAK2 activation and downstream signaling pathways. Blood 105:4604–4612

Vannucchi AM, Antonioli E, Guglielmelli P, Rambaldi A, Barosi G, Marchioli R, Marfisi RM, Finazzi G, Guerini V, Fabris F et al (2007) Clinical profile of homozygous JAK2 617V>F mutation in patients with polycythemia vera or essential thrombocythemia. Blood 110:840–846

Veerakumarasivam A, Scott HE, Chin SF, Warren A, Wallard MJ, Grimmer D, Ichimura K, Caldas C, Collins VP, Neal DE et al (2008) High-resolution array-based comparative genomic hybridization of bladder cancers identifies mouse double minute 4 (MDM4) as an amplification target exclusive of MDM2 and TP53. Clin Cancer Res 14:2527–2534

Velazquez L, Cheng AM, Fleming HE, Furlonger C, Vesely S, Bernstein A, Paige CJ, Pawson T (2002) Cytokine signaling and hematopoietic homeostasis are disrupted in Lnk-deficient mice. J Exp Med 195:1599–1611

Wattel E, Preudhomme C, Hecquet B, Vanrumbeke M, Quesnel B, Dervite I, Morel P, Fenaux P (1994) p53 mutations are associated with resistance to chemotherapy and short survival in hematologic malignancies. Blood 84:3148–3157

Do We Need Biological Studies for Patient Management?

2

Moosa Qureshi and Claire Harrison

Contents

M. Qureshi
Clinical Research Fellow in Haematology,
Guy's and St Thomas' NHS Foundation Trust,
Guy's Hospital, London, UK
e-mail: moosa.qureshi@gstt.nhs.uk

C. Harrison (✉)
Consultant Haematologist, Guy's and St Thomas'
NHS Foundation Trust, Guy's Hospital, London, UK
e-mail: claire.harrison@gstt.nhs.uk

2.1 Introduction

Management decisions for patients with MPN vary between the different disease entities and must include of course the achievement of an accurate diagnosis. For patients with essential thrombocythaemia (ET) and polycythaemia vera (PV), initial disease management most commonly focuses upon preventing thrombotic events, ideally without exacerbating the risk of bleeding. However, a further important management goal for both clinicians and patients is to reduce the risk of progression or transformation to more destructive disease entities. In this respect, clinicians will target treatment to reduce the risk of transformation to acute myeloid leukaemia (AML) and myelodysplasia (MDS). There is, thus far, no clear evidence that specific treatment can reduce the risk of transformation to post-ET or post-PV myelofibrosis (MF). For example, although studies of French patients entered into Polycythemia Vera Study Group (PVSG) trials suggest that hydroxycarbamide treatment and elevated platelet count may increase the risk of post-PV MF (Najean and Rain 1997), the PT-1 trial in ET suggests that risks of post-ET MF may be greater with anagrelide than hydroxycarbamide (Harrison et al. 2005). However, if a biological marker for accelerated risk of transformation was identified, then this would potentially facilitate better targeted care. For patients with established MF, whether arising de novo as primary MF (PMF) or following ET or PV, the risk of thrombosis and haemorrhage subsists. Indeed, a recent study (Barbui et al. 2010) suggests the risk of thrombosis in PMF is very similar to that for ET. More pressing in the management of MF, however, is the need to accurately separate patients by likely prognosis, and in this regard, biological studies may prove to contribute significantly. As we shall discuss in this chapter, there is also potential to use additional biological studies or markers to orientate treatment strategies and, indeed, to design novel therapeutics against disease-specific features (e.g. increased JAK2 activation), as well as to monitor response.

2.2   Attributes of Biological Studies

Research findings are often made by a small group of investigators either in the laboratory or with a specific patient cohort. There are a number of potential difficulties inherent in the process of translating these findings into a global health-care strategy. Clinicians will need to interpret and apply research data appropriately. For example, a positive result for the *JAK2* V617F mutation in a patient with a thrombocytosis does not always imply the presence of ET, PV or PMF. Alternative diagnostic entities may present this picture, such as chronic myelomonocytic anaemia or an MDS variant such as refractory anaemia with sideroblasts and thrombocytosis. Biological markers should therefore provoke careful evaluation in the context of history, examination and other investigations.

A further important factor is that the biological study or test should be sufficiently robust and reproducible in different clinical settings. This should be established prior to widespread adoption in clinical practice, and thenceforth in the longer term should be subject to ongoing quality control. In the UK, the National External Quality Assurance Scheme (NEQAS) serves this purpose by providing regular assessment exercises, peer-group comparison of results and assistance in the case of persistently unsatisfactory performance. These concerns regarding reliability and reproducibility are relevant for novel biological studies which can be undertaken by most laboratories as well as more specialised tests which are performed only in specialist centres either due to low volume, cost, or technical requirements.

2.3   Markers for Diagnosis

Diagnostic criteria for MPN were first developed under the auspices of the PVSG, and until the discovery of the *JAK2* V617F (James et al. 2005), mutation generally required a cardinal myeloproliferative feature and the exclusion of other causative mechanisms. For instance, a diagnosis of ET would typically involve a finding of thrombocytosis, followed by the exclusion of a reactive cause or another myeloid disease (MDS, PV, PMF, etc.) (Murphy et al. 1986). The World Health Organization (WHO) diagnostic criteria first introduced the concept of characteristic bone marrow histological features which would support a diagnosis of an MPN. These criteria have subsequently been modified to incorporate molecular markers such as *JAK2* V617F, *MPL* mutations and *JAK2* exon 12 mutations (Tefferi et al. 2009). The inclusion of these molecular markers greatly improves both the speed and certainty of diagnosis, thus having a positive impact upon patient management. However, it should be emphasised that these studies are incorporated into diagnostic criteria and do not replace them. Although over 95% of patients with PV will have one or more *JAK2* mutations, only 50–60% of patients with ET or PMF will have *JAK2* or *MPL* mutations. Furthermore, the robust application of diagnostic criteria should be followed for all patients, regardless of the results of molecular markers, to exclude concomitant conditions and the rare possibility of a false-positive molecular test. A significant number of additional molecular abnormalities have been defined, including mutations of *TET2, ASLXI, EZLH, IDH* and *Lnk* (as discussed in Chap. 1). These mutations are not generally employed as diagnostic markers in routine practice, and many are not as specific for MPN as *JAK2* and *MPL* mutations. The predisposition afforded by the *JAK2* 46/1 (GGCC) haplotype (Jones et al. 2009) is also not of routine diagnostic utility, nor should it be used to screen family members for potential to develop disease.

Under current WHO diagnostic criteria, it remains possible to make a robust diagnosis of MPN without performing tests beyond a full blood count, blood film and bone marrow biopsy. Certain patients with PV may require in addition an erythropoietin level and red cell mass test, whereas confirmation of a diagnosis of PMF may necessitate measurement of lactate dehydrogenase (LDH) levels. Hence biological studies are not imperative to achieve a diagnosis of MPN, but they are in routine and widespread use. A particular clinical scenario where testing for *JAK2* and *MPL* mutations may be of significant diagnostic utility is in the case of a patient with unexplained splanchnic vein thrombosis, where an occult MPN is a common predisposing factor and classical blood count abnormalities may be masked by haemodilution (Patel et al. 2006).

2.4 Prognosis and Disease Transformation

The prognosis for patients with MPN is variable; for patients with ET and PV, it is likely to exceed 20 years, whereas for PMF, the median prognosis is 10 years (Barbui et al. 2011). Leukaemic transformation is a poor prognostic factor for all diseases and is generally fatal, with the exception of a small minority of patients who remit with intensive chemotherapy and are able to undergo allogeneic transplantation (Mesa et al. 2005). For PMF, a number of prognostic scores, including the IPSS (Cervantes et al. 2009) and the dynamic IPSS (Passamonti et al. 2010; Gangat et al. 2011), have been developed and are discussed further in chapters 7 and 14 of this book. These prognostic evaluations do not at present include biological studies apart from cytogenetics. There are variable reports for the prognostic implication of allelic burden for *JAK2* V617F in PMF. Most recent publications suggest a poor prognosis with low allelic burden (Tefferi et al. 2008). However, the difficulties in quality assurance of this test, and the strength of the IPSS and dynamic IPSS, have precluded the inclusion of allelic burden as a standard prognostic marker.

For patients with ET and PV, prognosis is largely determined by the number of thrombotic complications (Lengfelder et al. 1998), and the utility of biological studies in defining the risk of their occurrence is discussed below. Transformation to MF or AML portends a markedly worse prognosis, but novel

biological studies do not contribute significantly to this assessment. Elevated *JAK2* V617F allelic burden has been associated with features of more advanced disease in PV, but it is not known whether it is predictive of progression in disease status. Of interest are reports that in patients with *JAK2* V617F mutation in chronic phase disease, leukaemic blasts in at least a half of cases are negative for the mutation (Campbell et al. 2006; Theocharides et al. 2007).

2.5 Thrombosis or Haemorrhage

Thrombotic events are particularly common clinical manifestations of MPN, and define risk stratification for patients with ET and PV. For these patients, the dominant predictors for thrombosis are age and a prior event, with increasing evidence of a role for leucocytosis (Barbui et al. 2011). For patients with PMF, recent data suggest that these patients do suffer from an increased risk of fatal and non-fatal cardiovascular events at a rate of 1.75% per patient-year, which is similar to that for patients with ET (Barbui et al. 2010). Risks for thrombosis in patients with PMF include age over 60 years and the presence of *JAK2* V617F, particularly for patients with leucocytosis ($>15 \times 10^9$/L). Recent biological studies at present do not contribute further to the assessment of thrombotic risk, although a meta-analysis does suggest an increased risk of thrombosis in *JAK2* V617F–positive patients with ET (Dahabreh et al. 2009). Haemorrhage is less frequent than thrombosis and is associated with extreme thrombocytosis, aspirin use and acquired von Willebrand's disease (Budde et al. 1984).

2.6 Treatment Strategy

Once a specific instance of MPN has been disease-risk stratified and associated health conditions taken into account, is there any impact of current biological studies in further deciding which particular therapy a patient would most benefit from? At the present time, there is no established evidence to advocate a particular therapeutic option on the basis of a patient's mutation status. A subgroup analysis of the PT-1 study has suggested that ET patients with the *JAK2* V617F mutation were less likely to have arterial thrombosis when treated with hydroxycarbamide and aspirin than with anagrelide and aspirin, whereas for patients without the *JAK2* V617F mutation, there was no difference in arterial thrombotic events when treated with either drug combination (Campbell et al. 2005). Given the association of *JAK2* V617F mutation with leucocytosis (Cheung et al. 2006), and the correlation both between leucocytosis and *JAK2* V617F mutation and between leucocytosis and thrombosis, the panmyelosuppressive action of hydroxycarbamide compared with the specific action of anagrelide to lower the platelet count suggests a mechanism to explain this observation. This finding has not been tested by other authors and has not translated into a general recommendation.

More recently, it is of significant interest that emerging data with regard to JAK inhibitor therapy, as a treatment initially for PMF, suggest that these agents appear to be equally effective in patients regardless of whether they have a *JAK2* mutation or not (Verstovsek et al. 2010). Thus, even with novel therapies, biological studies are not yet required to tailor treatment choice.

2.7 Monitoring Response

Response criteria to guide the management of ET, PV and PMF have been drawn up by expert consensus through the European Leukemia Net (ELN) (Barosi et al. 2009), European Myelofibrosis Network (EUMNET) (Barosi et al. 2005) and International Working Group for Myelofibrosis Research and Therapy (IWG-MRT) (Tefferi et al. 2006). Most recently, critical concepts and management recommendations have been developed by the ELN (Barbui et al. 2011). In general, these response criteria refer to control of blood counts, relief of anaemia or moderation of transfusion dependency, reduction in organomegaly (particularly splenomegaly), control of symptoms and resolution of bone marrow abnormalities on trephine biopsy. The presence or resolution of cytogenetic abnormalities is not generally referenced in these criteria. The only response criteria to reference biological studies are the ELN consensus criteria for response in ET and PV which include molecular response (Barosi et al. 2009). Here, the definition of molecular response is based on quantitative allele burden of the specific molecular abnormalities (e.g. *JAK2* V617F, exon 12 and *MPL* mutations) and acknowledges that sensitivity of detection varies according to the method used and that significant variation in consecutive samples from an individual patient is possible even without therapy. Consequently, the concept of molecular response is defined on the basis of detection levels, and partial response is applied only to patients with a baseline value of mutant allele burden greater than 10%. Implicit in these statements is the admission of technical difficulties in assessing molecular response.

Recently, the value of monitoring *JAK2* V617F and *MPL* 515L allele burden has been demonstrated in the setting of bone marrow transplant where monitoring of minimal residual disease guides the use of post-transplant immunotherapy (Kroger et al. 2007); the same group failed to find correlation with circulating CD34 cell number as a marker of minimal residual disease or predictor of relapse (Alchalby et al. 2011). Interestingly with regard to *JAK2* V617F allele burden, these authors conclude that knowledge of the *JAK2* V617F–mutated status, but not allele frequency, yields improved survival and that rapid clearance after allograft reduces the risk of relapse (Alchalby et al. 2010). For patient management outside the setting of transplantation, the clinical value of monitoring mutated allele burden has not been validated. For example, although Kildajian and colleagues demonstrated that Pegasys therapy in 40 newly diagnosed patients with PV was able to significantly reduce *JAK2* V617F allele burden, there was no clearly demonstrated reduction in thrombosis as the study had no control group and was not designed to demonstrate this endpoint (Kiladjian et al. 2006). A larger trial in progress is required to elucidate whether biologic modification translates into clinically meaningful response such as reduction in risk of thrombosis or disease evolution.

Thus, the use of biological studies to monitor response is currently restricted to the context of post-transplant immunotherapy and to clinical trials designed to assess the value of newer agents for disease management.

2.8   Summary and Conclusion

Significant advances in our understanding of the MPN have been underpinned by biological discoveries. In this chapter, we have discussed their current utility in patients' management, addressing the question "Do we need biological studies for patient management?" At present, we have identified that the main utility for these studies is in achieving a diagnosis, although a diagnosis may be achieved without recourse to these sometimes expensive tests. Advances in the field are at a stage where we are beginning to consider the use of minimal residual disease monitoring especially in the post-transplant setting. We have much to learn before these studies will fully complement accurate clinical evaluation and standard laboratory tests.

References

Alchalby H, Badbaran A et al (2010) Impact of JAK2V617F mutation status, allele burden, and clearance after allogeneic stem cell transplantation for myelofibrosis. Blood 116(18):3572–3581

Alchalby H, Lioznov M et al (2011) Circulating CD34(+) cells as prognostic and follow-up marker in patients with myelofibrosis undergoing allo-SCT. Bone Marrow Transplant. Epub Feb 2011

Barbui T, Carobbio A et al (2010) Thrombosis in primary myelofibrosis: incidence and risk factors. Blood 115(4):778–782

Barbui T, Barosi G et al (2011) Philadelphia-negative classical myeloproliferative neoplasms: critical concepts and management recommendations from European LeukemiaNet. J Clin Oncol 29(6):761–770

Barosi G, Bordessoule D et al (2005) Response criteria for myelofibrosis with myeloid metaplasia: results of an initiative of the European Myelofibrosis Network (EUMNET). Blood 106(8):2849–2853

Barosi G, Birgegard G et al (2009) Response criteria for essential thrombocythemia and polycythemia vera: result of a European LeukemiaNet consensus conference. Blood 113(20):4829–4833

Budde U, Schaefer G et al (1984) Acquired von Willebrand's disease in the myeloproliferative syndrome. Blood 64(5):981–985

Campbell PJ, Scott LM et al (2005) Definition of subtypes of essential thrombocythaemia and relation to polycythaemia vera based on JAK2 V617F mutation status: a prospective study. Lancet 366(9501):1945–1953

Campbell PJ, Baxter EJ et al (2006) Mutation of JAK2 in the myeloproliferative disorders: timing, clonality studies, cytogenetic associations, and role in leukemic transformation. Blood 108(10):3548–3555

Cervantes F, Dupriez B et al (2009) New prognostic scoring system for primary myelofibrosis based on a study of the International Working Group for Myelofibrosis Research and Treatment. Blood 113(13):2895–2901

Cheung B, Radia D et al (2006) The presence of the JAK2 V617F mutation is associated with a higher haemoglobin and increased risk of thrombosis in essential thrombocythaemia. Br J Haematol 132(2):244–245

Dahabreh IJ, Zoi K et al (2009) Is JAK2 V617F mutation more than a diagnostic index? A meta-analysis of clinical outcomes in essential thrombocythemia. Leuk Res 33(1):67–73

Gangat N, Caramazza D et al (2011) DIPSS plus: a refined Dynamic International Prognostic Scoring System for primary myelofibrosis that incorporates prognostic information from karyotype, platelet count, and transfusion status. J Clin Oncol 29(4):392–397

Harrison CN, Campbell PJ et al (2005) Hydroxyurea compared with anagrelide in high-risk essential thrombocythemia. N Engl J Med 353(1):33–45

James C, Ugo V et al (2005) A unique clonal JAK2 mutation leading to constitutive signalling causes polycythaemia vera. Nature 434(7037):1144–1148

Jones AV, Chase A et al (2009) JAK2 haplotype is a major risk factor for the development of myeloproliferative neoplasms. Nat Genet 41(4):446–449

Kiladjian JJ, Cassinat B et al (2006) High molecular response rate of polycythemia vera patients treated with pegylated interferon alpha-2a. Blood 108(6):2037–2040

Kroger N, Badbaran A et al (2007) Monitoring of the JAK2-V617F mutation by highly sensitive quantitative real-time PCR after allogeneic stem cell transplantation in patients with myelofibrosis. Blood 109(3):1316–1321

Lengfelder E, Hochhaus A et al (1998) Should a platelet limit of 600 x 10(9)/l be used as a diagnostic criterion in essential thrombocythaemia? An analysis of the natural course including early stages. Br J Haematol 100(1):15–23

Mesa RA, Li CY et al (2005) Leukemic transformation in myelofibrosis with myeloid metaplasia: a single-institution experience with 91 cases. Blood 105(3):973–977

Murphy S, Iland H et al (1986) Essential thrombocythemia: an interim report from the Polycythemia Vera Study Group. Semin Hematol 23(3):177–182

Najean Y, Rain JD (1997) Treatment of polycythemia vera: use of 32P alone or in combination with maintenance therapy using hydroxyurea in 461 patients greater than 65 years of age. The French Polycythemia Study Group. Blood 89(7):2319–2327

Passamonti F, Cervantes F et al (2010) A dynamic prognostic model to predict survival in primary myelofibrosis: a study by the IWG-MRT (International Working Group for Myeloproliferative Neoplasms Research and Treatment). Blood 115(9):1703–1708

Patel RK, Lea NC et al (2006) Prevalence of the activating JAK2 tyrosine kinase mutation V617F in the Budd-Chiari syndrome. Gastroenterology 130(7):2031–2038

Tefferi A, Barosi G et al (2006) International Working Group (IWG) consensus criteria for treatment response in myelofibrosis with myeloid metaplasia, for the IWG for Myelofibrosis Research and Treatment (IWG-MRT). Blood 108(5):1497–1503

Tefferi A, Lasho TL et al (2008) Low JAK2V617F allele burden in primary myelofibrosis, compared to either a higher allele burden or unmutated status, is associated with inferior overall and leukemia-free survival. Leukemia 22(4):756–761

Tefferi A, Thiele J et al (2009) The 2008 World Health Organization classification system for myeloproliferative neoplasms: order out of chaos. Cancer 115(17):3842–3847

Theocharides A, Boissinot M et al (2007) Leukemic blasts in transformed JAK2-V617F-positive myeloproliferative disorders are frequently negative for the JAK2-V617F mutation. Blood 110(1):375–379

Verstovsek S, Kantarjian H et al (2010) Safety and efficacy of INCB018424, a JAK1 and JAK2 inhibitor, in myelofibrosis. N Engl J Med 363(12):1117–1127

Part II

General Issues in the Management of MPNs

Critical Issues About the Diagnosis of MPNs: Bone Marrow Histopathology

3

Jürgen Thiele and Hans Michael Kvasnicka

Contents

J. Thiele (✉)
Institute of Pathology, University of Cologne,
Cologne, Germany
e-mail: j.thiele@uni-koeln.de

H.M. Kvasnicka
Senckenberg Institute of Pathology,
University of Frankfurt,
Frankfurt, Germany
e-mail: hans-michael.kvasnicka@kgu.de

3.1 Introduction

Although the revised 2008 World Health Organization (WHO) criteria (Swerdlow et al. 2008) for the diagnosis and classification of Philadelphia chromosome-negative chronic myeloproliferative neoplasms (MPNs) was defined by a panel of expert hematopathologists and clinicians (Tefferi et al. 2007), serious concern has been repeatedly expressed for its emphasis upon specific histological bone marrow (BM) features (Spivak and Silver 2008). On the other hand, contemporary diagnostic approach regards BM morphology as an integral part, in context with clinical findings and genetics (Tefferi and Vardiman 2008; Tefferi et al. 2009). Moreover, it should not be overlooked that preceding the original descriptions of BM characteristics in MPNs by the WHO (Jaffe et al. 2001), a number of authors had already endorsed some important issues that later were incorporated into this classification (Buhr et al. 1992, 1993; Dickstein and Vardiman 1993; Georgii et al. 1998; Kvasnicka et al. 1997; Thiele et al. 1989a, b, 1996, 1999). On the other hand, the majority of clinical trials usually followed the postulates of the Polycythemia Vera Study Group (PVSG) or related diagnostic guidelines (Barosi 1999; Murphy 1999; Pearson 1998; Wasserman 1986). This review tries to highlight not only histological BM features characterizing the main MPNs like polycythemia vera, essential thrombocythemia, and primary myelofibrosis according to the updated WHO criteria (Vardiman et al. 2009) but also

T. Barbui and A. Tefferi (eds.), *Myeloproliferative Neoplasms*, Hematologic Malignancies,
DOI 10.1007/978-3-642-24989-1_3, © Springer-Verlag Berlin Heidelberg 2012

more controversial issues like standardization as well as reproducibility of BM morphology that are significantly associated with accurate diagnosis.

3.2   Polycythemia Vera (PV)

Usually, in PV, hypercellularity of the BM is a characteristic feature (Dickstein and Vardiman 1993; Georgii et al. 1998; Thiele et al. 2001a, 2005a) due to a trilineage proliferation (so-called panmyelosis) involving nucleated erythroid precursors, megakaryocytes, as well as neutrophil granulopoiesis (Fig. 3.1a). Contrasting this finding in BM trephines described in the PVSG trial, there was a wide variation among individuals with about 13% of the cases showing a normal cellularity (Ellis and Peterson 1979; Ellis et al. 1986). In this context, one should be aware that in the elderly population of patients presenting with PV, the subcortical BM spaces are regularly transformed to adipose tissue, and any expansion of hematopoiesis toward this area implies hypercellularity when evaluated in a representative core biopsy performed at an orthograde direction (Thiele and Kvasnicka 2005a; Thiele et al. 2005c). Quantification of erythropoiesis in relation to neutrophil granulopoiesis reveals a clear shifting to the red cell lineage including many precursors (Fig. 3.1b). Particularly, the normally small and rounded islets of nucleated erythroid precursors display not only a conspicuous enlargement but also a tendency for merging into sheets (Fig. 3.1b). Megakaryocytes have been acknowledged to exhibit peculiar features that facilitate a distinction between PV and reactive erythrocytosis (Georgii et al. 1998; Thiele et al. 2001a). It is noteworthy that this lineage is characterized by a polymorphous aspect showing mature megakaryocytes of very different sizes, i.e., small- to medium-sized and large to giant forms are either dispersed or loosely clustered (Fig. 3.1a, c). All these findings are a significant extension to former descriptions by the PVSG in which 95% of the BM specimens demonstrated only an increase in megakaryocyte numbers (Ellis and Peterson 1979). A minor to moderate increase in reticulin

fibers (Fig. 3.1d) has been reported to be seen already at presentation in 10–20% of patients (Ellis and Peterson 1979; Georgii et al. 1998; Thiele et al. 2006). Until now, a conflict of opinion exists whether this feature is consistent with a later diagnosis and/or a more aggressive course of disease progressing into post-PV myelofibrosis (Barosi et al. 2008; Ellis et al. 1986). Discrimination (relative frequency and ranking) of standardized BM features in PV versus reactive erythrocytosis (Thiele and Kvasnicka 2005a) and the other MPN entities as well (Thiele et al. 2005a) resulted in a substantial prediction of group membership concerning correct diagnosis.

Concerning the endpoints in the evolution of the disease process in PV, the 2008 WHO classification recognizes explicitly a prodromal, so-called prepolycythemic stage (Swerdlow et al. 2008; Tefferi et al. 2007; Vardiman et al. 2009), that initially fails to present with a significant increase in the red cell mass or hemoglobin/hematocrit level (Kvasnicka and Thiele 2010; Ruggeri et al. 2003). Consequently, these cases are not conforming with the original or updated diagnostic criteria of the PVSG (Murphy 1999; Pearson 1998; Wasserman 1986). Histopathology of the BM displays some overlapping features to essential thrombocythemia (ET), especially concerning the prevalence of large to giant hyperlobulated megakaryocytes in addition to an only moderate increase in cellularity including erythropoiesis (Gianelli et al. 2008; Thiele et al. 2005b). For this reason, at onset differentiation from ET may be difficult, and further clinical and JAK2 mutation status investigations are needed (Gianelli et al. 2008; Kvasnicka and Thiele 2010).

The terminal endpoint is the so-called spent phase/postpolycythemic myeloid metaplasia according to the PVSG (Ellis et al. 1986; Murphy 1999) consistent with post-PV myelofibrosis (Barosi et al. 2008) with BM features revealing conspicuous changes. Contrasting manifest polycythemic PV, there is a prominence of a left-shifted neutrophil granulopoiesis associated with a reduction of erythroid precursors and an increase of a dense meshwork of reticulin fibers intermingled with collagen (Buhr et al. 2003; Ellis et al. 1986; Georgii et al. 1998; Thiele and

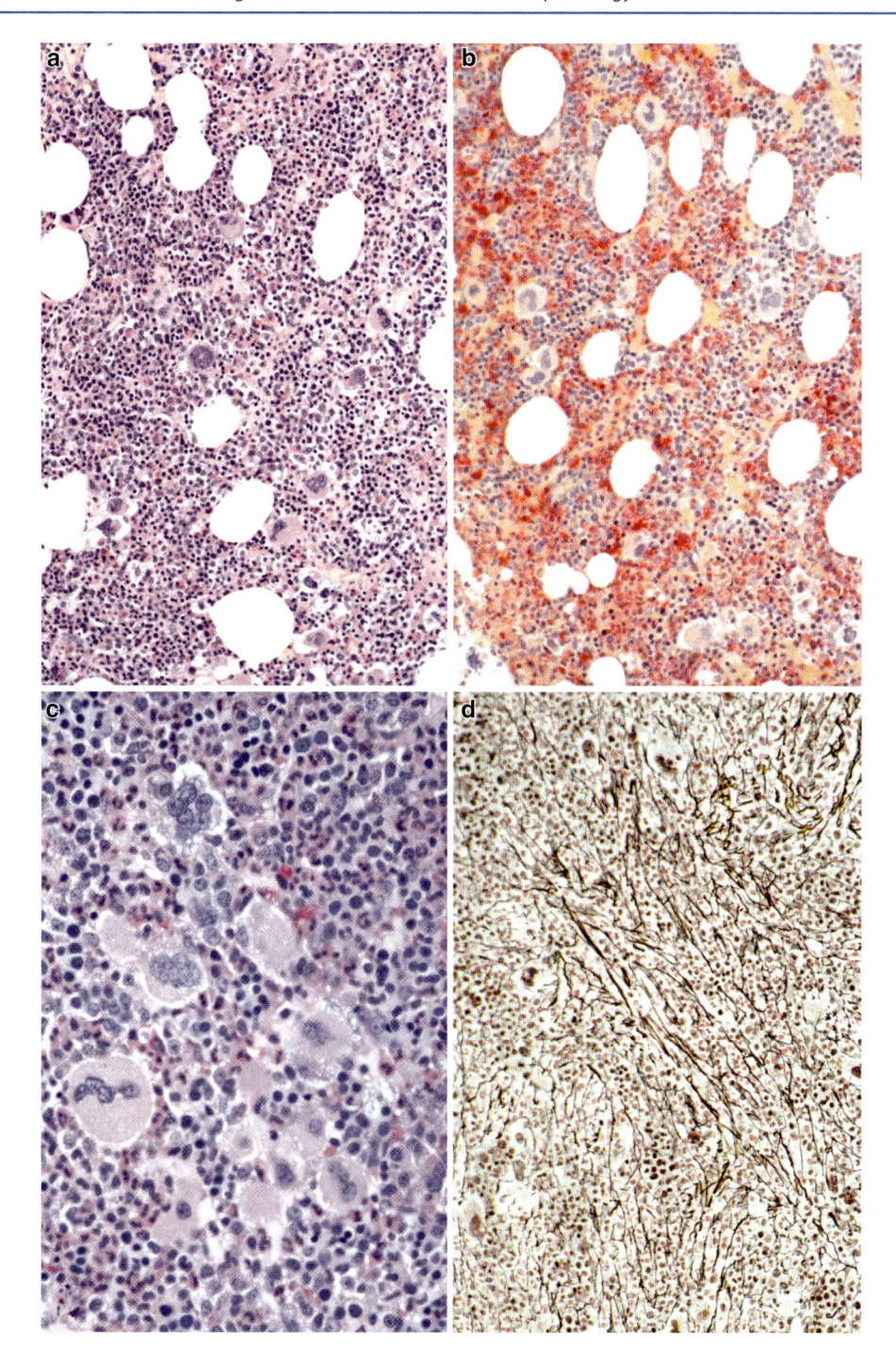

Fig. 3.1 Polycythemia vera. (**a**) Conspicuous hypercellularity for age with increase of all three cell lineages (panmyelosis) including extended islets of nucleated erythroid precursors and dispersed mature megakaryocytes. (**b**) Prominent enlargement of erythropoiesis surrounded by left-shifted neutrophil granulopoiesis (*red*). (**c**) Megakaryocytes of different size ranging from small to giant ones are increased and may be clustered, but fail to show maturation defects (compare with Fig. 3.3c). (**d**) Moderate increase in reticulin may be found in a number of patients already at diagnosis. Magnification: **a**, **b**, **d**, ×180; **c**, ×380. Staining: **a** = hematoxylin and eosin; **b** = AS-D-chloroacetate esterase reaction; **c** = periodic acid Schiff reagent (PAS); **d** = silver impregnation after Gomori

Kvasnicka 2005a). Overt collagen fibrosis resembling phenotypically primary myelofibrosis (PMF) is usually considered as the forerunner of myelodysplastic and leukemic transformation showing either severe maturation defects of cell lineages or more than 20% blasts (Thiele and Kvasnicka 2005a; Thiele et al. 2006; Vardiman et al. 2009).

3.3 Essential Thrombocythemia (ET)

In BM biopsy specimens derived from ET patients, usually neither a relevant increase in overall cellularity (Fig. 3.2a) nor a significant proliferation of a left-shifted neutrophil granulo- or erythropoiesis is detectable (Fig. 3.2b). The majority of cases present with an inconspicuous appearance of these cell lineages. On the other hand, randomly distributed or loosely clustered large to giant mature megakaryocytes with deeply folded nuclei (so-called staghorn type) surrounded by correspondingly mature cytoplasm (Fig. 3.2c) are the outstanding features (Buhr et al. 1992; Florena et al. 2004; Georgii et al. 1998; Gianelli et al. 2006; Thiele et al. 1989a, 2005d; Thiele and Kvasnicka 2006b). Usually, there is no increase in BM fibers (Fig. 3.2d). Only in a small subfraction of patients (about 5%) minor, i.e., grade 1, reticulin fibrosis (Thiele et al. 2005c) according to WHO may be observed (Barbui et al. 2011; Georgii et al. 1998; Kreft et al. 2005; Thiele et al. 2002). Until now, it is not clear if this feature may be associated with a later diagnosis/performance of the biopsy in this very small cohort of patients. According to the WHO criteria (Swerdlow et al. 2008; Tefferi et al. 2007), any substantial increase in reticulin or occurrence of collagen fibers is not compatible with ET at onset contrasting terminal stages of disease (Barosi et al. 2008). Presence of BM fibrosis as well as proliferation of neutrophil granulopoiesis and abnormalities of the megakaryocytic cell lineage raises the possibility of PMF (Gianelli et al. 2006; Thiele et al. 2000, 2003). It has to be realized that significant differences are encountered in the diagnosis of ET when following the guidelines of the PVSG (Murphy et al. 1997) compared to those of the

WHO (Thiele and Kvasnicka 2003b). Because the PVSG unfortunately failed to render a detailed description of BM features characterizing ET on the one hand, but allows a certain amount of fibrosis among their diagnostic parameters on the other hand (Murphy et al. 1997; Murphy 1999; Pearson 1998), discrimination from early/prefibrotic stages of PMF with presenting thrombocythemia (so-called false ET) is not feasible (Florena et al. 2004; Gianelli et al. 2006; Thiele et al. 1989b, 2000, 2011; Thiele and Kvasnicka 2003b, 2006b). A clear-cut differentiation between ET and early/prefibrotic PMF is an essential issue for the outcome including progression to overt myelofibrosis, transformation to leukemia, as well as survival (Barbui et al. 2011; Thiele et al. 2002, 2006; Thiele and Kvasnicka 2006b). Further differentiation includes initial/early stages of PV clinically presenting with overt thrombocythemia and therefore mimicking ET (Gianelli et al. 2006; Thiele et al. 2005b). In these cases, BM shows a mild hypercellularity due to trilineage proliferation (panmyelosis) including large to giant megakaryocytes with hyperlobulated nuclei (Kvasnicka and Thiele 2010). Transformation of WHO-diagnosed ET into acute leukemia (AML) is a rare event with a cumulative incidence of 0.7% at 10 years (Barbui et al. 2011), compared to the reported incidence of 8.3% when following the PVSG criteria (Girodon et al. 2010). Consequently, frequency of AML transformation occurred significantly less (range 1.4–3.0%) when investigating cohorts that included also fractions of WHO-diagnosed ET patients (Palandri et al. 2009; Passamonti et al. 2008; Wolanskyj et al. 2006). Similarly, risk of post-ET myelofibrosis (Barosi et al. 2008) is also significantly dependent on the applied diagnostic criteria. Following the PVSG guidelines (Murphy et al. 1997), the 10-year risk was found to range from 8.3% to 9.7% (Cervantes et al. 2002; Chim et al. 2005), whereas the WHO-classified ET patients revealed a corresponding rate of only 0.8% (Barbui et al. 2011). Again, series that consisted of a mixture of either PVSG- or WHO-defined ET patients revealed a higher incidence of myelofibrosis ranging between 3.8% and 4.9% (Palandri et al. 2009; Passamonti et al. 2008; Wolanskyj et al. 2006).

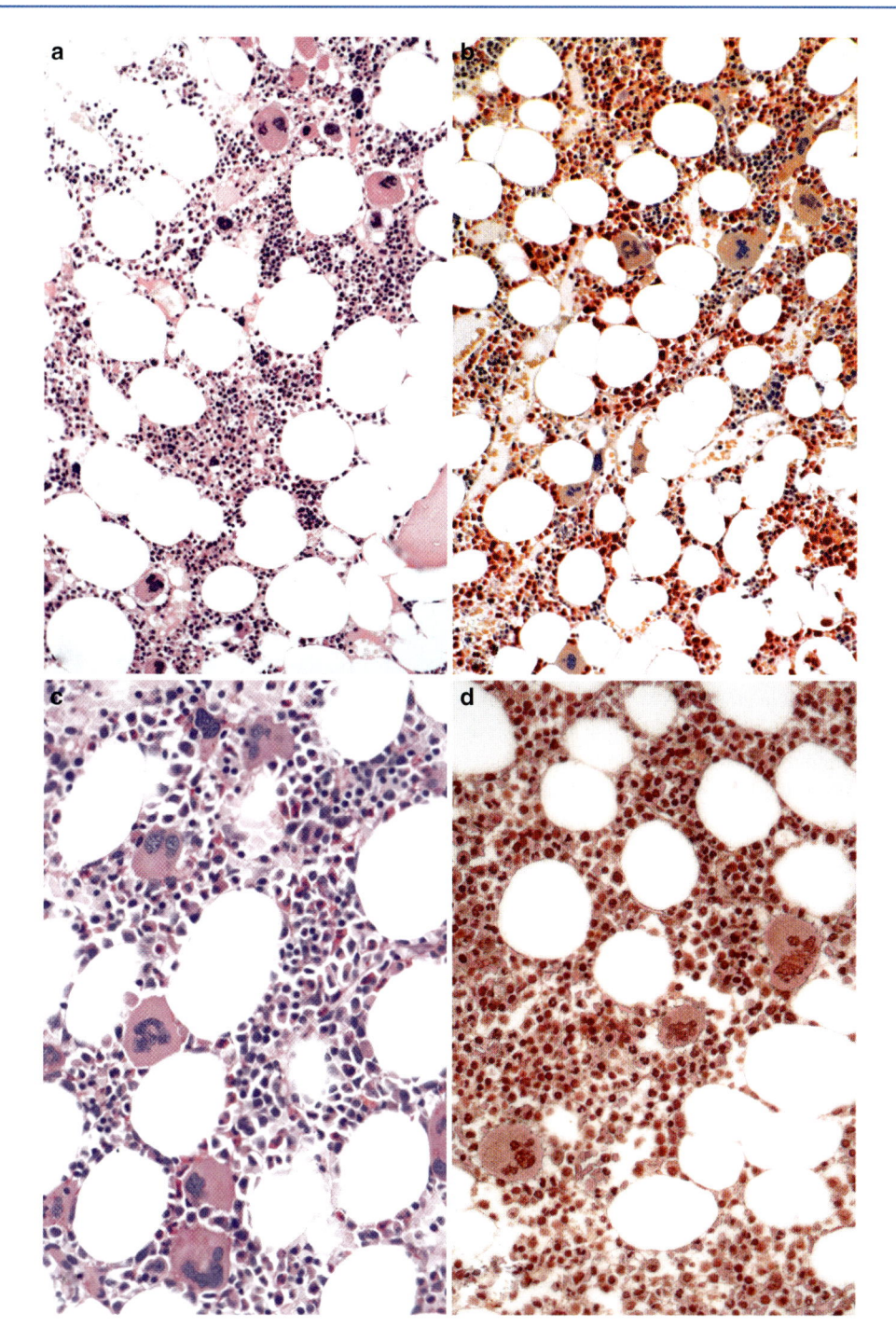

Fig. 3.2 Essential thrombocythemia. (**a**) Normal age-matched cellularity, except for a prominent increase in large to giant megakaryocytes loosely clustered or dispersed throughout the bone marrow space. (**b**) No proliferation or significant left shift of neutrophil granulopoiesis or erythropoiesis surrounding giant mature megakaryocytes. (**c**) Conspicuous increase in large megakaryocytes without maturation defects showing hyperlobulated, occasionally staghorn-like nuclei. (**d**) No increase in reticulin fibers, but giant megakaryocytes with deep foldings of their nuclei. Magnification: **a**, **b**, **c**, ×180; **d**, ×380. Staining: **a**=hematoxylin and eosin; **b**=AS-D-chloroacetate esterase reaction; **c**=periodic acid Schiff reagent (PAS); **d**=silver impregnation after Gomori

This impact of BM morphology and accurate classification on complications and outcome of ET is reflected by corresponding data on survival (Barbui et al. 2011; Kvasnicka and Thiele 2006; Thiele et al. 2006).

3.4 Primary Myelofibrosis (PMF)

Concerning BM morphology in PMF in large series clinicians have reported a striking variability in hematological findings at the time of first presentation (Cervantes et al. 1998; Gangat et al. 2011; Tefferi 2000). This conspicuously wide spectrum of clinical manifestations is paralleled by BM features that in the beginning may show a hypercellularity with no or only minor increase in reticulin fibers or, in advanced stages, specimens presenting with a hypocellular marrow and overt collagen fibrosis and osteosclerosis (Buhr et al. 2003; Dickstein and Vardiman 1995; Kvasnicka et al. 1997; Thiele et al. 1989a, 2003; Thiele and Kvasnicka 2005b, 2006a) consistent with classical myelofibrosis with myeloid metaplasia (Barosi 1999; Cervantes and Barosi 2005). The concept of an early stage of PMF characterized among others by the BM fiber content raises the salient question of progression or a stepwise evolution of the disease process. This important issue has been settled by scrutinized clinicopathological follow-up studies involving sequential BM biopsy specimens with grading of myelofibrosis and reference to hematological findings (Buhr et al. 2003; Kreft et al. 2005; Thiele et al. 2003; Thiele and Kvasnicka 2006a). Consequently, this finding of developing myelofibrosis and accompanying clinical presentations was adopted by the WHO classification (Swerdlow et al. 2008; Tefferi et al. 2007).

In the early/prefibrotic stage at the initial endpoint of disease evolution, histopathology of the BM is characterized by hypercellularity (Fig. 3.3a) consisting of a prominent neutrophil granulocytic and megakaryocytic proliferation (Fig. 3.3b) which is often associated with a slight to moderate reduction of nucleated red cell precursors (Buhr et al. 2003; Florena et al. 2004; Gianelli et al. 2006; Kreft et al. 2005; Thiele et al.

2001b, 2003; Thiele and Kvasnicka 2004, 2005b). Most important in this setting are conspicuous abnormalities of the megakaryocytic cell lineage (Fig. 3.3a, c, d). These include megakaryocyte arrangement and localization in the marrow space (histotopography with endosteal-paratrabecular dislocation, forming of dense or loose clusters) and a high variability in size (small and giant forms) (Fig. 3.3a). Moreover, there are significant aberrations of nuclear organization (marked hypolobulation, irregular folding, condensed chromatin patterns) generating bulbous or so-called cloud-like/balloon-shaped nuclei, increased nuclear-cytoplasmic ratio (maturation defect), as well as increased numbers of bare (denuded) nuclei (Fig. 3.3c). At this so-called hypercellular early stage of PMF, there is no or only grade 1 reticulin fibrosis (Thiele and Kvasnicka 2005b) detectable (Fig. 3.3d), and because of the remarkable megakaryocyte proliferation, differentiation from ET is a key issue (Buhr et al. 1992; Florena et al. 2004; Gianelli et al. 2006; Thiele et al. 2000, 2001b; Thiele and Kvasnicka 2003a, b).

The other, well-known, i.e., significantly advanced to terminal endpoints characterizing the evolution of PMF are represented by the classical clinical features of myelofibrosis with myeloid metaplasia (Barosi 1999; Cervantes and Barosi 2005; Tefferi 2000). These were renamed overt fibrotic PMF (Swerdlow et al. 2008; Tefferi et al. 2007). Contrasting the early stages, BM cellularity is variable with areas of patchy hematopoiesis that may be separated by adipose tissue or gross fibrosis causing a streaming effect (Fig. 3.4a). Although neutrophil granulopoiesis as well as erythropoiesis are usually reduced in the overall hypocellular BM, there may still be some areas of residual hematopoiesis detectable (Fig. 3.4b). Similar to the early stages but often more pronounced abnormalities are prevalent in the clustered megakaryocyte (Fig. 3.4c) that together with precursors of the other cell lineages are often localized along as well as in the dilated marrow sinuses. A grossly fibrotic BM matrix with a dense increase in reticulin and collagen conforming with grades 2 and 3 myelofibrosis (Thiele et al. 2005c) is recognizable (Fig. 3.4d), often associated with osteosclerosis, i.e., new bone

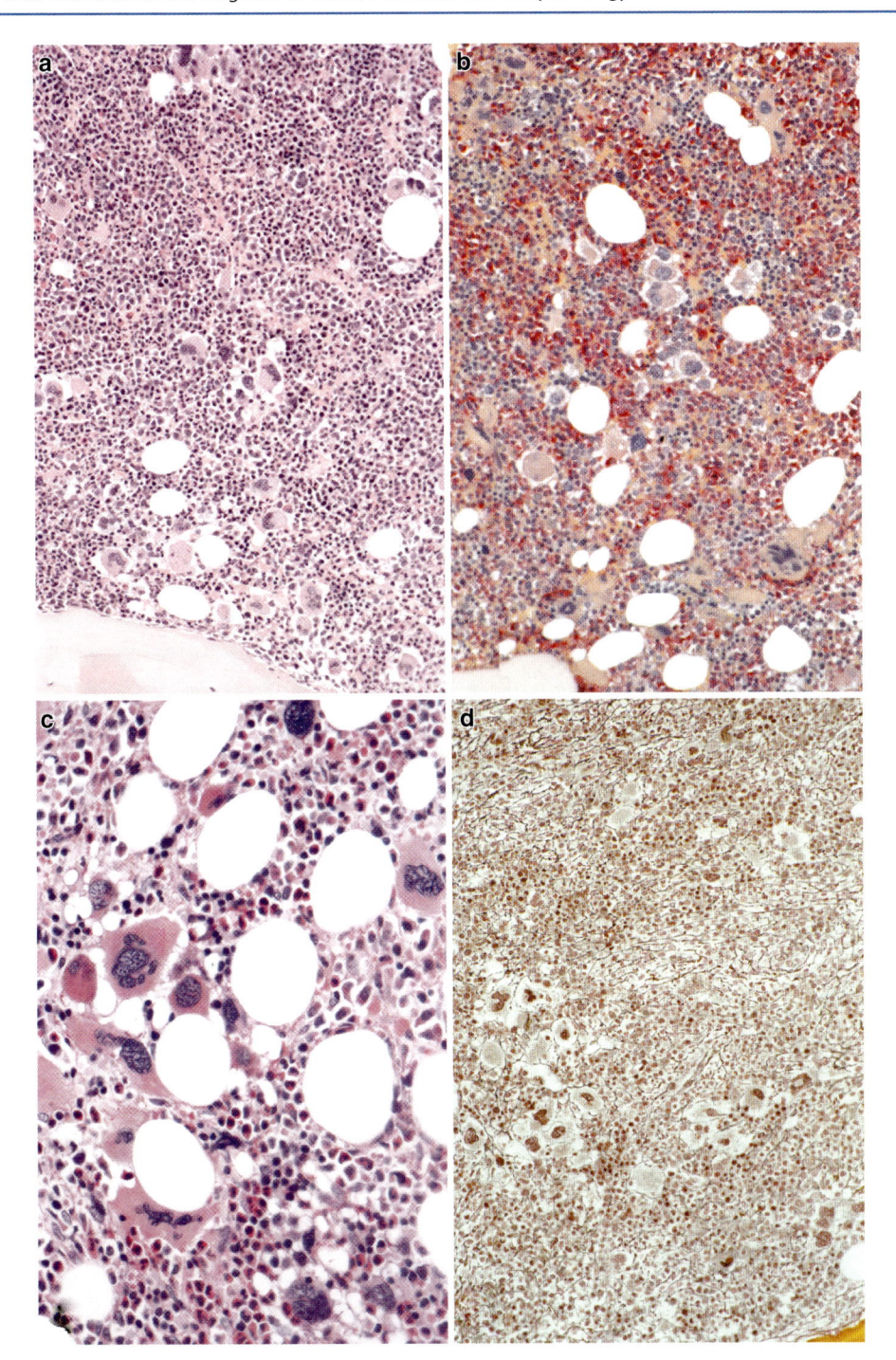

Fig. 3.3 Early/prefibrotic primary myelofibrosis. (**a**) Remarkable hypercellularity for advanced age revealing large clusters of megakaryocytes abnormally dislocated toward the trabecular bone. (**b**) In addition to megakaryocyte proliferation, there is a conspicuous increase in neutrophil granulopoiesis (*red*) accompanied by reduction of nucleated erythroid precursors. (**c**) Clustered small to giant megakaryocytes show a prevalence of striking maturation defects including cloud-like, hypolobulated, and hyperchromatic nuclei with only some irregular foldings. (**d**) Only minimal increase in reticulin fibers. Magnification: **a**, **b**, **d**, ×180; **c**, ×380. Staining: **a**=hematoxylin and eosin; **b**=AS-D-chloroacetate esterase reaction; **c**=periodic acid Schiff reagent (PAS); **d**=silver impregnation after Gomori

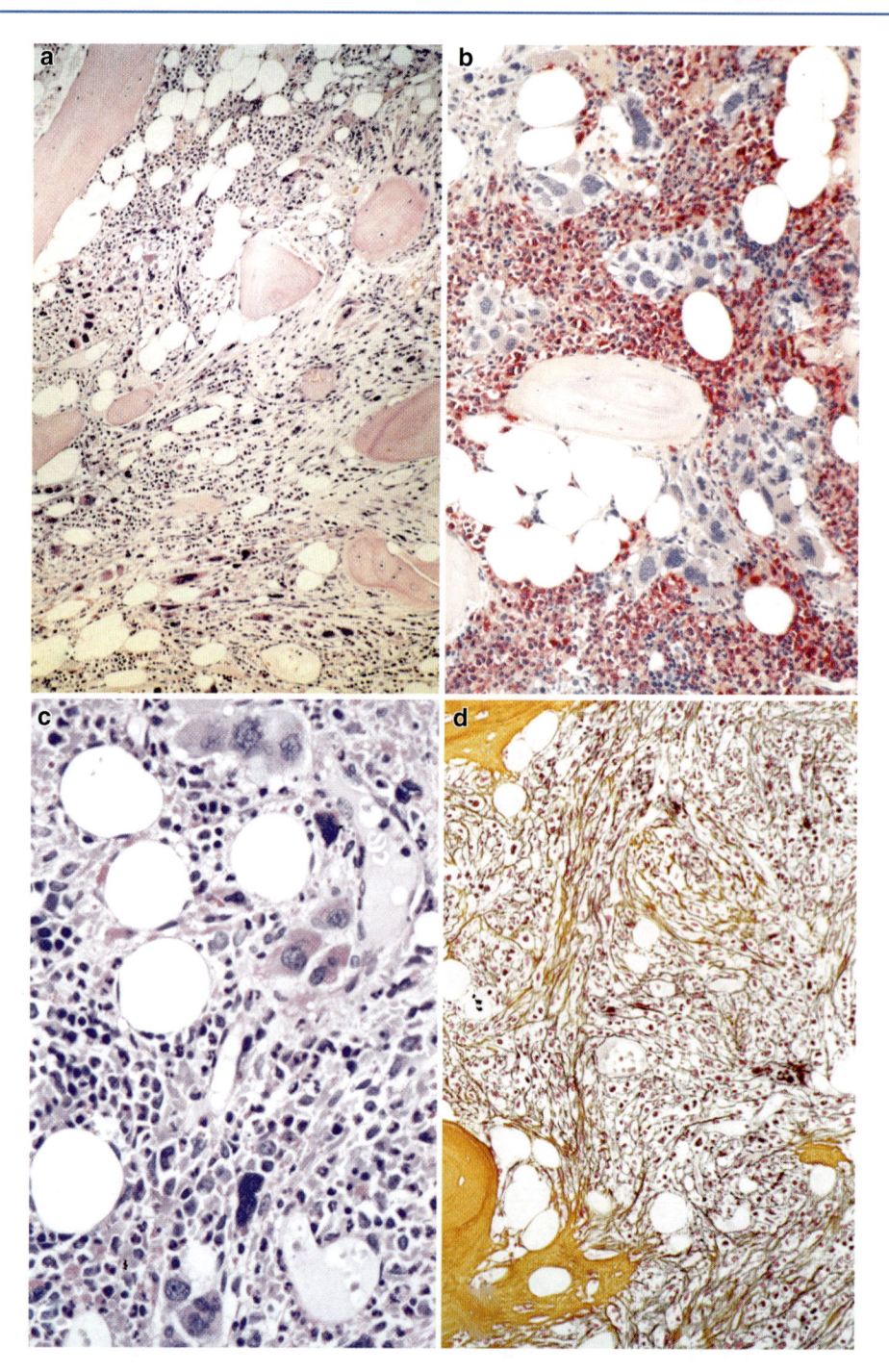

Fig. 3.4 Advanced primary myelofibrosis. (**a**) Reduced cellularity with streaming-like pattern of residual hematopoiesis including atypical megakaryocytes in addition to initial osteosclerosis (new bone formation). (**b**) In other areas, there may be still a patchy hematopoiesis with densely clustered megakaryocytes surrounded by neutrophil granulopoiesis (*red*) but only a very few erythrocyte precursors. (**c**) Clustered megakaryocytes are lying along a dilated sinus and reveal severe aberrations of maturation including cloud-like, dense, or abnormally lobulated nuclei. (**d**) Overt myelofibrosis showing bundles of collagen (*yellow*) between a dense network of reticulin and osteosclerosis. Magnification: **a**, **b**, **d**, ×180; **c**, ×380. Staining: **a** = hematoxylin and eosin; **b** = AS-D-chloroacetate esterase reaction; **c** = periodic acid Schiff reagent (PAS); **d** = silver impregnation after Gomori

formation (Buhr et al. 1993, 2003; Dickstein and Vardiman 1993; Georgii et al. 1998; Thiele et al. 2003, 2005d, 2006; Thiele and Kvasnicka 2005b). In advanced or terminal PMF, the BM is not only characterized by an overt reticulin and collagen myelofibrosis but also by a dramatic alteration concerning the vascular architecture including frequency and shape of the vessels. Contrasting the early/prefibrotic stages without, or minor, reticulin following the progression of fibrosis, a significant increase in quantity of the microvasculature is noticeably associated with marked luminal dilatation and tortuosity (Kvasnicka and Thiele 2004; Thiele et al. 1992). Although restricted to overt (classical) PMF or post-ET and post-PV myelofibrosis in comparison with other MPN entities, ample evidence has been produced regarding the significant enhancement of vascular proliferation (Arora et al. 2004; Boveri et al. 2008; Lundberg et al. 2000; Mesa et al. 2000; Ni et al. 2006). These remarkable changes were assumed to be in keeping with a complex functional network existing between fibrillo- and neoangiogenesis (Boiocchi et al. 2011; Boveri et al. 2008; Ni et al. 2006). In terminal stages, the BM may be almost totally effaced by collagen fibrosis associated with pronounced osteosclerosis and/or increased dysplastic changes of hematopoietic cells and blastic transformation, clinically causing BM failure and AML (Cervantes and Barosi 2005; Tefferi 2000).

3.5 Standardization of the WHO Morphological Criteria

The complex composition of BM tissue, particularly its changes associated with a malignant hematopoietic process warrants special care concerning the recognition of characteristic histological patterns that may be readily assigned to certain disease entities. Hematopathologists and clinicians are aware of the unwanted impact of subjectivity and therefore insist on reproducible morphological BM interpretations as a fundamental tool for an accurate discrimination of conditions that require elaborate up-to-date treatment regimens. A basal requirement is

certainly the selection and definition of as many BM constituents as possible followed by a systematically conducted categorization of their most prominent alterations and semiquantitative grading of features (Florena et al. 2004; Thiele and Kvasnicka 2003a; Thiele et al. 2005a, d). Regarding the situation in the three main entities of MPNs under discussion, standardized features of discriminating impact for generating a diagnostic histopathological pattern are shown in Table 3.1. In this context, it should be emphasized that apart from their incidence, these features exert a variable impact on differential diagnosis. While iron deposits or lymphoid nodules have little discriminative power, overall cellularity in concert with the listed alterations of granulo-, erythro-, and megakaryopoiesis as well as BM fiber content present the most important determinants to create a characteristic histological BM pattern as demonstrated for the conflicting differentiation between early/prefibrotic PMF and ET (Fig. 3.5). Concerning the crucial parameter of hematopoietic cellularity, changes associated with age have to be explicitly regarded (Table 3.2) including especially the subcortical marrow spaces (Thiele et al. 2005c). Altogether, Table 3.1 may serve as a checking list to create a constellation of morphological features exerting a discriminating impact in order to achieve an accurate diagnosis. In this scheme, exact grading of BM fibrosis is a crucial point because as reviewed by Kuter et al. (2007), essentially two different scoring systems exist (Table 3.3). In most studies, a four-graded scheme was used occasionally with slight modification of the most frequently applied scoring systems (Bauermeister 1971; Manoharan et al. 1979). On the other hand, the revised 2008 WHO classification (Tefferi et al. 2007; Vardiman et al. 2009) adopted a more simplified three-graded system (Thiele et al. 2005c) that has been proven to be of clinical relevance (Thiele and Kvasnicka 2006a; Vener et al. 2008). Concerning all these features, it has to be emphasized that not a single morphological constituent of the BM or its alteration characterizes a specific subtype of MPNs, but only a synoptical view of a large number of components creates a certain pattern. This approach

Table 3.1 Discriminating features according to WHO morphological criteria generating histological patterns in initially performed bone marrow biopsy specimens as modified from Thiele and Kvasnicka (2009)

	PV, %	ET, %	PMF, % Prefibrotic/early stage	Overt fibrotic stage
I. Cellularity (age-matched) increased	100	10–20	80–100	10–20
II. Neutrophil granulopoiesis				
Increased quantity	80–100	≤10	50–80	0
Left shifting	50–80	≤10	20–50	10–20
III. Erythropoiesis				
Increased quantity	100	≤10	≤10	0
Left shifting	80–100	≤10	10–20	≤10
IV. Megakaryopoiesis				
Increased quantity	50–80	80–100	50–80	20–50
Size:				
Small	20–50	0	20–50	20–50
Medium	20–50	10–20	10–20	10–20
Large	20–50	20–50	20–50	10–20
Giant	10–20	20–50	10–20	≤20
Histotopography				
Endosteal translocation	10–20	10–20	20–50	20–50
Cluster formation:				
Size:				
Small (at least 3)	10–20	10–20	50–80	50–80
Large (more than 7)	≤10	0	20–50	20–50
Quality:				
Dense	≤10	0	20–50	50–80
Loose	20–50	20–50	50–80	10–20
Nuclear features:				
Hypolobulation (bulbous)	10–20	≤10	50–80	50–80
Hyperlobulation (staghorn-like)	50–80	50–80	≤10	0
Maturation defects	0	0	50–80	80–100
Naked nuclei	20–50	20–50	50–80	80–100
V. Fibers				
1. Increased reticulin	10–20	0	20–50	80–100
2. Increased collagen	0	0	0	50–100
VI. Osteosclerosis	0	0	0	20–50
VII. Iron deposits	0	20–50	10–20	≤10
VIII. Lymphoid nodules present	10–20	0	10–20	≤10

Semiquantitative evaluation (relative incidence): 0 usually absent, ≤10 rare, 10–20 slight, 20–50 moderate, 50–80 manifest, 80–100 overt
PV polycythemia vera, *ET* essential thrombocythemia, *PMF* primary myelofibrosis

resembles the recognition of the various colorful particles included in a mosaic pavement forming a complex picture.

Finally, the possibility of unclassifiable entities has to be addressed. Their frequency ranges from 5% to 10%, and incidence significantly depends

WHO-Classification

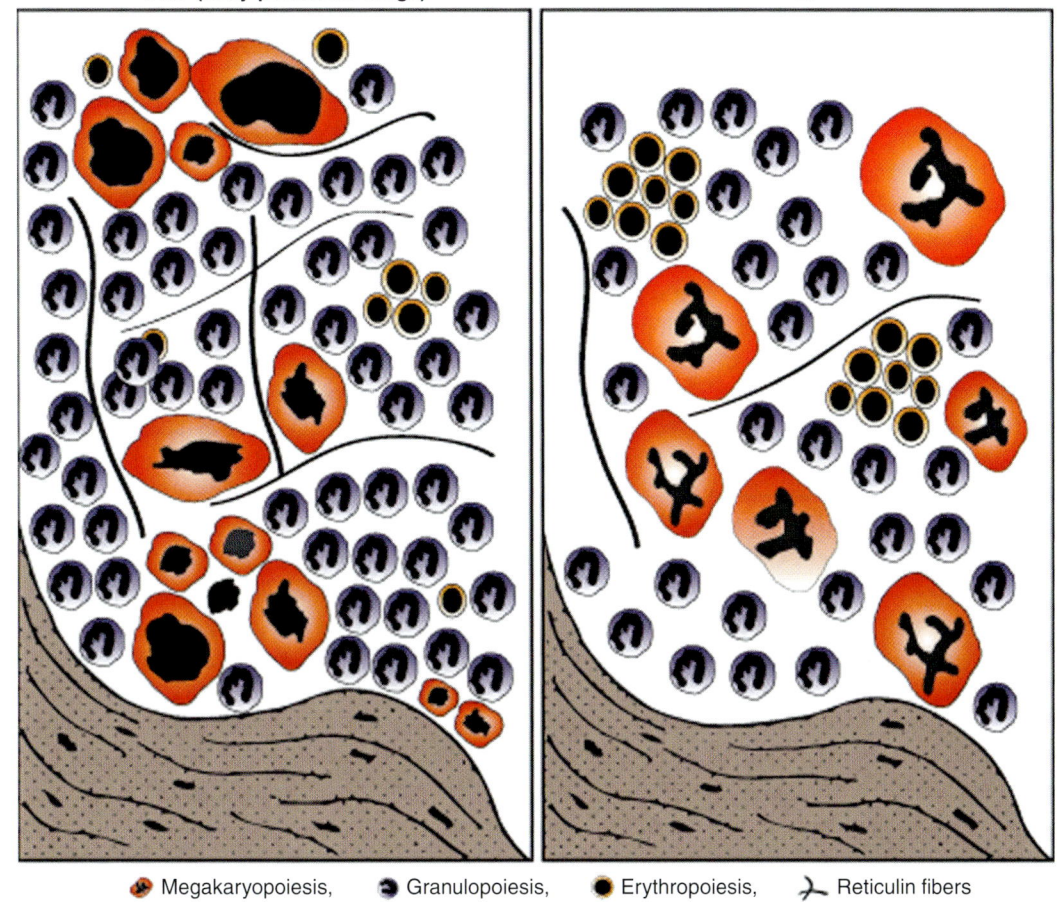

| PMF (early-prefibrotic stage) | ET |

🔴 Megakaryopoiesis,   🔵 Granulopoiesis,   ⚫ Erythropoiesis,   ⋏ Reticulin fibers

Characteristic features:

- Marked to moderate increase in age-matched cellularity

- Pronounced proliferation of neutrophil granulopoiesis and reduction of erythroid precursors

- Dense or loose clustering and frequent endosteal translocation of medium sized to giant megakaryocytes with hyperchromatic, hypolobulated, bulbous, or irregularly folded nuclei and an aberrant nuclear/cytoplasmic ratio

- No or no significant increase in reticulin fibers

- No or only slight increase in age-matched cellularity

- No significant increase or left-shift in neutrophil granulopoiesis and erythropoiesis

- Dispersed or loosely clustered large to giant mature megakaryocytes with hyperlobulated or deeply folded nuclei

- No or very rarely minor increase in reticulin fibers

Fig. 3.5 Schematic presentation of characteristic histological bone marrow patterns and morphological criteria in early/prefibrotic primary myelofibrosis (*PMF*) versus essential thrombocythemia (*ET*) generated from semiquantitative evaluations of prominent diagnostic features as listed in Table 3.1 (Modified from Thiele et al. (2011))

Table 3.2 Normal ranges of bone marrow cellularity for selected age groups (years) as adapted from the literature (Thiele et al. 2005c)

Age	% Hematopoietic area
20–30	60–70
40–60	40–50
≥70	30–40
≥80	10–20

not only on the experience of the investigator but particularly on the examination of a representative, properly sized (at least 1.5 cm) biopsy specimen performed at clinical diagnosis, and before any relevant therapy (Vardiman et al. 2009).

3.6 Reproducibility of the WHO Morphological Criteria

Concerning the reproducibility of the WHO-defined histological criteria regarding MPNs (Vardiman et al. 2009), a conflict of opinion has to be discussed. In this context, among several pathologists controversy is especially focused on the crucial discrimination between ET and early stage PMF presenting with an elevated platelet count (false ET). Independently from the Cologne

group, an increasing number of authorities were able to confirm the reliability of morphological BM features as proposed by the WHO (Boiocchi et al. 2011; Koopmans et al. 2011; Florena et al. 2004; Gianelli et al. 2006, 2008; Kreft et al. 2005; Vener et al. 2008). Additionally, in subsequently performed central reviews, involving more than 1,400 patients and a large number of local pathologists from different institutions, a more than 80% concordance was revealed (Barbui et al. 2011; Thiele et al. 2011). This rate of agreement is comparable with or even better than results of blinded histological panel evaluations by international study groups subtyping malignant B- and T-cell lymphomas (Diebold et al. 2002; Lones et al. 2000; Rüdiger et al. 2002) and Hodgkin's disease (Glaser et al. 2001) as well as cytological classifications of myelodysplastic syndromes (Mufti et al. 2008). Contrasting these confirmatory studies, a blinded semiquantitative evaluation of certain BM features among three hematologists/pathologists questions explicitly these results (Wilkins et al. 2008). Noteworthy is that the 370 BM biopsy specimens investigated were derived from the UK-PT1 trial (Harrison et al. 2005) and that the study design and performance are unfortunately impaired by a number of inconsistencies. Among others, these

Table 3.3 Standard (Bauermeister 1971; Manoharan et al. 1979) and European Consensus (Thiele et al. 2005c) criteria for grading of myelofibrosis

Fibrosis grade[a]	Standard grading of reticulin fibrosis	European Consensus grading of myelofibrosis
0	Occasional fine and coarse individual fibers only; or foci of perivascular fiber network associated with benign lymphoid nodules	Scattered linear reticulin with no intersections (crossovers) corresponding to normal bone marrow
1	Fine fiber network (with occasional coarse fibers) throughout most of the section; or focal increase in reticulin away from vessels and benign lymphoid nodules	Loose network of reticulin with many intersections, especially in perivascular areas
2	Diffuse fiber network with an increase in scattered fibers	Diffuse and dense increase in reticulin with extensive intersections, occasionally with only focal bundles of collagen, and/or focal osteosclerosis
3	Diffuse, often coarse fiber network with no evidence of collagenization (negative trichrome stain)	Diffuse and dense increase in reticulin with extensive intersections with coarse bundles of collagen, often associated with significant osteosclerosis
4	Diffuse, coarse fiber network with areas of collagenization (positive trichrome stain)	Not applicable

[a]Fiber density should be assessed in hematopoietic (cellular) areas

impairments include a lack of a clear-cut standardization of the 16 evaluated BM parameters strictly according to WHO (Thiele and Kvasnicka 2003a, 2009; Thiele et al. 2005a). Remarkable was further a failing intraobserver evaluation (self-assessment) during the long period of examination with the unwanted bias of a learning effect. Moreover, the small size of evaluated biopsy specimens (≥ 0.5 cm), contrasting the minimally requested length of ≥ 1.5 cm (Thiele et al. 2005c; Vardiman et al. 2009) precludes an accurate recognition of localized features like clusters or a more exact grading of fibrosis and assessment of age-matched cellularity. Finally, the very poor reproducibility of basic BM features that may have served as controls for reliability like quantity of erythropoiesis raises serious concerns. Although this series of patients was explicitly defined to be consistent with ET according to the diagnostic criteria of the PVSG (Murphy et al. 1997; Pearson 1998), in a conspicuously wide range from 37% to 76% among the panelists, higher levels of BM fibrosis (probably grades 3 and 4) on a four-graded scale (Table 3.3) and new bone formation (osteosclerosis) were found (Wilkins et al. 2008). This result regarding the semiquantitative scoring of a basic parameter like BM fibrosis among the panelists is not compatible with a consistent evaluation strictly applying standardized parameters. Comparable findings were reiterated in a study of the same group on 361 patients with ET mostly (82%) derived from the UK-PT1 trial (Harrison et al. 2005) reporting that about 60% of cases showed an increased BM fibrosis at disease onset, including more than 20% with moderate to overt myelofibrosis (Campbell et al. 2009). Although the PVSG criteria for ET (Murphy et al. 1997; Pearson 1998) do allow a certain amount of BM fibrosis at presentation, the 80 patients with outright myelofibrosis, i.e., grades 3 and 4 (Table 3.3), are hardly consistent with these diagnostic guidelines. Concerning outcome, Campbell et al. (2009) reported that 11 of 226 patients diagnosed with ET, who showed reticulin fibrosis grades ≥ 2, developed overt myelofibrosis after 68 months of follow-up, contrasting none of 135 patients with reticulin grade ≤ 1. Additionally, a greater propor-

tion of patients with so-called ET and reticulin grades ≥ 2 presented with splenomegaly, a higher white blood cell count and increased marrow granulocytic cellularity as compared to patients with reticulin grade ≤ 1. According to a number of experts, at presentation, ET is not characterized by BM fibrosis or osteosclerosis, and contrasting PMF, progression into overt myelofibrosis or leukemia is a rather rare event occurring after many years (Barbui et al. 2011; Kreft et al. 2005; Thiele et al. 2002, 2006). For this reason, it may be assumed that a considerable number of cases reported in the three papers of the English group (Campbell et al. 2009; Harrison et al. 2005; Wilkins et al. 2008) including overlapping cohorts of patients are more likely consistent with thrombocythemic manifestations of PMF (Thiele et al. 2009, 2011).

In another study critical to the WHO classification, two pathologists tried to reproduce the relevant criteria on 127 BM biopsy specimens with ET originally diagnosed according to PVSG (Murphy et al. 1997; Pearson 1998) resulting in a significant discordance of 35% among the panelists (Brousseau et al. 2010). The overall conclusion of these authors was that a discrimination between ET and early/prefibrotic PMF according to WHO criteria is impaired by subjectivity and of questionable clinical relevance. This argument has not only been refuted by large multicenter studies (Barbui et al. 2011; Thiele et al. 2011) but also by a number of inconsistencies characterizing this semiquantitative evaluation on BM samples grossly comparable with the investigation by Wilkins et al. (2008). The selection of the specimens up to 3 years after clinical diagnosis, with no data on the biopsy size and particularly the disturbing finding that 54% of the patients claimed explicitly by the authors to present WHO-defined ET showed a minor to moderate reticulin fibrosis, is rather confusing. Following strictly the WHO classification of MPNs, in ET incidence of minor reticulin fibrosis (grade 1, Table 3.3), is very rare and observed in less than 5% (Barbui et al. 2011; Thiele et al. 2002, 2006). Finally, statistical analysis of morphological features (semiquantitative scoring system) and clinical data including outcome did not take the significant disparity in the number of cases in both groups (ET 102 patients versus PMF 18 patients) into account (Brousseau et al. 2010). Altogether, there is a striking prevalence of authors and relevant studies that endorse the histological WHO criteria including an increasing number of reports in favor of a reproducibility of entities, especially concerning ET and early/prefibrotic PMF to a substantial extent (Thiele et al. 2011).

Finally, to enhance the reliability of reproducing these features in accordance with the WHO classification, hematopathologists involved in this field should be provided with a training set of characteristic slides and/or attend corresponding tutorials/workshops as is usually done in the case of other hematological malignancies (subtyping of malignant lymphomas, myelodysplastic syndromes, etc.).

Conclusion

Histopathological diagnosis, particularly discrimination of the different MPN entities, is significantly based on standardized morphological features and recognition of distinctive BM patterns generating concordant results among pathologists as first step toward clinical studies. By regarding these postulates on treatment-naive and representative BM biopsy specimens, early stages of PMF presenting with thrombocythemia (false ET) are clearly separated from true ET. Persuasive evidence has been provided that this distinction exerts a significant clinical impact on the outcome concerning progression to myelofibrosis, leukemic transformation, and survival. Histological data, particularly regarding BM fibrosis derived from the UK-PT1 study and related investigations, suggest that these partially overlapping cohorts consist of a heterogeneous series of patients with a significant prevalence of PMF.

References

Arora B, Ho CL, Hoyer JD et al (2004) Bone marrow angiogenesis and its clinical correlates in myelofibrosis with myeloid metaplasia. Haematologica 89:1454–1458

Barbui T, Thiele J, Passamonti F et al (2011) Survival and disease progression in essential thrombocythemia are significantly influenced by accurate morphologic diagnosis: an international study of 1,104 patients. J Clin Oncol 29:3179–3184

Barosi G (1999) Myelofibrosis with myeloid metaplasia: diagnostic definition and prognostic classification for clinical studies and treatment guidelines. J Clin Oncol 17:2954–2970

Barosi G, Mesa RA, Thiele J et al (2008) Proposed criteria for the diagnosis of post-polycythemia vera and post-essential thrombocythemia myelofibrosis: a consensus statement from the International Working Group for Myelofibrosis Research and Treatment. Leukemia 22:437–438

Bauermeister DE (1971) Quantitation of bone marrow reticulin – a normal range. Am J Clin Pathol 56:24–31

Boiocchi L, Vener C, Savi F et al (2011) Increased expression of vascular endothelial growth factor receptor 1 correlates with VEGF and microvessel density in Philadelphia chromosome-negative myeloproliferative neoplasms. J Clin Pathol 64:226–231

Boveri E, Passamonti F, Rumi E et al (2008) Bone marrow microvessel density in chronic myeloproliferative disorders: a study of 115 patients with clinicopathological and molecular correlations. Br J Haematol 140:162–168

Brousseau M, Parot-Schinkel E, Moles MP et al (2010) Practical application and clinical impact of the WHO histopathological criteria on bone marrow biopsy for the diagnosis of essential thrombocythemia versus prefibrotic primary myelofibrosis. Histopathology 56:758–767

Buhr T, Georgii A, Schuppan O et al (1992) Histologic findings in bone marrow biopsies of patients with thrombocythemic cell counts. Ann Hematol 64:286–291

Buhr T, Georgii A, Choritz H (1993) Myelofibrosis in chronic myeloproliferative disorders. Incidence among subtypes according to the Hannover Classification. Pathol Res Pract 189:121–132

Buhr T, Buesche G, Choritz H et al (2003) Evolution of myelofibrosis in chronic idiopathic myelofibrosis as evidenced in sequential bone marrow biopsy specimens. Am J Clin Pathol 119:152–158

Campbell PJ, Bareford D, Erber WN et al (2009) Reticulin accumulation in essential thrombocythemia: prognostic significance and relationship to therapy. J Clin Oncol 27:2991–2999

Cervantes F, Barosi G (2005) Myelofibrosis with myeloid metaplasia: diagnosis, prognostic factors, and staging. Semin Oncol 32:395–402

Cervantes F, Pereira A, Esteve J et al (1998) The changing profile of idiopathic myelofibrosis: a comparison of the presenting features of patients diagnosed in two different decades. Eur J Haematol 60:101–105

Cervantes F, Alvarez-Larran A, Talarn C et al (2002) Myelofibrosis with myeloid metaplasia following essential thrombocythaemia: actuarial probability, presenting characteristics and evolution in a series of 195 patients. Br J Haematol 118:786–790

Chim CS, Kwong YL, Lie AK et al (2005) Long-term outcome of 231 patients with essential thrombocythemia: prognostic factors for thrombosis, bleeding, myelofibrosis, and leukemia. Arch Intern Med 165: 2651–2658

Dickstein JI, Vardiman JW (1993) Issues in the pathology and diagnosis of the chronic myeloproliferative disorders and the myelodysplastic syndromes. Am J Clin Pathol 99:513–525

Dickstein JI, Vardiman JW (1995) Hematopathologic findings in the myeloproliferative disorders. Semin Oncol 22:355–373

Diebold J, Anderson JR, Armitage JO et al (2002) Diffuse large B-cell lymphoma: a clinicopathologic analysis of 444 cases classified according to the updated Kiel classification. Leuk Lymphoma 43:97–104

Ellis JT, Peterson P (1979) The bone marrow in polycythemia vera. Pathol Annu 14(Pt 1):383–403

Ellis JT, Peterson P, Geller SA et al (1986) Studies of the bone marrow in polycythemia vera and the evolution of myelofibrosis and second hematologic malignancies. Semin Hematol 23:144–155

Florena AM, Tripodo C, Iannitto E et al (2004) Value of bone marrow biopsy in the diagnosis of essential thrombocythemia. Haematologica 89:911–919

Gangat N, Caramazza D, Vaidya R et al (2011) DIPSS plus: a refined Dynamic International Prognostic Scoring System for primary myelofibrosis that incorporates prognostic information from karyotype, platelet count, and transfusion status. J Clin Oncol 29: 392–397

Georgii A, Buesche G, Kreft A (1998) The histopathology of chronic myeloproliferative diseases. Baillieres Clin Haematol 11:721–749

Gianelli U, Vener C, Raviele PR et al (2006) Essential thrombocythemia or chronic idiopathic myelofibrosis? A single-center study based on hematopoietic bone marrow histology. Leuk Lymphoma 47:1774–1781

Gianelli U, Iurlo A, Vener C et al (2008) The significance of bone marrow biopsy and JAK2V617F mutation in the differential diagnosis between the "early" prepolycythemic phase of polycythemia vera and essential thrombocythemia. Am J Clin Pathol 130:336–342

Girodon F, Dutrillaux F, Broseus J et al (2010) Leukocytosis is associated with poor survival but not with increased risk of thrombosis in essential thrombocythemia: a population-based study of 311 patients. Leukemia 24: 900–903

Glaser SL, Dorfman RF, Clarke CA (2001) Expert review of the diagnosis and histologic classification of Hodgkin disease in a population-based cancer registry: interobserver reliability and impact on incidence and survival rates. Cancer 92:218–224

Harrison CN, Campbell PJ, Buck G et al (2005) Hydroxyurea compared with anagrelide in high-risk essential thrombocythemia. N Engl J Med 353:33–45

Jaffe E, Harris N, Stein H et al (2001) WHO classification of tumours of haematopoietic and lymphoid tissues. IARC Press, Lyon

Koopmans SM, Bot FJ, Lam KH et al (2011) Reproducibility of histologic classification in nonfibrotic myeloproliferative neoplasia. AM J Clin Pathol 136: 618–624

Kreft A, Buesche G, Ghalibafian M et al (2005) The incidence of myelofibrosis in essential thrombocythaemia, polycythaemia vera and chronic idiopathic myelofibrosis: a retrospective evaluation of sequential bone marrow biopsies. Acta Haematol 113:137–143

Kuter DJ, Bain B, Mufti G et al (2007) Bone marrow fibrosis: pathophysiology and clinical significance of increased bone marrow stromal fibres. Br J Haematol 139:351–362

Kvasnicka HM, Thiele J (2004) Bone marrow angiogenesis: methods of quantification and changes evolving in chronic myeloproliferative disorders. Histol Histopathol 19:1245–1260

Kvasnicka HM, Thiele J (2006) The impact of clinicopathological studies on staging and survival in essential thrombocythemia, chronic idiopathic myelofibrosis, and polycythemia rubra vera. Semin Thromb Hemost 32:362–371

Kvasnicka HM, Thiele J (2010) Prodromal myeloproliferative neoplasms: the 2008 WHO classification. Am J Hematol 85:62–69

Kvasnicka HM, Thiele J, Werden C et al (1997) Prognostic factors in idiopathic (primary) osteomyelofibrosis. Cancer 80:708–719

Lones MA, Auperin A, Raphael M et al (2000) Mature B-cell lymphoma/leukemia in children and adolescents: intergroup pathologist consensus with the revised European-American Lymphoma Classification. Ann Oncol 11:47–51

Lundberg LG, Lerner R, Sundelin P et al (2000) Bone marrow in polycythemia vera, chronic myelocytic leukemia, and myelofibrosis has an increased vascularity. Am J Pathol 157:15–19

Manoharan A, Horsley R, Pitney WR (1979) The reticulin content of bone marrow in acute leukaemia in adults. Br J Haematol 43:185–190

Mesa RA, Hanson CA, Rajkumar SV et al (2000) Evaluation and clinical correlations of bone marrow angiogenesis in myelofibrosis with myeloid metaplasia. Blood 96:3374–3380

Mufti GJ, Bennett JM, Goasguen J et al (2008) Diagnosis and classification of myelodysplastic syndrome: International Working Group on Morphology of myelodysplastic syndrome (IWGM-MDS) consensus proposals for the definition and enumeration of myeloblasts and ring sideroblasts. Haematologica 93:1712–1717

Murphy S (1999) Diagnostic criteria and prognosis in polycythemia vera and essential thrombocythemia. Semin Hematol 36:9–13

Murphy S, Peterson P, Iland H et al (1997) Experience of the Polycythemia Vera Study Group with essential thrombocythemia: a final report on diagnostic criteria, survival, and leukemic transition by treatment. Semin Hematol 34:29–39

Ni H, Barosi G, Hoffman R (2006) Quantitative evaluation of bone marrow angiogenesis in idiopathic myelofibrosis. Am J Clin Pathol 126:241–247

Palandri F, Catani L, Testoni N et al (2009) Long-term follow-up of 386 consecutive patients with essential thrombocythemia: safety of cytoreductive therapy. Am J Hematol 84:215–220

Passamonti F, Rumi E, Arcaini L et al (2008) Prognostic factors for thrombosis, myelofibrosis, and leukemia in essential thrombocythemia: a study of 605 patients. Haematologica 93:1645–1651

Pearson TC (1998) Diagnosis and classification of erythrocytoses and thrombocytoses. Baillieres Clin Haematol 11:695–720

Rüdiger T, Weisenburger DD, Anderson JR et al (2002) Peripheral T-cell lymphoma (excluding anaplastic large-cell lymphoma): results from the Non-Hodgkin's Lymphoma Classification Project. Ann Oncol 13:140–149

Ruggeri M, Tosetto A, Frezzato M et al (2003) The rate of progression to polycythemia vera or essential thrombocythemia in patients with erythrocytosis or thrombocytosis. Ann Intern Med 139:470–475

Spivak JL, Silver RT (2008) The revised World Health Organization diagnostic criteria for polycythemia vera, essential thrombocytosis, and primary myelofibrosis: an alternative proposal. Blood 112:231–239

Swerdlow S, Campo E, Harris N et al (2008) WHO classification of tumours of haematopoietic and lymphoid tissues. IARC Press, Lyon

Tefferi A (2000) Myelofibrosis with myeloid metaplasia. N Engl J Med 342:1255–1265

Tefferi A, Vardiman JW (2008) Classification and diagnosis of myeloproliferative neoplasms: the 2008 World Health Organization criteria and point-of-care diagnostic algorithms. Leukemia 22:14–22

Tefferi A, Thiele J, Orazi A et al (2007) Proposals and rationale for revision of the World Health Organization diagnostic criteria for polycythemia vera, essential thrombocythemia, and primary myelofibrosis: recommendations from an ad hoc international expert panel. Blood 110:1092–1097

Tefferi A, Skoda R, Vardiman JW (2009) Myeloproliferative neoplasms: contemporary diagnosis using histology and genetics. Nat Rev Clin Oncol 6:627–637

Thiele J, Kvasnicka HM (2003a) Diagnostic differentiation of essential thrombocythaemia from thrombocythaemias associated with chronic idiopathic myelofibrosis by discriminate analysis of bone marrow features – a clinicopathological study on 272 patients. Histol Histopathol 18:93–102

Thiele J, Kvasnicka HM (2003b) Chronic myeloproliferative disorders with thrombocythemia: a comparative study of two classification systems (PVSG, WHO) on 839 patients. Ann Hematol 82:148–152

Thiele J, Kvasnicka HM (2004) Prefibrotic chronic idiopathic myelofibrosis – a diagnostic enigma? Acta Haematol 111:155–159

Thiele J, Kvasnicka HM (2005a) Diagnostic impact of bone marrow histopathology in polycythemia vera (PV). Histol Histopathol 20:317–328

Thiele J, Kvasnicka HM (2005b) Hematopathologic findings in chronic idiopathic myelofibrosis. Semin Oncol 32:380–394

Thiele J, Kvasnicka HM (2006a) Grade of bone marrow fibrosis is associated with relevant hematological findings-a clinicopathological study on 865 patients with chronic idiopathic myelofibrosis. Ann Hematol 85:226–232

Thiele J, Kvasnicka HM (2006b) Clinicopathological criteria for differential diagnosis of thrombocythemias in various myeloproliferative disorders. Semin Thromb Hemost 32:219–230

Thiele J, Kvasnicka HM (2009) The 2008 WHO diagnostic criteria for polycythemia vera, essential thrombocythemia, and primary myelofibrosis. Curr Hematol Malig Rep 4:33–40

Thiele J, Zankovich R, Steinberg T et al (1989a) Agnogenic myeloid metaplasia (AMM) – correlation of bone marrow lesions with laboratory data: a longitudinal clinicopathological study on 114 patients. Hematol Oncol 7:327–343

Thiele J, Zankovich R, Steinberg T et al (1989b) Primary (essential) thrombocythemia versus initial (hyperplastic) stages of agnogenic myeloid metaplasia with thrombocytosis – a critical evaluation of clinical and histomorphological data. Acta Haematol 81:192–202

Thiele J, Rompcik V, Wagner S et al (1992) Vascular architecture and collagen type IV in primary myelofibrosis and polycythaemia vera: an immunomorphometric study on trephine biopsies of the bone marrow. Br J Haematol 80:227–234

Thiele J, Kvasnicka HM, Werden C et al (1996) Idiopathic primary osteo-myelofibrosis: a clinico-pathological study on 208 patients with special emphasis on evolution of disease features, differentiation from essential thrombocythemia and variables of prognostic impact. Leuk Lymphoma 22:303–317

Thiele J, Kvasnicka HM, Boeltken B et al (1999) Initial (prefibrotic) stages of idiopathic (primary) myelofibrosis (IMF) – a clinicopathological study. Leukemia 13:1741–1748

Thiele J, Kvasnicka HM, Zankovich R et al (2000) Relevance of bone marrow features in the differential diagnosis between essential thrombocythemia and early stage idiopathic myelofibrosis. Haematologica 85:1126–1134

Thiele J, Kvasnicka HM, Muehlhausen K et al (2001a) Polycythemia rubra vera versus secondary polycythemias. A clinicopathological evaluation of distinctive features in 199 patients. Pathol Res Pract 197:77–84

Thiele J, Kvasnicka HM, Zankovich R et al (2001b) Clinical and morphological criteria for the diagnosis of prefibrotic idiopathic (primary) myelofibrosis. Ann Hematol 80:160–165

Thiele J, Kvasnicka HM, Schmitt-Graeff A et al (2002) Follow-up examinations including sequential bone marrow biopsies in essential thrombocythemia (ET): a retrospective clinicopathological study of 120 patients. Am J Hematol 70:283–291

Thiele J, Kvasnicka HM, Schmitt-Gräff A et al (2003) Dynamics of fibrosis in chronic idiopathic (primary) myelofibrosis during therapy: a follow-up study on 309 patients. Leuk Lymphoma 44:549–553

Thiele J, Kvasnicka HM, Diehl V (2005a) Standardization of bone marrow features – does it work in hematopathology for histological discrimination of different disease patterns? Histol Histopathol 20:633–644

Thiele J, Kvasnicka HM, Diehl V (2005b) Initial (latent) polycythemia vera with thrombocytosis mimicking essential thrombocythemia. Acta Haematol 113:213–219

Thiele J, Kvasnicka HM, Facchetti F et al (2005c) European consensus for grading of bone marrow fibrosis and assessment of cellularity. Haematologica 90:1128–1132

Thiele J, Kvasnicka HM, Orazi A (2005d) Bone marrow histopathology in myeloproliferative disorders – current diagnostic approach. Semin Hematol 42:184–195

Thiele J, Kvasnicka HM, Vardiman J (2006) Bone marrow histopathology in the diagnosis of chronic myeloproliferative disorders: a forgotten pearl. Best Pract Res Clin Haematol 19:413–437

Thiele J, Kvasnicka HM, Vardiman JW et al (2009) Bone marrow fibrosis and diagnosis of essential thrombocythemia. J Clin Oncol 27:e220–e221; author reply e222–e223

Thiele J, Kvasnicka HM, Mullauer L et al (2011) Essential thrombocythemia versus early primary myelofibrosis: a multicenter study to validate the WHO classification. Blood 117:5710–5718

Vardiman JW, Thiele J, Arber DA et al (2009) The 2008 revision of the WHO classification of myeloid neoplasms and acute leukemia: rationale and important changes. Blood 114:937–951

Vener C, Fracchiolla NS, Gianelli U et al (2008) Prognostic implications of the European consensus for grading of bone marrow fibrosis in chronic idiopathic myelofibrosis. Blood 111:1862–1865

Wasserman LR (1986) Polycythemia Vera Study Group: a historical perspective. Semin Hematol 23:183–187

Wilkins BS, Erber WN, Bareford D et al (2008) Bone marrow pathology in essential thrombocythemia: interobserver reliability and utility for identifying disease subtypes. Blood 111:60–70

Wolanskyj AP, Schwager SM, McClure RF et al (2006) Essential thrombocythemia beyond the first decade: life expectancy, long-term complication rates, and prognostic factors. Mayo Clin Proc 81:159–166

Critical Issues About the Diagnosis of Myeloproliferative Neoplasms: World Health Organization Classification

4

Mary Frances McMullin

Contents

M.F. McMullin
Department of Haematology, 'C' Floor,
Belfast City Hospital, Queen's University Belfast,
Belfast, Northern Ireland, UK
e-mail: m.mcmullin@qub.ac.uk

4.1 Polycythaemia Vera

Polycythaemia vera (PV) is a primary bone marrow disorder where excessive numbers of red blood cells are produced. A somatic gain-of-function mutation of the *Janus Kinase* (*JAK*) 2 gene is present in most cases. The disease may present in a latent form where there is only a borderline erythrocytosis, the classical overt polycythaemia form and finally may progress to a spent or post-polycythaemic myelofibrotic disorder (post-PV MF).

The World Health Organization (WHO) has now defined diagnostic criteria for PV (Thiele et al. 2008a).

The *major criteria* are

1. Haemoglobin >18.5 g/dl in men, 16.5 g/dl in women or other evidence of increased red cell volume.

    (This is further defined as haemoglobin or haematocrit >99th percentile of method specific reference range for age, sex, altitude of residence or haemoglobin >17 g/dl if associated with a documented and sustained increase of at least 2 g/dl from an individual's baseline value that cannot be attributed to correction of iron deficiency, or elevated red cell mass >25% above mean normal predicted value).

2. Presence of *JAK*2V617F or other functionally similar mutation such as *JAK*2 exon 12 mutation.

The *minor criteria* are

1. Bone marrow biopsy showing hypercellularity for age with tri-lineage growth (panmyelosis) with prominent erythroid, granulocytic and megakaryocytic proliferation
2. Serum erythropoietin (EPO) level below the reference range for normal
3. Endogenous erythroid colony (EEC) formation in vitro

Diagnosis requires the presence of both major criteria and one minor criterion or the presence of the first major criterion and two of the minor criteria.

There are a number of issues with each of these criteria which must be considered when the criteria are being used to make the diagnosis in routine practice.

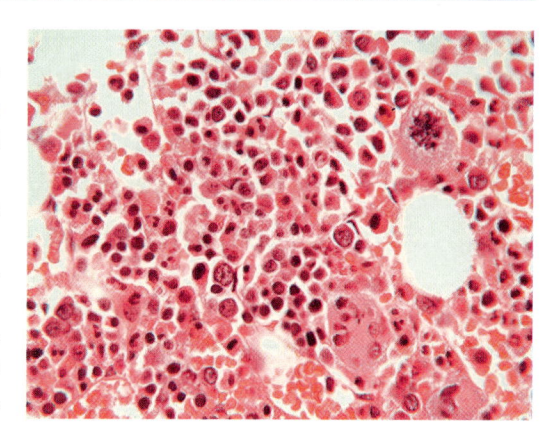

Fig. 4.1 Trephine in polycythaemia vera showing tri-lineage hypercellularity (Image courtesy of Dr. R. Cuthbert)

4.1.1 Haemoglobin

Haemoglobin levels for the diagnosis have been defined with important caveats. Haemoglobins are defined as above the 99th percentile for the measurement used or a sustained increase from baseline not due to iron deficiency or other 'evidence of increased red cell mass'. This attempts to include a variety of situations where the haemoglobin is significantly increased. However, there are a number of issues with this which may be of importance.

The true measurement of an erythrocytosis is an increased red cell mass. This does not always equate to an increased haemoglobin or haematocrit as shown by the study of Johansson where in both males and females, a raised haemoglobin was not always consistent with an absolute erythrocytosis by red cell mass measurement, and conversely, haemoglobins below the cut-off level could be present with an absolute erythrocytosis (Johansson et al. 2005).

Iron deficiency is also excluded, and this means that the patient presenting with an obvious iron deficiency will need to be considered carefully. Judicious and carefully monitored administration of iron may be indicated, but it may also be correct from a therapeutic point of view to withhold iron and in such a patient the

haemoglobin would not make the diagnostic criteria.

4.1.2 *JAK2* Mutations

In 2005, the *JAK2* V617F mutation was described in the majority of patients who were then classified with PV (Baxter et al. 2005; James et al. 2005; Kralovics et al. 2005; Levine et al. 2005). This is a gain-of-function acquired mutation in a bone marrow clone which leads to a constitutively active JAK2 protein. In a further group of patients with erythrocytosis, different mutations in exon 12 of the *JAK2* gene were discovered (Scott et al. 2007; Percy et al. 2007). These mutations can be detected in the peripheral blood with increasingly sensitive techniques, and it is possible to detect the presence of small clones (Chen et al. 2007).

This criterion which has completely altered the new WHO diagnostic criteria for PV is a crucial major criterion and in clinical practice is increasingly an initial diagnostic test for investigating and confirming a diagnosis of a patient with raised haemoglobin.

4.1.3 Bone Marrow Biopsy

The bone marrow biopsy showing defined tri-lineage hypercellularity is a minor criterion (Fig. 4.1). Much of the work in coming to the histopathological interpretations has been done in retrospective and unblinded settings (Hussein et al. 2007). There are also patients with congenital erythrocytosis/polycythaemia with mutations in the *von Hippel–Lindau* gene who have had their bone marrow interpreted as consistent with PV (Gordeuk et al. 2005), so the discriminatory power of the described bone marrow changes may not be sufficient. Widespread prospective use may be difficult, requiring very specific expertise, and this haematopathology experience may not be widely available. It may also be difficult to persuade patients and justify the expense of the widespread use of bone marrow biopsy to add to the diagnostic pathways in those who fulfil other criteria using less invasive tests.

4.1.4 Erythropoietin Level

The EPO level in a patient can be below the normal range, normal or elevated. A below normal levels suggests a primary bone marrow problem with production of increased red cells and is usually seen in cases of PV and as such is a useful discriminating test. However, the assay is only of limited availability, and the result may be influenced by other factors such as venesection and secondary causes of erythrocytosis such as smoking.

4.1.5 Endogenous Erythroid Colonies

The growth of EECs from the peripheral blood demonstrating in a patient with PV that erythroid colonies grow in the absence of added EPO is a skilled technique, requires 2 weeks of culture for each sample, and is only available in a very few centres. It can be standardised and quality controlled between centres, but this requires considerable technical effort (Dobo et al. 2004). Therefore, while this is a useful research tool and can be useful in those with the skills, it is unlikely to be used in any widespread fashion. The addition of this test as a minor criterion does not seem to add anything to the diagnostic process but

merely acknowledges an old test (Prchal and Axelrad 1974) which was of use in the past before more practical, easy to perform and generally applicable tests became available.

4.1.6 Diagnostic Issues

The commentary above elucidates some of the issues with the individual tests which are required to make a diagnosis of PV in the WHO criteria, but the criteria require both major and one minor criterion or the first major criterion plus two minor criteria to make the diagnosis. Is this necessary and sufficient for this diagnosis?

If both major criteria are present does the addition of a minor criterion add anything? It can be argued that it does not. A patient with both major criteria present has been shown to have a clonal erythrocytosis and as such a PV-type disorder. The addition of minor criteria complements this diagnosis and acknowledges tests which have been used to discriminate in cases in the past before the discovery of the acquired clonal markers, but they do not actually add anything from the point of view of confirming the diagnosis. In clinical practice, there will be increasing reluctance to do invasive tests or those which are difficult to carry out if they do not add to the diagnostic process.

The other alternative set of criteria, the first major criterion and two minor criteria, is present to give a set of criteria for the diagnosis of PV in a case where no mutation in *JAK*2 can be detected. With the discovery of exon 12 mutations (Scott et al. 2007) and increasingly sensitive techniques, this situation is becoming vanishingly rare, and it could not be argued that if a *JAK*2 clone has not been discovered then it is necessary to look with a more sensitive technique. It must be questioned if there is truly such an entity as *JAK*2 mutation negative PV.

4.1.7 Latent Polycythaemia Vera

The WHO authors allude to the situation which is referred to as latent PV or a pre-polycythaemia phase. This is the situation where a patient is discovered to have a *JAK*2 mutation, a subnormal EPO level or typical EECs but does not fulfil the PV criteria. It is to be expected that these patients will go onto develop PV. One cannot set diagnostic criteria as by definition the issue is that they do not fulfil the necessary criteria, but these individuals require ongoing observation.

4.1.8 Post-Polycythaemia Vera Myelofibrosis

Patients with PV often develop an end-stage disease where they have anaemia and other cytopenias, extramedullary haematopoiesis, ineffective haematopoiesis, increasing splenomegaly and bone marrow fibrosis. This has been known by many different terms in the literature, and the criteria for describing this phase have been confusing. The WHO set defined criteria for this condition which are set out as follows:

Diagnostic criteria for post-polycythaemic myelofibrosis
Required criteria
1. Documentation of a previous diagnosis of WHO-defined PV
2. Bone marrow fibrosis grade 2–3 (on a 3 scale) or grade 3–4 (on a 0–4 scale)

Additional criteria (two are required)
1. Anaemia or sustained loss of either phlebotomy (in the absence of cytoreductive therapy) or cytoreductive treatment requirement for erythrocytosis. (anaemia defined as a haemoglobin below the reference range for the appropriate age, sex, gender and altitude considerations)
2. Leukoerythroblastic peripheral blood picture
3. Increasing splenomegaly defined as either an increase in palpable splenomegaly of >5 cm from baseline (distance from the left costal margin) or the appearance of newly palpable splenomegaly
4. Development of >1 of 3 constitutional symptoms: >10% weight loss in 6 months, night sweats, unexplained fever (>37.5°C)

These criteria are very helpful in categorising patients who fallen into this group with this constellation of signs and symptoms.

4.2 Primary Myelofibrosis

The revised WHO criteria for primary myelofibrosis (PMF) are divided into major and minor criteria (Thiele et al. 2008b). To make the diagnosis, all three major criteria must be present and two minor criteria:

Major criteria
1. Presence of megakaryocyte proliferation and atypia (small to large megakaryocytes with an aberrant nuclear/cytoplasmic ratio and hyperchromatic, bulbous or irregularly folded nuclei and dense clustering), usually accompanied by reticulin and/or collagen fibrosis, or in the absence of significant reticulin fibrosis, the megakaryocyte changes must be accompanied by an increased bone marrow cellularity characterised by granulocyte proliferation and often decreased erythropoiesis (i.e. prefibrotic cellular-phase disease).
2. Not meeting WHO criteria for polycythaemia vera, *BCR-ABL 1+* chronic myelogenous leukaemia, myelodysplastic syndrome or other myeloid neoplasms.
3. Demonstration of *JAK*2 V617F or other clonal marker (e.g. *MPL* W515K/L) or in the absence of a clonal marker, no evidence that the bone marrow fibrosis or other changes are secondary to infection, autoimmune disorder or other chronic inflammatory condition, hairy cell leukaemia or other lymphoid neoplasm, metastatic malignancy or other toxic (chronic) myelopathies.

Minor criteria
1. Leukoerythroblastosis
2. Increase in serum lactate dehydrogenase level (which can be borderline or marked)
3. Anaemia
4. Splenomegaly

4.2.1 Histopathology

The histopathological features of myelofibrosis are clearly defined and included in the criteria. These are megakaryocyte proliferation and atypia and described further as small to large megakaryocytes with an aberrant nuclear/cytoplasmic ratio and

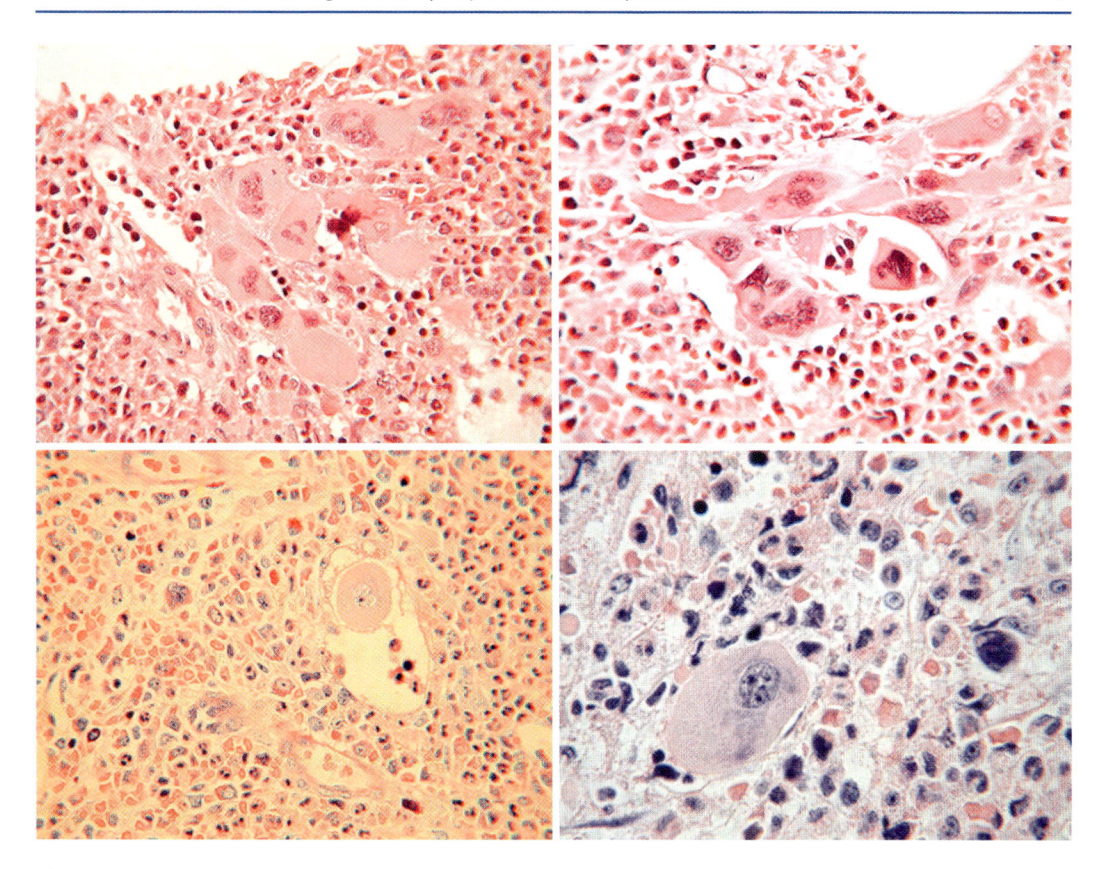

Fig. 4.2 Trephine in primary myelofibrosis showing dense clustering, hyperchromatic, bulbous and irregularly folded nuclei (Image courtesy of Dr. R. Cuthbert)

hyperchromatic, bulbous or irregularly folded nuclei and dense clustering. It is stated that these megakaryocyte changes are usually accompanied by reticulin and/or collagen fibrosis. The grading of fibrosis must be done carefully and reproducibly, and there are agreed scoring systems for this (Thiele et al. 2005). Figure 4.2 demonstrates some of these changes.

4.2.2 Prefibrotic Myelofibrosis

The previous version WHO classification distinguished 'prefibrotic' myelofibrosis from 'fibrotic' myelofibrosis. This revision incorporates the described entity within major criterion 1. Prefibrotic myelofibrosis is defined as a cellular phase of the disorder where there is no fibrosis seen but megakaryocyte proliferation and atypia accompanied by an increased bone marrow cellularity characterised by granulocyte proliferation and often decreased erythropoiesis. These changes have been defined in published literature mainly originating from the Cologne group in multiple retrospective analyses of an archive of trephine biopsies (Thiele et al. 1996, 1999, 2011; Thiele and Kvasnicka 2003a, b). It is claimed that the entity of prefibrotic myelofibrosis is distinct from essential thrombocythaemia (ET) and can and must be distinguished by the histopathological changes. However, several studies have now found that the histopathological differences are subjective and not reproducible (Wilkins et al. 2008; Brousseau et al. 2010), so there is considerable doubt about the existence of an entity of prefibrotic myelofibrosis.

The diagnostic criteria require all three major criteria plus two of the minor criteria to make the diagnosis so the presence of the so-called prefibrotic changes alone would not be sufficient without at least two of leukoerythroblastosis, raised lactate dehydrogenase, anaemia or splenomegaly. It is hoped that there would be some other features to support making a diagnosis of PMF. Nevertheless, the WHO continues to discriminate a category of prefibrotic myelofibrosis which cannot be identified reproducibility and is not of diagnostic or therapeutic benefit but could be dangerous for patients. If myelofibrosis is considered a more serious disorder with a worse prognosis, patients may be advised to have higher risk procedures like bone marrow transplant if a fibrotic process is considered to be the main pathology.

4.2.3 Myelofibrosis: An Accelerated Phase of Polycythaemia Vera or Essential Thrombocythaemia

The WHO discusses how myelofibrosis is characterised over time by increasing reticulin, collagen fibrosis and osteosclerosis. The disorder transforms to an acute leukaemia with increasing percentages of blasts present. PV and ET also transform to myelofibrosis over time and are indistinguishable from PMF. The evolution of the diseases over time is poorly understood. However, considering all the disorders, it may be logical to consider myelofibrosis as an accelerated phase of the myeloproliferative disorders with PV and ET as the chronic phases and all ultimately ending in a leukaemia transformation (Campbell and Green 2005).

4.3 Essential Thrombocythaemia

The WHO has defined a set of criteria which are required for the diagnosis of ET (Thiele et al. 2008c). To make the diagnosis, all four criteria must be fulfilled:

1. Sustained platelet count $\geq 450 \times 10^9/L$ (sustained during the work-up process)
2. Bone marrow biopsy specimen showing proliferation mainly of the megakaryocytic lineage with increased numbers of enlarged, mature megakaryocytes. No significant increase or left shift of neutrophil granulopoiesis or erythropoiesis

3. Not meeting WHO criteria for polycythaemia vera, primary myelofibrosis, *BCR-ABL*1 positive chronic myelogenous leukaemia or myelodysplastic syndrome of other myeloid neoplasm
4. Demonstration of *JAK*2 V617F of other clonal marker, or in the absence of *JAK*2 V617F, no evidence for reactive thrombocytosis

In criterion 3, there are defined criteria for the excluded diagnoses. To exclude PV, there is a requirement for failure of iron replacement therapy to increase haemoglobin level to the PV range in the presence of decreased serum ferritin. PV diagnosis is based on haemoglobin and haematocrit. Red cell mass measurement is not required. Exclusion of PMF requires the absence of the relevant reticulum fibrosis, collagen fibrosis, peripheral blood leukoerythroblastosis or markedly hypercellular marrow accompanied by megakaryocyte morphology that is typical for PMF including small to large megakaryocytes with an aberrant nuclear/cytoplasmic ratio and hyperchromatic, bulbous or irregularly folded nuclei and dense clustering. Exclusion of chronic myeloid leukaemia (CML) requires the absence of *BCR-ABL*1. Exclusion of myelodysplastic syndrome requires absence of dyserythropoiesis and dysgranulopoiesis.

A reactive thrombocytosis must also be excluded, and the causes of this which have to be eliminated include iron deficiency, splenectomy, surgery, infection, inflammation, connective tissue disease, and metastatic cancer and lymphoproliferative disorders. It is noted that a condition associated with a reactive thrombocytosis may not exclude the possibility of ET if the first three criteria are met.

4.3.1 Platelet Count

Compared to the previous set of WHO criteria for ET, these criteria require a lower platelet count of $450 \times 10^9/L$ rather than the higher limit of $600 \times 10^9/L$. This will include all individuals with a platelet count above the 95th percentile for normal counts and means that the other diagnostic criteria need to be considered. However, it does

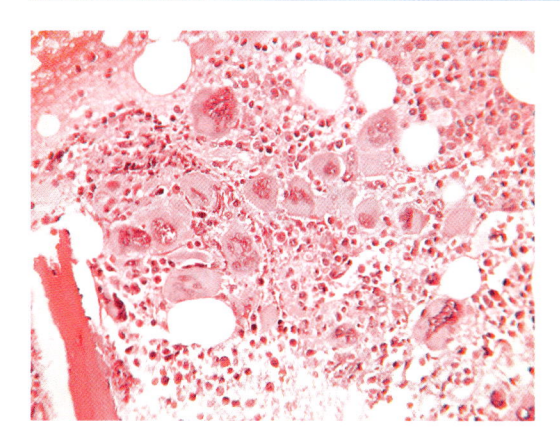

Fig. 4.3 Trephine in essential thrombocythaemia with megakaryocytes clustering with large forms which have abundant mature cytoplasm and deeply lobulated nuclei (Image courtesy of Dr. R. Cuthbert)

seem logical as there is no longer a group with sustained platelet counts above the upper limit but below the 600×10^9/L limit who did not fit the previous criteria.

4.3.2 Haematopathology

Haematopathological changes in ET and the distinction from prefibrotic myelofibrosis have been described by pathologists in large retrospective series with clearly defined cases (Thiele et al. 1996, 1999, 2011; Thiele and Kvasnicka 2003a, b). Changes include proliferation of megakaryocytes with large forms which have abundant mature cytoplasm and hyperlobulated or deeply lobulated (staghorn-like) nuclei (Fig. 4.3). Megakaryocytes may be clustered or dispersed throughout the marrow. Proliferation of erythroid and granulocytic precursors is minor. Reticulin should be essentially normal, and any significant increase in reticulin fibrosis excludes the diagnosis. These various histopathological changes are described by the WHO, but no guidance is given on the importance of the various features. In a study of a cohort of patients, three experienced haematopathologists assessed the morphologic features and overall diagnosis according to the described WHO criteria. There was substantial interobserver variability for overall diagnosis and individual cellular characteristics including megakaryocyte morphology. Analysis suggested that cellularity, megakaryocyte clustering and degree of fibrosis were the three underlying processes which describe the morphologic patterns in the bone marrow in ET. Reticulin grade was the major factor which all three haematopathologists used to assign WHO classification. The conclusions from this study were that even experienced haematopathologists need special training to distinguish subtypes of ET, and therefore the general use of the WHO criteria in routine practice is difficult, or the criteria are not sufficiently robust to describe subtypes of ET (Wilkins et al. 2008).

Recently, a large retrospective study looked at over 1,000 patients who had been classified as ET prior to 2002 using the Polycythemia Vera Study Group criteria. The bone marrow biopsies in conjunction with clinical and laboratory data were reviewed by the local experts and by the haematopathology expert who originally described prefibrotic myelofibrosis. Using all this data, the experts reclassified 16% of those evaluable who were originally labelled ET as prefibrotic myelofibrosis. Outcomes were then looked at, and those labelled prefibrotic myelofibrosis had worse outcomes. Age, leucocyte count anaemia and thrombosis history were independent risk factors for survival (Barbui et al. 2011). This study shows that there may be factors within a group of ET patients which are associated with poorer outcomes, but it does not prove the existence of a distinct independent pathological entity which can be identified reproducibly by haematopathologists.

4.3.3 Diagnostic Issues

The major point to note is that with these criteria, ET remains a diagnosis of exclusion. In the presence of a raised platelet count, typical histological changes must be observed, but other myeloproliferative and reactive causes have to be excluded.

The WHO criteria rely heavily on histopathology. However, there will be patients in whom it will be very difficult to undertake a bone marrow trephine in order to complete a diagnostic process. A patient with a persistent markedly raised platelet count with a clonal marker has a strong indication of a diagnosis of ET, and the clinician and patient may be very reluctant to undertake a biopsy. This perhaps should always be undertaken in a younger patient of if there is any doubt, but in routine practice, there will be patients where it may not be justified.

The WHO criteria distinguish between PV and JAK2 V617F positive ET. There may be overlap between these disorders as iron levels, sex EPO levels and other factors may influence the clinical presentation (Campbell et al. 2005). The two disorders may represent a biological continuum rather than distinct entities. The long tradition of defining by splitting up the disorders may not be accurate, and in the future, the preference may be to consider the disorders on a spectrum rather than as separate. The therapeutic relevance of the distinction is not yet clear.

4.4   MPN in Children

Myeloproliferative disorders are very rare in children. The applicability of the revised WHO criteria to cases of MPN in children may not be appropriate. This is demonstrated in a series of 45 unselected children, 13 with PV and 32 with ET. Applying WHO criteria to this group, 1 familial erythrocytosis and all 12 familial thrombocytosis would have been classified as PV or ET according to the WHO criteria. The *JAK* V617F mutation was also present in a smaller number of sporadic cases of PV than would be expected in an adult series (Teofilli et al. 2007). When considering children, criteria need to exclude familial forms and consider that pathogenetic lesions found in adults are only present in a minority of children.

Conclusion

The revised WHO criteria for MPNs are useful in categorising and defining the different disorders. The criteria continue to emphasise differences in bone marrow morphology between disorders, and these differences have been developed mainly in small groups of patients and in retrospective settings. The criteria need to be developed and validated further so that they can be generally applicable.

References

Barbui T, Thiele J, Passamonti F et al (2011) Survival, leukemic transformation and fibrotic progression in essential thrombocythaemia are significantly influenced by accurate morphologic diagnosis: an international study of 1,104 patients. J Clin Oncol July 11, 29(23):3179–3184

Baxter EJ, Scott LM, Campbell PJ et al (2005) Acquired mutation of the tyrosine kinase JAK2 in human myeloproliferative disorders. Lancet 365:1054–1061

Brousseau M, Parot-Schindel E, Moles M-P et al (2010) Practical application and clinical impact of the WHO histopathological criteria on bone marrow biopsy for the diagnosis of essential thrombocythaemia versus prefibrotic primary myelofibrosis. Histopathology 56: 758–767

Campbell PJ, Green AR (2005) The myeloproliferative disorders. N Engl J Med 355:2452–2466

Campbell PJ, Scott LM, Buck G et al (2005) Definition of subtypes of essential thrombocythaemia and relation of polycythaemia vera based on *JAK*2 V617F mutation status: a prospective study. Lancet 366:1945–1953

Chen Q, Lu P, Jones AV et al (2007) Amplification refractory mutation system, a highly sensitive and simple polymerase chain reaction assay, for the detection of JAK2 V617F mutation in chronic myeloproliferative disorders. J Mol Diagn 9(2):272–276

Dobo I, Donnard M, Girodon F et al (2004) Standardization and comparison of endogenous erythroid colony assays performed with bone marrow or blood progenitors for the diagnosis of polycythaemia vera. Hematol J 5:161–167

Gordeuk VR, Stockton DW, Prchal JT (2005) Congenital polycythemias/erythrocytoses. Haematologica 90: 109–116

Hussein K, Bock O, Kreipe H (2007) Histological and molecular classification of chronic myeloproliferative disorders in the age of JAK2: persistence of old questions despite new answers. Pathobiology 74:72–80

James C, Ugo V, Le Couedic J-P et al (2005) A unique clonal JAK2 mutation leading to constitutive signalling causes polycythaemia vera. Nature 434: 1144–1148

Johansson PL, Soodabeh S-K, Kutti J (2005) An elevated venous haemoglobin concentration cannot be used as a surrogate marker for absolute erythrocytosis: a study of patients with polycythaemia vera and apparent polycythaemia. Br J Haematol 129:701–705

Kralovics R, Passamonti F, Buser AS et al (2005) A gain-of-function mutation of JAK2 in myeloproliferative disorders. N Engl J Med 352:1779–1790

Levine RL, Wadleigh M, Cools J et al (2005) Activating mutation in the tyrosine kinase. JAK2 in polycythemia vera, essential thrombocythemia, and myeloid metaplasia with myelofibrosis. Cancer Cell 7:387–397

Percy MJ, Scott LM, Erber WN et al (2007) The frequency of *JAK*2 exon 12 mutations in idiopathic erythrocytosis patients with low serum erythropoietin. Haematologica 92(12):1607–1614

Prchal JF, Axelrad AA (1974) Bone-marrow responses in polycythemia vera. N Engl J Med 290:1382

Scott LM, Tong W, Levine RL et al (2007) *JAK2* exon 12 mutations in Polycythemia Vera and idiopathic erythrocytosis. N Engl J Med 356:459–468

Teofilli L, Giona F, Martini M et al (2007) The revised WHO diagnostic criteria for Ph-negative myeloproliferative diseases are not appropriate for the diagnostic screening of childhood polycythaemia vera and essential thrombocythaemia. Blood 110:3384–3386

Thiele J, Kvasnicka HM (2003a) Chronic myeloproliferative disorders with thrombocythaemia: a comparative study of two classification systems (PVSG, WHO) on 839 patients. Ann Hematol 82:148–152

Thiele J, Kvasnicka HM (2003b) Diagnostic differentiation of essential thrombocythaemia from thrombocythaemias associated with chronic idiopathic myelofibrosis by discriminate analysis of bone marrow features – a clinicopathological study on 272 patients. Histol Histopathol 18:93–102

Thiele J, Kvasnicka HM, Werden C et al (1996) Idiopathic primary osteo-myelofibrosis: a clinico-pathological study on 208 patients with special emphasis on evolution of disease features, differentiation from essential thrombocythaemia and variables of prognostic impact. Leuk Lymphoma 22:303–317

Thiele J, Kvasnicka HM, Boeltken B et al (1999) Initial (prefibrotic) stages of idiopathic (primary) myelofibrosis (IMF) – a clinicopathological study. Leukemia 13: 1741–1748

Thiele J, Kvasnicka HM, Facchetti F et al (2005) European consensus on grading bone marrow fibrosis and assessment of cellularity. Haematologica/Hematol J 90:1128–1132

Thiele J, Kvasnicka HM, Orazi A et al (2008a) Polycythaemia Vera. In: Swerdlow SH et al (eds) WHO Classification of tumours of haematopoietic and lymphoid tumours, 4th edn. International Agency for Research on Cancer, Lyon, pp 40–43

Thiele J, Kvasnicka HM, Tefferi A et al (2008b) Primary myelofibrosis. In: Swerdlow SH et al (eds) WHO Classification of tumours of haematopoietic and lymphoid tumours, 4th edn. International Agency for Research on Cancer, Lyon, pp 44–47

Thiele J, Kvasnicka HM, Orazi A et al (2008c) Essential thrombocythaemia. In: Swerdlow SH et al (eds) WHO Classification of tumours of haematopoietic and lymphoid tumours, 4th edn. International Agency for Research on Cancer, Lyon, pp 48–50

Thiele J, Kvasnicka HM, Mullauer L et al (2011) Essential thrombocythaemia versus primary myelofibrosis: a multicenter study to validate the WHO classification. Blood 117(21):5710–5718

Wilkins BS, Erber WN, Bareford D et al (2008) Bone marrow pathology in essential thrombocythemia: interobserver reliability and utility for identifying disease subtypes. Blood 111:60–69

Patient's Information and Examinations Needed Before Planning Therapy in the Myeloproliferative Neoplasms

5

Francisco Cervantes and Juan-Carlos Hernández-Boluda

Contents

5.1 Introduction

Patient communication represents an important element of the clinical work of the treating physicians, with this especially applying to individuals with neoplastic diseases, as it is the case of the myeloproliferative neoplasms (MPNs). In the current Internet era, an increasing number of patients seek for information in the network, and, very often, misinterpretation of the information found raises additional doubts and creates more uncertainties. In MPN patients, concerns about the nature of the disease, the symptoms and complications that can derive from it, and the prognosis and life expectancy are common, as well as the possibility that the disease could be inherited. Once they are informed on these important aspects, they usually want to know on the available therapeutic options, if progress is being made in the understanding of their disease and if this will eventually translate into the availability of better treatment options in the next future. Moreover, since a substantial proportion of MPN patients are young individuals and, for most of them, the expected survival is close to normal, information on the possibility of creating a family and the risks associated with this process is a frequent request. The present chapter tries to summarize the more relevant information to be provided to MPN patients.

5.2 Patient Information Before Planning Therapy

The first topic to address in an interview with a patient that has been diagnosed with a myeloproliferative neoplasm (MPN) and his or her family could be to explain the neoplastic nature of these diseases. This having been said, it is advisable to explicitly distinguish these disorders from

F. Cervantes (✉)
Hematology Department, Hospital Clínic,
IDIBAPS, University of Barcelona, Barcelona, Spain
e-mail: fcervan@clinic.ub.es

J.-C. Hernández-Boluda
Hematology Department, Hospital Clínico, Valencia,
Spain

T. Barbui and A. Tefferi (eds.), *Myeloproliferative Neoplasms*, Hematologic Malignancies,
DOI 10.1007/978-3-642-24989-1_5, © Springer-Verlag Berlin Heidelberg 2012

leukemia, a much more feared condition, and this especially applies to patients with polycythemia vera (PV) or essential thrombocythemia (ET), two disorders that, when properly managed, are associated with a life expectancy not substantially different from that of the general population (Passamonti et al. 2004). Beside, the lack of a causative agent in most MPNs cases must also be highlighted. Patients might be interested in knowing that the annual incidence of ET and PV is low, from one to three new cases per 100,000 inhabitants per year, whereas primary myelofibrosis (PMF) is even less frequent (Johansson et al. 2004). However, because life expectancy, particularly in patients with ET and PV, is long, the prevalence of these diseases is severalfold higher.

A typical concern of a MPN patient is the possibility that the disease might be heritable. This issue can be clarified by indicating that the MPNs originate from an acquired somatic mutation in the hematopoietic stem cells, not present therefore in the germ line (Campbell and Green 2006), and that the majority of cases of MPNs are of sporadic appearance. However, it can be added that there is occasional occurrence of MPNs among members of the same family and that an increased incidence of MPNs has been observed among first-degree relatives of patients with MPNs (Landgren et al. 2008; Rumi et al. 2007). This does not mean that specific laboratory tests should be performed to the patient's relatives in order to rule out the presence of one such disorder, unless indicated by a history suggesting an MPN (for instance, being aware of persistent thrombocytosis or polyglobulia, or a history of aquagenic pruritus, microvascular disturbances or recurrent thrombosis). Moreover, if the patient asks about the existence of biological data supporting a predisposition to develop an MPN, it can be said that an increased frequency of a special genetic background, the so-called haplotype 46/1 of the JAK2 gene, has been recently found in MPN patients and their first-grade relatives (Jones et al. 2009) but, again, no specific test to screen for this haplotype should be performed to the patient's relatives out of the research setting.

Information on the genetic abnormalities most commonly encountered in MPNs can also be disclosed, but always making it clear that genetic is not synonymous of hereditary, since, as already mentioned, the genetic abnormalities typical of the MPNs are acquired and, as such, while they are present in the hematopoietic cells, they are not in the cells of other organs or tissues of the patient. In this sense, it can be indicated that the most frequent molecular abnormality in the MPNs consists of a mutation in the JAK2 gene, which is detected in around 95% of PV patients and in 50% to 60% of patients with ET or PMF (Tefferi 2010). In addition, that activating mutations in the MPL gene are found in about 4% of patients with ET and in 10% of those with PMF, but not in PV (Tefferi 2010). Of note, it can be mentioned that, for the time being, there is no universal agreement on the possibility that the presence of the JAK2 or MPL mutations might affect the thrombotic risk, the patients' survival, or the frequency of leukemic transformation of the disease (Barbui et al. 2011).

The onset of the MPNs is often a gradual process, with many patients (especially those with ET and, to a lesser extent, PV) being currently diagnosed by chance while having blood tests done for other reasons. Because of this, it might be helpful to educate the patient on identifying the signs and symptoms that could be related to the MPN. Thus, patients should be aware of the possibility of suffering microvascular disturbances either at diagnosis or during the disease evolution, including dizziness, transient ischemic attacks or other neurological symptoms, transient visual abnormalities, acral paresthesia, erythromelalgia, or others. These manifestations should not be overlooked, since they are generally sensitive to low-dose aspirin and might precede a major thrombotic event. Large vessel thrombosis and mucocutaneous bleeding can occur in all three MPNs, but they appear mainly in PV and ET (Landolfi et al. 2008). With regard to bleeding, patients must be recommended to avoid the intake of aspirin at standard dosage in order to minimize the risk of this complication (Tartaglia et al. 1986; Willoughby and Pearson 1998). PMF patients are more often symptomatic at diagnosis, with roughly one-third of them complaining of either constitutional symptoms, anemic symptoms, and discomfort or pain in the upper left part of the abdomen due to the splenomegaly, respectively. Pruritus, typically exacerbated by hot water, is a particularly distressing symptom that preferentially occurs in patients with PV but can also be noted in a minority of patients with ET and PMF.

5.3 Prognostic Information

The prognosis of MPNs should be underscored to patients as soon as the diagnosis is established. In this sense, while PMF is associated with a substantial reduction in life expectancy, it must be stressed that ET affects more the patients' quality of life than their survival, whereas PV is associated with both a substantial morbidity derived from thrombosis but also with a certain reduction in the patients' life expectancy (Passamonti et al. 2004; Rozman et al. 1991; Wolanskyj et al. 2006). When the survival of PMF patients has been compared with that of age- and sex-matched individuals from the general population, a substantial reduction in life expectancy has been observed (Cervantes et al. 2009; Rozman et al. 1991), mainly due to evolution to acute leukemia, infection, bleeding, portal hypertension, and heart failure. Despite this, life expectancy of PMF patients is widely variable and younger patients without adverse prognostic factors (anemia, constitutional symptoms, circulating blast cells) can be reassured by telling them that their predicted outcome is favorable (Cervantes et al. 1997). Patients with PV and ET have to understand that their life expectancy is mainly affected by vascular complications, especially thrombosis, although there is also a small risk of transformation to either myelofibrosis or leukemia, particularly in PV. Transformation to acute leukemia in PV and ET is exceedingly infrequent in cytoreductive treatment-naïf patients and can increase slightly depending on the treatment administered (Kiladjian et al. 2006; Murphy et al. 1997). With regard to thrombosis, in PV, the incidence is 18 per 1,000 person-years, being about 5 per 1,000 person-years for the evolution to myelofibrosis and leukemia, whereas in ET, it is 12 per 1,000 person-years, being 1.6 per 1,000 person-years for evolution to myelofibrosis and 1.2 per 1,000 person-years for leukemic transformation

(Passamonti et al. 2004). Therefore, given that thrombosis is the more frequent complication of PV and ET, patients must be informed that the treatment strategy is based on their thrombosis risk (and, to a lesser extent, their bleeding risk), with advanced age and a previous history of thrombosis being the two major predictors for such complication. In this regard, a point to be stressed in order to minimize the risk of thrombosis is the importance of an appropriate control of generic cardiovascular risk factors, including arterial hypertension, diabetes mellitus, hyperlipidemia, and obesity, as well as strict smoking cessation. Patients, particularly those managed without cytoreductive drugs, should understand that the platelet count per se does not correlate with the risk of thrombosis. However, they should know that extreme thrombocytosis ($\geq 1.500 \times 10^9$/L) is used as an indication for cytoreductive therapy, due to the bleeding tendency associated with the appearance of acquired von Willebrand disease (Buss et al. 1985).

5.4 Examinations Needed for Prognostic Stratification and Treatment Monitoring

A detailed history of the patient's health habits, comorbidities, and concomitant therapies is mandatory. In particular, direct inquisition about the possible presence of the above-mentioned cardiovascular risk factors and past history of thrombohemorrhagic complications is essential since such information constitutes the basis for risk stratification in treatment decision-making for these patients (Tefferi and Vainchenker 2011). A thorough investigation of the family history should be part of the initial work-up, in order to evaluate potential familial predisposition to the MPNs, as well as the possibility of inherited thrombophilia, which would highly increase the thrombotic risk (Ruggeri et al. 2002). Attention should also be paid to collect relevant information on prognostic clinical factors, such as presence of constitutional symptoms (including weight loss, night sweats, and more rarely, low-grade temperature) in PMF and PV or the need for red blood cell transfusions in PMF.

Table 5.1 Definition of clinicohematologic response in ET and PV according to the criteria of the European LeukemiaNet

Response grade	Essential thrombocythemia	Polycythemia vera
Complete response (CR)	1. Platelet count ≤400×10⁹/L	1. Hematocrit <45% without phlebotomy
	2. No disease-related symptoms	2. Platelet count ≤400×10⁹/L
	3. Normal spleen size on imaging	3. Leukocyte count ≤10×10⁹/L
	4. Leukocyte count ≤10×10⁹/L	4. Normal spleen size on imaging
		5. No disease-related symptoms
Partial response (PR)	In the absence of CR, platelet count ≤600×10⁹/L or decrease >50% from baseline	In the absence of CR, hematocrit <45% without phlebotomy or response in 3 or more of the other criteria
No response	Any response that does not satisfy PR	Any response that does not satisfy PR

Physical examination will assess the patient's general clinical condition and check for possible signs of the disease, such as facial plethora or enlarged spleen or liver. Complete blood counts with a manual differential will provide prognostic information on variables potentially increasing the thrombotic risk (leukocytosis), or associated with higher bleeding risk (extreme thrombocytosis) or shorter survival (anemia, excessive leukocytosis, circulating blood blasts) (Cervantes et al. 2009). Although detection of *JAK2* or *MPL* mutations is very important for the diagnosis of the MPNs, their prognostic value has not been fully established yet (Barbui et al. 2011). Cytogenetic studies are not usually required in PV and ET at presentation, since abnormalities are rarely found in these two diseases (Diez-Martin et al. 1991; Gangat et al. 2009), but they can provide relevant prognostic information in PMF. In this sense, an abnormal karyotype is observed in about a third of PMF patients at diagnosis, and a negative influence on survival has been noted for trisomy 8, deletion of 12p, and abnormalities in chromosomes 5, 7, and 17, while, on the contrary, the sole detection of deletions of 13q and 20q is associated with an outcome comparable to that of patients with a normal diploid karyotype (Hussein et al. 2010; Tam et al. 2009). A bone marrow biopsy is not usually required to establish the diagnosis of PV, but it is mandatory for PMF and is also essential to differentiate ET from PMF. Moreover, an increase in the reticulin fiber content at ET diagnosis has been associated with a higher incidence of myelofibrotic transformation (Campbell et al. 2009).

Treatment monitoring should adopt the European LeukemiaNet criteria for PV and ET, which were proposed for defining the clinicohematologic response (Table 5.1) (Barosi et al. 2009), and the criteria established by the International Working Group for Myeloproliferative Neoplasms Research and Treatment for myelofibrosis (Tefferi et al. 2006) (Table 5.2). Complete blood counts and regular biochemical tests should be frequently obtained during the first 3 months of initiation of treatment to allow for drug dose titration. There is no formal indication to routinely monitor *JAK2* allele burden during treatment, unless the therapeutic intervention may induce molecular responses (i.e., interferon-α or hemopoietic stem cell transplantation). Similarly, bone marrow studies are not required for response assessment (with the exception of allogeneic transplantation or trials with experimental drugs in myelofibrosis), although they may be performed during follow-up if clinically indicated, such as in case of suspicion of transformation to myelofibrosis of PV or ET.

5.5 General Information on Therapy

Although several drugs are currently available to effectively control the MPNs, for the time being, none of them have curative potential. However, patients should understand that the current goal of treatment is not to cure the MPN but to avoid the development of complications and to improve the patients' quality of life by relieving the disease-related symptoms. To date,

Table 5.2 International Working Group (IWG) consensus criteria for treatment response in myelofibrosis

Complete remission (CR)	1. Complete resolution of disease-related symptoms and signs including palpable hepatosplenomegaly
	2. Peripheral blood count remission (Hb $\geq$ 110 g/L, platelet count $\geq$ 100 $\times$ 10⁹/L, neutrophil count $\geq$ 1.0 $\times$ 10⁹/L). All 3 blood counts should be no higher than the upper normal limit
	3. Normal leukocyte differential including disappearance of nucleated red blood cells, blasts, and immature myeloid cells in the peripheral smear, in the absence of splenectomy[a]
	4. Bone marrow histologic remission defined as the presence of age-adjusted normocellularity, no more than 5% myeloblasts, and an osteomyelofibrosis grade no higher than one[b]
Partial remission (PR)	All of the above criteria for CR except bone marrow histologic remission A repeat bone marrow biopsy is required in the assessment of PR
Clinical improvement (CI)	Requires one of the following in the absence of both disease progression and CR/PR assignment (CI response is validated only if it lasts for no fewer than 8 weeks):
	1. A minimum 20 g/L Hb increase or becoming transfusion independent (applicable only for patients with baseline Hb < 100 g/L)[c]
	2. Either a minimum 50% reduction in palpable splenomegaly of a spleen that is at least 10 cm at baseline or a spleen that is palpable at more than 5 cm at baseline becomes not palpable[d]
	3. A minimum 100% increase in platelet count and an absolute platelet count of at least 50 $\times$ 10⁹/L (applicable only for patients with baseline platelets <50 $\times$ 10⁹/L)
	4. A minimum 100% increase in neutrophil count and neutrophils of at least 0.5 $\times$ 10⁹/L (applicable only for patients with baseline absolute neutrophil count <1 $\times$ 10⁹/L)
Progressive disease (PD)	Requires one of the following[e]:
	1. Progressive splenomegaly defined by the appearance of a previously absent splenomegaly that is palpable at greater than 5 cm below the left costal margin or a minimum 100% increase in palpable distance for baseline splenomegaly of 5–10 cm or a minimum 50% increase in palpable distance for baseline splenomegaly of greater than 10 cm
	2. Leukemic transformation confirmed by a bone marrow blast count of at least 20%
	3. An increase in peripheral blood blast percentage of at least 20% that lasts for at least 8 weeks
Stable disease (SD)	None of the above
Relapse	Loss of CR, PR, or CI

[a]CR does not require absence of morphologic abnormalities of red cells, platelets, and neutrophils
[b]In patients with CR, a complete cytogenetic response is defined as failure to detect a cytogenetic abnormality in cases with a preexisting abnormality. A partial cytogenetic response is defined as 50% or greater reduction in abnormal metaphases. In both cases, at least 20 bone marrow– or peripheral blood–derived metaphases should be analyzed. A major molecular response is defined as the absence of a specific disease-associated mutation in peripheral blood granulocytes of previously positive cases. In the absence of a cytogenetic/molecular marker, monitoring for treatment-induced inhibition of endogenous myeloid colony formation is encouraged. Finally, baseline and posttreatment bone marrow slides are to be stained at the same time and interpreted at one sitting by a central review process
[c]Transfusion dependency is defined by a history of at least 2 units of red blood cell transfusions in the last month for a hemoglobin level of less than 85 g/L that was not associated with clinically overt bleeding. Similarly, during protocol therapy, transfusions for a hemoglobin level of 85 g/L or more are discouraged unless it is clinically indicated
[d]In splenectomized patients, palpable hepatomegaly is substituted with the same measurements
[e]A decrease in hemoglobin level of 20 g/L or more, a 100% increase in transfusion requirement, and new development of transfusion dependency, each lasting for more than 3 months after the discontinuation of protocol therapy, can be considered disease progression

the only curative strategy for the MPNs is allo-geneic stem cell transplantation, but its utility is limited by the relatively high treatment-related mortality and morbidity (Kroger et al. 2009). For this reason, transplantation is only an option for patients with myelofibrosis (either PMF or post-PV/ET myelofibrosis) with intermediate-2 or high-risk features either at diagnosis (Cervantes et al. 2009) or during follow-up (Gangat et al. 2011), whenever their clinical condition is reasonably good and an appropriate donor is available.

In general, treatment is dictated by the baseline or evolutive risk factors of the MPN, as well as by the patient's age and general condition. The differ-ent therapeutic options must be discussed with the patient, along with comments regarding how both the disease and its treatment might affect the patient's quality of life (Barbui et al. 2011). All patients should be reinforced to follow a healthy diet and exercise regularly, whenever possible. A strict control of cardiovascular risk factors is strongly encouraged, with this including smoking cessation. Combined oral contraceptive pill must be avoided since this drug has been associated with an increased risk of venous thrombosis in women with ET, particularly thromboses that involve splanchnic sites (Gangat et al. 2006). By contrast, hormone replacement therapy seems safe in this setting (Gangat et al. 2006). Aquagenic pruritus can occa-sionally be controlled by avoidance of precipitating conditions, but several drugs may be effective to manage the more disabling cases, mainly antihista-mines, paroxetine, interferon-α, and the currently in clinical trials JAK2 inhibitors (Tefferi and Fonseca 2002; Verstovsek et al. 2010).

It is worthy to remind PV patients not to take iron supplements, as this will cause the hemoglo-bin level to rise rapidly. Low-dose aspirin is rou-tinely used in PV and ET to prevent clotting from overactive platelets, unless contraindicated. Patients should understand that aspirin does not reduce the number of platelets but inactivate them for a period of 5–7 days. Therefore, they should be aware of the need to contact his or her hema-tologist in case of active bleeding or surgery while receiving this drug. In patients who must undergo surgery, antiplatelet therapy must be stopped 7–10 days before. A high incidence of thrombotic and hemorrhagic complications has been observed in MPN patients submitted to sur-gical procedures (Ruggeri et al. 2008). Therefore, to minimize the risk of such complications, in case of elective surgery, normalization of the hematocrit and the platelet counts by cytoreduc-tive therapy is recommended and, for all patients, prophylaxis of postoperative thrombosis with low molecular weight heparin (LMWH) manda-tory. A particularly risky intervention is splenec-tomy in PMF since, even in experienced hands, it has been associated with a perioperative mortal-ity of 9%, mainly derived from hemoperitoneum, infection, or thrombosis (especially in the spleno-portal vein tract) (Tefferi et al. 2000). In this set-ting, treatment with heparin or antiplatelet drugs had no apparent effect on adverse outcomes, although there was a trend for heparin efficacy in the prevention of venous thromboembolism.

Treatment of arterial and venous thrombosis in MPN subjects should not differ from that rec-ommended in the general population (Landolfi et al. 2008). However, the optimal duration of anticoagulation is uncertain, due to the lack of studies addressing this issue in the MPNs. An exception to this would be splanchnic vein throm-bosis, for which long-life anticoagulation is usu-ally recommended (Barbui et al. 2011).

Hydroxyurea is currently the most effective drug for preventing thrombosis in high-risk ET and PV patients (Cortelazzo et al. 1995; Fruchtman et al. 1997). However, some patients may be reluctant to use this drug due to fear regarding its possible leukemogenicity. In this sense, it must be remarked that, whereas the potential leukemogenic effect of hydroxyurea in MPN patients remains a matter of controversy, to date, no data supporting such hypothesis in either ET or PV are available from controlled studies (Finazzi et al. 2005; Harrison et al. 2005).

5.6 Information on Pregnancy

Information on the management of pregnancy in the setting of MPNs is limited (Harrison 2005). Despite this, the available data indicate that there is an increased risk of miscarriage and thrombosis during pregnancy in ET and PV, including preeclampsia, placental abruption, intrauterine death or stillbirth, and intrauterine growth retardation; venous thrombosis may also occur, especially in the postpartum period (Passamonti et al. 2007). However, a successful outcome may still be achieved in about a half of the patients with correct planning and close follow-up. On the contrary, due to reduced survival and risk of disease progression in the midterm, pregnancy is not recommended for women with PMF. If a properly informed patient is willing to become pregnant, a preconception meeting should be held to delineate the overall management of pregnancy, which should include a multidisciplinary team. Some factors might help to identify women at high risk of pregnancy-related complications, such as previous major thrombosis, a history of severe pregnancy or obstetric complications or having genetic thrombophilia.

Treatment options include no therapy, phlebotomy, aspirin, LMWH, and interferon-α. Although evidence for therapeutic guidelines is limited, management recommendations on this topic are available (Barbui et al. 2011; Harrison et al. 2010). In brief, low-risk pregnancy can be managed with phlebotomies in PV to maintain normal hematocrit values, low-dose aspirin throughout the pregnancy (unless contraindicated), and LMWH during the weeks following delivery, while management of high-risk pregnancy must be more aggressive, including LMWH during the pregnancy and postdelivery, low-dose aspirin in the absence of a bleeding history, and cytoreduction with interferon in case of previous major thrombosis, recurrent miscarriage, serious obstetric problems, or marked thrombocytosis. It is important to inform the patient that chemotherapy (in practice, hydroxyurea) and anagrelide are contraindicated during pregnancy due to their teratogenic potential. For this reason, interferon-α is the drug of choice for those women wishing pregnancy who require administration of cytoreductive therapy.

References

Barbui T, Barosi G, Birgegard G, Cervantes F, Finazzi G, Griesshammer M, Harrison C, Hasselbalch HC, Hehlmann R, Hoffman R, Kiladjian JJ, Kroger N, Mesa R, McMullin MF, Pardanani A, Passamonti F, Vannucchi AM, Reiter A, Silver RT, Verstovsek S, Tefferi A (2011) Philadelphia-negative classical myeloproliferative neoplasms: critical concepts and management recommendations from European LeukemiaNet. J Clin Oncol 29:761–770

Barosi G, Birgegard G, Finazzi G, Griesshammer M, Harrison C, Hasselbalch HC, Kiladjian JJ, Lengfelder E, McMullin MF, Passamonti F, Reilly JT, Vannucchi AM, Barbui T (2009) Response criteria for essential thrombocythemia and polycythemia vera: result of a European LeukemiaNet consensus conference. Blood 113:4829–4833

Buss DH, Stuart JJ, Lipscomb GE (1985) The incidence of thrombotic and hemorrhagic disorders in association with extreme thrombocytosis: an analysis of 129 cases. Am J Hematol 20:365–372

Campbell PJ, Green AR (2006) The myeloproliferative disorders. N Engl J Med 355:2452–2466

Campbell PJ, Bareford D, Erber WN, Wilkins BS, Wright P, Buck G, Wheatley K, Harrison CN, Green AR (2009) Reticulin accumulation in essential thrombocythemia: prognostic significance and relationship to therapy. J Clin Oncol 27:2991–2999

Cervantes F, Pereira A, Esteve J, Rafel M, Cobo F, Rozman C, Montserrat E (1997) Identification of 'short-lived' and 'long-lived' patients at presentation of idiopathic myelofibrosis. Br J Haematol 97:635–640

Cervantes F, Dupriez B, Pereira A, Passamonti F, Reilly JT, Morra E, Vannucchi AM, Mesa RA, Demory JL, Barosi G, Rumi E, Tefferi A (2009) New prognostic scoring system for primary myelofibrosis based on a study of the International Working Group for Myelofibrosis Research and Treatment. Blood 113:2895–2901

Cortelazzo S, Finazzi G, Ruggeri M, Vestri O, Galli M, Rodeghiero F, Barbui T (1995) Hydroxyurea for patients with essential thrombocythemia and a high risk of thrombosis. N Engl J Med 332:1132–1136

Diez-Martin JL, Graham DL, Petitt RM, Dewald GW (1991) Chromosome studies in 104 patients with polycythemia vera. Mayo Clin Proc 66:287–299

Finazzi G, Caruso V, Marchioli R, Capnist G, Chisesi T, Finelli C, Gugliotta L, Landolfi R, Kutti J, Gisslinger H, Marilus R, Patrono C, Pogliani EM, Randi ML, Villegas A, Tognoni G, Barbui T (2005) Acute leukemia in polycythemia vera: an analysis of 1638 patients enrolled in a prospective observational study. Blood 105:2664–2670

Fruchtman SM, Mack K, Kaplan ME, Peterson P, Berk PD, Wasserman LR (1997) From efficacy to safety: a Polycythemia Vera Study group report on hydroxyurea in patients with polycythemia vera. Semin Hematol 34:17–23

Gangat N, Wolanskyj AP, Schwager SM, Mesa RA, Tefferi A (2006) Estrogen-based hormone therapy and thrombosis risk in women with essential thrombocythemia. Cancer 106:2406–2411

Gangat N, Tefferi A, Thanarajasingam G, Patnaik M, Schwager S, Ketterling R, Wolanskyj AP (2009) Cytogenetic abnormalities in essential thrombocythemia: prevalence and prognostic significance. Eur J Haematol 83:17–21

Gangat N, Caramazza D, Vaidya R, George G, Begna K, Schwager S, Van Dyke D, Hanson C, Wu W, Pardanani A, Cervantes F, Passamonti F, Tefferi A (2011) DIPSS plus: a refined Dynamic International Prognostic Scoring System for primary myelofibrosis that incorporates prognostic information from karyotype, platelet count, and transfusion status. J Clin Oncol 29:392–397

Harrison C (2005) Pregnancy and its management in the Philadelphia negative myeloproliferative diseases. Br J Haematol 129:293–306

Harrison CN, Campbell PJ, Buck G, Wheatley K, East CL, Bareford D, Wilkins BS, van der Walt JD, Reilly JT, Grigg AP, Revell P, Woodcock BE, Green AR (2005) Hydroxyurea compared with anagrelide in high-risk essential thrombocythemia. N Engl J Med 353:33–45

Harrison CN, Bareford D, Butt N, Campbell P, Conneally E, Drummond M, Erber W, Everington T, Green AR, Hall GW, Hunt BJ, Ludlam CA, Murrin R, Nelson-Piercy C, Radia DH, Reilly JT, Van der Walt J, Wilkins B, McMullin MF (2010) Guideline for investigation and management of adults and children presenting with a thrombocytosis. Br J Haematol 149:352–375

Hussein K, Pardanani AD, Van Dyke DL, Hanson CA, Tefferi A (2010) International Prognostic Scoring System-independent cytogenetic risk categorization in primary myelofibrosis. Blood 115:496–499

Johansson P, Kutti J, Andreasson B, Safai-Kutti S, Vilen L, Wedel H, Ridell B (2004) Trends in the incidence of chronic Philadelphia chromosome negative (Ph-) myeloproliferative disorders in the city of Goteborg, Sweden, during 1983–99. J Intern Med 256:161–165

Jones AV, Chase A, Silver RT, Oscier D, Zoi K, Wang YL, Cario H, Pahl HL, Collins A, Reiter A, Grand F, Cross NC (2009) JAK2 haplotype is a major risk factor for the development of myeloproliferative neoplasms. Nat Genet 41:446–449

Kiladjian JJ, Rain JD, Bernard JF, Briere J, Chomienne C, Fenaux P (2006) Long-term incidence of hematological evolution in three French prospective studies of hydroxyurea and pipobroman in polycythemia vera and essential thrombocythemia. Semin Thromb Hemost 32:417–421

Kroger N, Holler E, Kobbe G, Bornhauser M, Schwerdtfeger R, Baurmann H, Nagler A, Bethge W, Stelljes M, Uharek L, Wandt H, Burchert A, Corradini P, Schubert J, Kaufmann M, Dreger P, Wulf GG, Einsele H, Zabelina T, Kvasnicka HM, Thiele J, Brand R, Zander AR, Niederwieser D, de Witte TM (2009) Allogeneic stem cell transplantation after reduced-intensity conditioning in patients with myelofibrosis: a prospective, multicenter study of the Chronic Leukemia Working Party of the European Group for Blood and Marrow Transplantation. Blood 114:5264–5270

Landgren O, Goldin LR, Kristinsson SY, Helgadottir EA, Samuelsson J, Bjorkholm M (2008) Increased risks of polycythemia vera, essential thrombocythemia, and myelofibrosis among 24,577 first-degree relatives of 11,039 patients with myeloproliferative neoplasms in Sweden. Blood 112:2199–2204

Landolfi R, Di Gennaro L, Falanga A (2008) Thrombosis in myeloproliferative disorders: pathogenetic facts and speculation. Leukemia 22:2020–2028

Murphy S, Peterson P, Iland H, Laszlo J (1997) Experience of the Polycythemia Vera Study Group with essential thrombocythemia: a final report on diagnostic criteria, survival, and leukemic transition by treatment. Semin Hematol 34:29–39

Passamonti F, Rumi E, Pungolino E, Malabarba L, Bertazzoni P, Valentini M, Orlandi E, Arcaini L, Brusamolino E, Pascutto C, Cazzola M, Morra E, Lazzarino M (2004) Life expectancy and prognostic factors for survival in patients with polycythemia vera and essential thrombocythemia. Am J Med 117:755–761

Passamonti F, Randi ML, Rumi E, Pungolino E, Elena C, Pietra D, Scapin M, Arcaini L, Tezza F, Moratti R, Pascutto C, Fabris F, Morra E, Cazzola M, Lazzarino M (2007) Increased risk of pregnancy complications in patients with essential thrombocythemia carrying the JAK2 (617V>F) mutation. Blood 110:485–489

Rozman C, Giralt M, Feliu E, Rubio D, Cortes MT (1991) Life expectancy of patients with chronic nonleukemic myeloproliferative disorders. Cancer 67:2658–2663

Ruggeri M, Gisslinger H, Tosetto A, Rintelen C, Mannhalter C, Pabinger I, Heis N, Castaman G, Missiaglia E, Lechner K, Rodeghiero F (2002) Factor V Leiden mutation carriership and venous thromboembolism in polycythemia vera and essential thrombocythemia. Am J Hematol 71:1–6

Ruggeri M, Rodeghiero F, Tosetto A, Castaman G, Scognamiglio F, Finazzi G, Delaini F, Mico C, Vannucchi AM, Antonioli E, De Stefano V, Za T, Gugliotta L, Tieghi A, Mazzucconi MG, Santoro C, Barbui T (2008) Postsurgery outcomes in patients with polycythemia vera and essential thrombocythemia: a retrospective survey. Blood 111:666–671

Rumi E, Passamonti F, Della Porta MG, Elena C, Arcaini L, Vanelli L, Del Curto C, Pietra D, Boveri E, Pascutto C, Cazzola M, Lazzarino M (2007) Familial chronic myeloproliferative disorders: clinical phenotype and evidence of disease anticipation. J Clin Oncol 25:5630–5635

Tam CS, Abruzzo LV, Lin KI, Cortes J, Lynn A, Keating MJ, Thomas DA, Pierce S, Kantarjian H, Verstovsek S (2009) The role of cytogenetic abnormalities as a prognostic marker in primary myelofibrosis: applicability at the time of diagnosis and later during disease course. Blood 113:4171–4178

Tartaglia AP, Goldberg JD, Berk PD, Wasserman LR (1986) Adverse effects of antiaggregating platelet therapy in the treatment of polycythemia vera. Semin Hematol 23:172–176

Tefferi A (2010) Novel mutations and their functional and clinical relevance in myeloproliferative neoplasms: JAK2, MPL, TET2, ASXL1, CBL, IDH and IKZF1. Leukemia 24:1128–1138

Tefferi A, Fonseca R (2002) Selective serotonin reuptake inhibitors are effective in the treatment of polycythemia vera-associated pruritus. Blood 99:2627

Tefferi A, Vainchenker W (2011) Myeloproliferative neoplasms: molecular pathophysiology, essential clinical understanding, and treatment strategies. J Clin Oncol 29:573–582

Tefferi A, Mesa RA, Nagorney DM, Schroeder G, Silverstein MN (2000) Splenectomy in myelofibrosis with myeloid metaplasia: a single-institution experience with 223 patients. Blood 95:2226–2233

Tefferi A, Barosi G, Mesa RA, Cervantes F, Deeg HJ, Reilly JT, Verstovsek S, Dupriez B, Silver RT, Odenike O, Cortes J, Wadleigh M, Solberg LA Jr, Camoriano JK, Gisslinger H, Noel P, Thiele J, Vardiman JW, Hoffman R, Cross NC, Gilliland DG, Kantarjian H (2006) International Working Group (IWG) consensus criteria for treatment response in myelofibrosis with myeloid metaplasia, for the IWG for Myelofibrosis Research and Treatment (IWG-MRT). Blood 108:1497–1503

Verstovsek S, Kantarjian H, Mesa RA, Pardanani AD, Cortes-Franco J, Thomas DA, Estrov Z, Fridman JS, Bradley EC, Erickson-Viitanen S, Vaddi K, Levy R, Tefferi A (2010) Safety and efficacy of INCB018424, a JAK1 and JAK2 inhibitor, in myelofibrosis. N Engl J Med 363:1117–1127

Willoughby S, Pearson TC (1998) The use of aspirin in polycythaemia vera and primary thrombocythaemia. Blood Rev 12:12–22

Wolanskyj AP, Schwager SM, McClure RF, Larson DR, Tefferi A (2006) Essential thrombocythemia beyond the first decade: life expectancy, long-term complication rates, and prognostic factors. Mayo Clin Proc 81:159–166

Mechanisms of Thrombogenesis

6

Anna Falanga, Laura Russo,
and Marina Marchetti

Contents

6.1 Introduction

The life expectancy of patients with polycythemia vera (PV) and essential thrombocythemia (ET) is strongly affected by disease-related hemostatic complications, including thrombosis and, to a lesser extent, hemorrhages. Reported incidence of thrombosis ranges from 12% to 39% in PV and from 11% to 25% in ET (Elliott and Tefferi 2005; Harrison 2005). The clinical manifestation of thrombosis varies from microcirculatory disturbances to most serious complications, like arterial and venous thromboses (Table 6.1).

Arterial thrombosis, which accounts for 60–70% of the events, includes ischemic stroke, acute myocardial infarction, and peripheral arterial occlusion. Events involving the venous system are represented by deep venous thrombosis of the lower extremities, pulmonary embolism, and intra-abdominal (hepatic, portal, and mesenteric) and cerebral vein thrombosis. The prevalence of the latter is unusually high among patients with PV or ET and is often the presenting feature of these diseases before diagnosis. Typical, but not exclusive, of ET is the involvement of the microcirculatory system and it manifests as erythromelalgia, transient ischemic attacks, visual or hearing transitory defects, recurrent headache, and peripheral paresthesia.

ET and PV management remains highly dependent on the patient's thrombotic risk (Finazzi and Barbui 2008; Tefferi 2011). Since the use of myelosuppressive drugs (hydroxyurea) can reduce the rate of thromboses and hemorrhages in these subjects but can also accelerate the rate of leukemic transformation, a risk-oriented management strategy is highly recommended in these patients. Older age (>60 years) and previous thrombosis are well-established cardiovascular risk factors for thrombosis in these patients. The absence of both of these two risk factors identifies the low-risk patients. There is great attention in moving beyond these recognized risk factors, particularly in the young or asymptomatic low- and intermediate-risk individuals not without risk of thrombosis. Recently, the impact of new risk factors, such as leukocytosis and JAK2V617F mutational status

A. Falanga (✉) • L. Russo • M. Marchetti
Division of Immunohematology and Transfusion
Medicine, Ospedali Riuniti di Bergamo, Bergamo, Italy
e-mail: annafalanga@yahoo.com; laurarusso78@yahoo.it;
marina.r.marchetti@gmail.com

T. Barbui and A. Tefferi (eds.), *Myeloproliferative Neoplasms*, Hematologic Malignancies,
DOI 10.1007/978-3-642-24989-1_6, © Springer-Verlag Berlin Heidelberg 2012

Table 6.1 Hemostatic disturbances described in patients with ET and PV

Arterial thrombosis
Myocardial infarction
Unstable angina
Ischaemic stroke
Transient ischaemic attack
Acute peripheral and visceral thromboembolism
Venous thrombosis
Deep venous thrombosis (legs and arms)
Pulmonary embolism
Fatal cerebral sinus and venous thrombosis
Unusual sites venous thrombosis (visceral vein thrombosis and cerebral sinus and venous thrombosis)
Superficial venous thrombosis
Micro-circulation disturbancies
Erythromelalgia
Seizures
Migraine
Vertigo
Tinnitus
Scintillating scotomas
Amaurosis fugax

and/or mutational burden, is under active investigation.

Even in the absence of thrombotic manifestation, ET and PV patients present with a hypercoagulable state, which is a laboratory finding of increased levels of plasma biomarkers of hemostatic system activation (Falanga et al. 1994, 2000; Posan et al. 1998; Wieczorek et al. 1995). Thus, an acquired thrombophilic state develops in these patients, who are prone to vascular complications, but the mechanisms ultimately responsible for activation of blood coagulation and the increased thrombotic tendency in ET and PV have not yet been elucidated.

6.2 Pathogenesis of Thrombosis

The pathogenesis of thrombosis and of the activation of blood coagulation in ET and PV is complex. Among other factors, a prominent role is played by abnormalities of the erythrocytes, platelets, and leukocytes, arising from the clonal proliferation of hematopoietic progenitor cells. These abnormalities involve not only quantitative

changes in the number of these cells, which cause hyperviscosity secondary to the increased blood cell mass, but also qualitative changes in the molecular characteristics of these cells. Prothrombotic factors expressed by transformed vascular cells (i.e., platelets, red blood cells, and leukocytes) include: (a) the production of procoagulant and proteolytic properties, (b) the secretion of inflammatory cytokines, and (c) the expression of adhesion molecules. In addition, the endothelial injury, caused by both hyperviscosity and by leukocyte-derived proteases (i.e., elastase, cathepsin G, and myeloperoxidase), may also predispose to thrombosis by upregulating endothelial adhesion molecules, which mediate platelet and leukocyte adhesion to vascular cells, and localize the secretion of thrombogenic and angiogenic peptides released by inflammatory cells. Recently, other two possible mechanisms of systemic hypercoagulability have been identified: an increased production of procoagulant microparticles and the occurrence of an acquired activated protein C resistance.

6.2.1 Red Blood Cell Abnormalities

6.2.1.1 Erythrocytosis

The prothrombotic effect of an elevated hematocrit has been clearly demonstrated in PV patients by the observation that at progressively higher hematocrit values, there is an increase of thrombotic risk (Pearson and Wetherley-Mein 1978). Hematocrit around the generally accepted upper limit of normal may be an important factor in the causation of occlusive vascular diseases, particularly in the cerebral circulation, as it determines an increase in blood viscosity (Adams et al. 2010). It has been observed that at high hematocrit values (47–53%), the cerebral blood flow is significantly lower than at hematocrit values in a lower range (36–46%). In addition, the reduction of hematocrit by venesection increases the flow by a mean of 50% largely due to a reduction in viscosity (Thomas et al. 1977). In untreated PV subjects, most thrombotic accidents occur in the cerebral circulation, particularly sensitive to blood hyperviscosity (Kwaan and Wang 2003).

At high shear rates, the raise of the red cell mass displaces the platelets toward the vessel wall, thus facilitating shear-induced platelet activation and further enhancing the increased platelet–platelet interactions (Huang and Hellums 1993; Turitto and Weiss 1983). In addition, at low shear rates, as it occurs in venous flow, hyperviscosity can increase the thrombotic risk by causing a major disturbance of blood flow. A proper management of blood hyperviscosity is essential but does not abolish the in vivo platelet activation and the increased thrombotic risk existing in PV subjects (Landolfi et al. 1992).

6.2.1.2   Red Blood Cell Functional Disorders

In addition to increased red blood cell count, in ET and PV biochemical changes in the cell membrane and content (Turitto and Weiss 1980) of these cells have been reported. These changes may independently impair blood flow also through the formation of red blood cell aggregates which have the potential to directly block blood flow in small vessels, thus contributing to cause ischemia and infarct, especially in the cerebral blood flow, and to facilitate platelet–leukocyte interaction with the vessel wall (Pearson and Lipowsky 2000; Yedgar et al. 2002).

6.2.2   Platelet Abnormalities

6.2.2.1   Thrombocytosis

The role of thrombocytosis in the pathogenesis of thrombotic events is controversial. Although clinical improvement of microcirculatory disturbances and/or improved platelet function after control of thrombocytosis have been reported, no clear correlation of thrombocytosis with risk of major cardiovascular events has been demonstrated (Elliott and Tefferi 2005; Harrison 2005). For example, both in the PVSG and the ECLAP (Landolfi et al. 2004) prospective study, the platelet count did not predict for thrombosis occurrence. Finally, the results of the only randomized trial to date (the primary thrombocythemia 1 [PT1] study), which randomized high-risk ET patients to hydroxyurea (a global myelosuppressive agent)

or anagrelide (a platelet-only-reducing agent), showed that, despite similar control of platelet count by either drug, indicated that the composite primary end point (arterial or venous thrombosis, serious hemorrhage, or death from vascular causes) occurred more often in recipients of anagrelide plus aspirin than in those receiving hydroxyurea plus aspirin (Harrison et al. 2005). The global effects of hydroxyurea on other blood cell populations, i.e., leukocytes, other than platelets, might underlie the correlation between control of platelet count and reduction of thrombosis rate observed in the first prospective study in high-risk patients with ET by Cortelazzo et al. (1995). Differently, in primary myelofibrosis (PMF), a condition characterized by less frequent cardiovascular events than in PV or ET, a correlation between thrombocytosis and thrombosis was found (Cervantes et al. 2006).

Extreme thrombocytosis (i.e., platelets $>1,500 \times 10^9$/L), on the other hand, can favor hemorrhagic rather than thrombotic manifestations in ET patients (Cortelazzo et al. 1995). This paradox has been attributed to the possible occurrence of an acquired von Willebrand syndrome, due to an increased clearance of the large von Willebrand factor multimers from plasma (Landolfi et al. 2006). Although generally asymptomatic, the same phenomenon has been reported occasionally in secondary thrombocytosis, particularly after splenectomy. Platelet count reduction proved successful in normalizing the plasma von Willebrand multimer pattern and in reducing bleeding tendency (Elliott and Tefferi 2005; Harrison 2005; Schafer 2004).

6.2.2.2   Platelet Functional Abnormalities

While the data on the role of thrombocytosis in the pathogenesis of thrombosis in ET and PV are not conclusive, there are several other lines of evidence for a contribution of platelets to thrombotic risk. For example, in patients with ET, a role of platelets in mediating microvessel occlusions (i.e., erythromelalgia) is suggested by the prompt relief of symptoms with aspirin, the normalization of tests measuring in vivo platelet activation (Michiels et al. 2006). In contrast to the inefficacy of coumadin, control of platelet function with low-dose aspirin and reduction of platelet counts to normal prevented the recurrence of microvascular circulation disturbances in the endarterial microvasculature of the cerebral, coronary, and peripheral circulation. Furthermore, low-dose aspirin significantly reduced the risk of cardiovascular events in PV as demonstrated by the ECLAP randomized clinical trial. Patients randomized to receive aspirin had a 60% reduction of combined end point of nonfatal acute myocardial infarction, nonfatal stroke, or death from cardiovascular causes (Landolfi et al. 2004).

The peculiar characteristics of thrombohemorrhagic diathesis in ET and PV prompted the design of many in vitro studies to demonstrate and characterize possible platelet abnormalities. In the past, numerous platelet defects have been identified in ET and PV patients. The majority of these observations were related to a decreased functionality and included abnormal platelet aggregation, reduced levels of membrane adhesion molecules (i.e., glycoproteins Ib, IIb/IIIa, IV, and VI), acquired storage pool disease, and defective platelet metabolism (i.e., abnormal arachidonic acid metabolism) (Landolfi et al. 1995; Schafer 1984). To the opposite, more recent studies have shown that platelets from these patients circulate in an activated status, as assessed by the detection of increased expression on their surface of P-selectin and tissue factor (Arellano-Rodrigo et al. 2006; Falanga et al. 2005b). An enhanced in vivo platelet activation in ET and PV patients is further suggested by the finding of increased levels of platelet activation products both in plasma (i.e., beta-thromboglobulin and platelet factor 4) and urine (i.e., thromboxane (Tx) A2 metabolites 11-dehydro-TxB2 and 2,3-dinor-TxB2) (Jensen et al. 2000; Landolfi et al. 1992).

Once activated, platelets provide a catalytic surface for the generation of thrombin, which further amplifies platelet activation. Recently, our group demonstrated in patients with ET and PV, and particularly in those carriers of the JAK2V617F mutation, an increased thrombin generation capacity of platelets, which was associated to the occurrence of platelet activation. The cytoreductive therapy with hydroxyurea significantly affects this prothrombotic phenotype (Panova-Noeva et al. 2011).

6.2.3 White Blood Cell Abnormalities

6.2.3.1 Leukocytosis

In the recent years, many retrospective studies have identified leukocytosis as a potential risk factor for arterial and venous thromboses in patients with ET and PV (Carobbio et al. 2008, 2007; Landolfi et al. 2007; Palandri et al. 2011). In addition, leukocytosis was also identified as a risk factor for recurrent arterial thrombosis in young (i.e., <60 years) ET and PV patients (HR for arterial recurrence 3.35, 95% CI 1.22–9.19) (De Stefano et al. 2010). Of note, in sickle cell patients, an increased baseline white cell count has been found to be an independent risk factor for acute chest syndrome and cerebral infarction, and quantitative and qualitative reductions in leukocytes during hydroxyurea treatment were correlated with a better disease outcome (Stuart and Nagel 2004). Differently, a retrospective study showed that leukocytosis at diagnosis (defined by a cutoff level of either 15 or 9.4×10^9/L) did not appear to influence the risk of thrombosis in low-risk ET or PV patients (Gangat et al. 2009). Prospective clinical studies with stratification of patients according to their baseline leukocyte counts are needed to definitely classified leukocytosis as a prognostic risk factor.

6.2.3.2 Leukocyte Qualitative Abnormalities

Leukocytes can contribute to the pathogenesis of thrombosis in ET and PV through recently discovered mechanisms of activation and interaction with platelets and endothelial cells and the coagulation system. In addition, leukocytes may contribute to inflammatory processes in atherosclerotic plaques and, in this way, increase the probability of vascular events (Falanga et al. 2005a; Marchetti and Falanga 2008). As neutrophils represent the most abundant proportion of the circulating leukocytes in ET and PV, a role for neutrophils in thrombosis has been hypothesized. Neutrophils have a central role in the inflammatory response

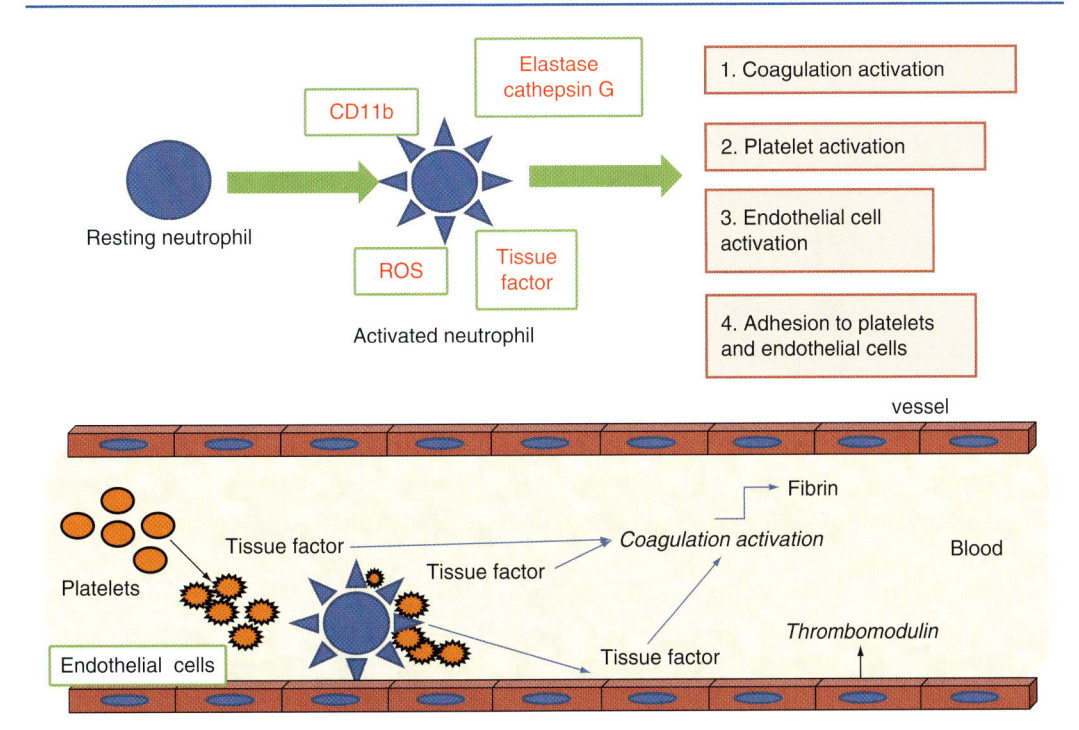

Fig. 6.1 Interaction of neutrophils with the hemostatic system. Molecules which specifically increase during the acute and chronic inflammatory disease (i.e., N-formyl-methionyl-leucyl-phenylalanine or fMLP, complement factors, cytokines, and growth factors) can activate the biological and metabolic functions of neutrophils, including adhesion and migration through the endothelium, phagocytosis, and oxidative killing. These activities represent the neutrophil response to inflammatory injury. On the other hand, activated neutrophils can also affect the hemostatic system through the same pathways. Particularly, the release of proteolytic enzymes (i.e., elastase, cathepsin G) and of reactive oxygen species (*ROS*) can activate/damage platelets and endothelial cells and impair some coagulation proteins. Elastase can proteolytically inactivate several plasma physiological inhibitors of blood coagulation and, on the other side, cleave and activate some procoagulant factors (i.e., factor V and factor X). Both elastase and cathepsin G can cause the detachment or lysis of endothelial cells and also modify endothelial cell functions involved in thromboregulation. The adhesion of neutrophils to other blood cells allows the formation of a close microenvironment where the enzymes released by neutrophils are protected against plasma inhibitors and can consequently easily act on their substrates. In addition, cathepsin G is a very potent platelet agonist. Activated platelets express P-selectin and TF and release microparticles. The increased expression of CD11b on neutrophil surface allows the adhesion of neutrophils to endothelial cells and platelets and the assembly of coagulation proteases on the neutrophil surface. Finally, neutrophils can express TF, even though the origin of neutrophil TF is not yet clarified, and provide an alternative pathway for thrombin generation

and also in linking the inflammatory response to the activation of blood coagulation (Falanga et al. 2005a). Once activated, neutrophils produce reactive oxygen species (ROS), release proteolytic enzymes from their cytoplasmic azurophilic granules (elastase, cathepsin G), and express higher and functional levels of the β2 integrin Mac-1 (or CD11b) on their cell surface (Fig. 6.1). All of these molecules can affect the hemostatic system and induce a prothrombotic condition (Falanga et al. 2005a; Afshar-Kharghan and Thiagarajan 2006). Notably, the fact that activated neutrophils can induce a hypercoagulable state in vivo has been well demonstrated by a study of a group of healthy donors administered granulocyte colony-stimulating factor (G-CSF) for the mobilization and collection of peripheral blood progenitor cells (Falanga et al. 1999). G-CSF caused the activation of neutrophils in these subjects, which was associated with a parallel increment in plasma levels of markers of activation of blood coagulation and endothelium. These effects were transient, as they

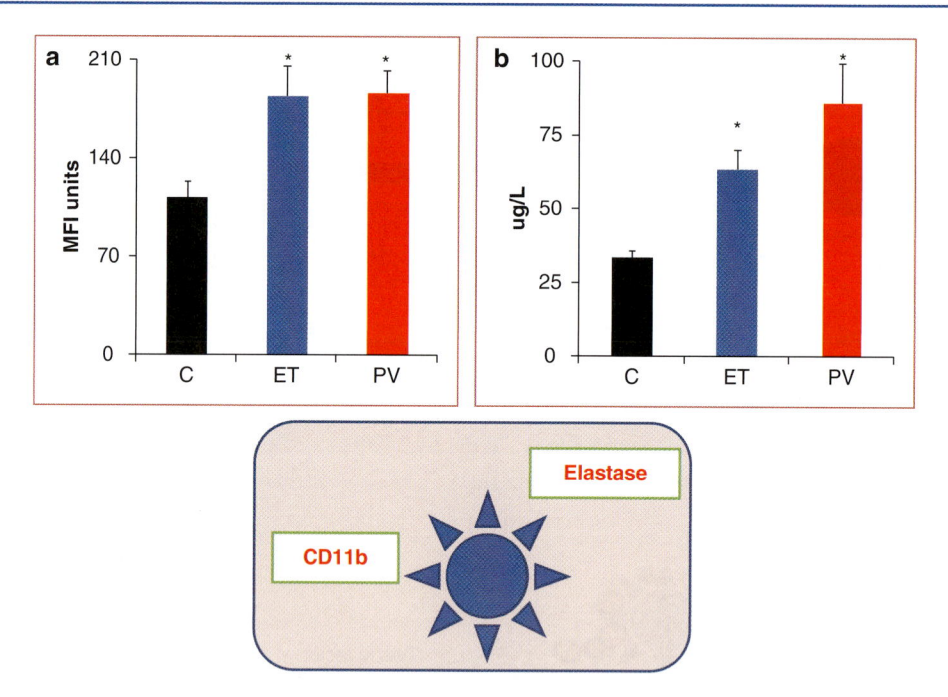

Fig. 6.2 Neutrophil activation. Cytofluorometric analysis of the expression of CD11b on the neutrophil cell surface (*panel A*) and measurement of neutrophil elastase concentration in plasma (*panel B*) showed a significant increment of this activation marker in patients with *ET* and *PV* compared to healthy control subjects (*C*). * $p < 0.05$ versus C (Modified from Falanga et al. (2000))

persisted as long as the growth factor was administered (i.e., 5–6 days), and normalized after G-CSF withdrawal.

In patients with ET and PV, the occurrence of neutrophil activation was demonstrated by the detection of specific phenotypical changes (increment in CD11b) and by the measurement of increased plasma concentration of neutrophil granule proteases (i.e., elastase and myeloperoxidase) (Falanga et al. 2000, 2005b) (Fig. 6.2). The abnormalities of neutrophils directly correlated with the increase in plasma levels of biomarkers of blood coagulation and vascular endothelium activation, supporting a possible involvement of neutrophils in the pathogenesis of the hypercoagulable state in these disorders. Several studies have described increased levels of circulating platelet/neutrophil aggregates in ET and PV patients and have attributed this phenomenon to both platelet (Jensen et al. 2001; Alvarez-Larran et al. 2004; Villmow et al. 2002) and neutrophil activation (Falanga et al. 2005b). Interestingly, in ET patients receiving aspirin, the increments in

CD11b expression and in neutrophil/platelet aggregates induced after in vitro neutrophil activation were significantly lower versus nonaspirin-receiving ET subjects, suggesting that aspirin treatment may inhibit the interaction between neutrophils and platelets.

6.2.4 JAK2V617F Mutation

The demonstration of the acquired gain-of-function V617F mutation in the tyrosine kinase JAK2 gene (Baxter et al. 2005; Kralovics et al. 2005; Levine et al. 2005; Zhao et al. 2005) has greatly influenced the diagnostic and therapeutic approach in MPN patients. Several studies have implicated JAK2V617F mutation in the increased thrombotic tendency observed in ET and PV patients. A recent metanalysis that included 21 studies involving patients with ET and 6 studies with PMF showed that in ET patients, the presence of JAK2V617F mutation was associated with a significant twofold

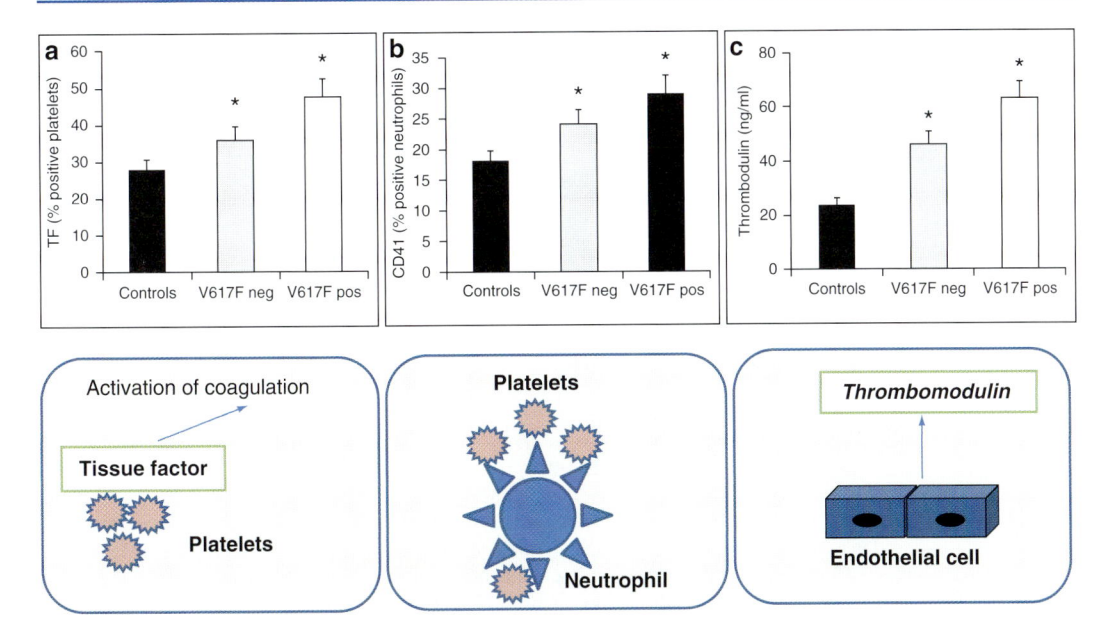

Fig. 6.3 ET patients with the JAK2V617F mutation and hemostatic system activation. ET patients carrying the JAK2V617F mutation present with significant higher expression of *TF* on platelet surface (*panel A*), circulating neutrophil/platelet aggregates (*panel B*), and plasma levels of the endothelial cell activation marker thrombomodulin (*panel C*). * $p < 0.05$ versus controls (Modified from Falanga et al. (2007))

increased risk of thrombosis (OR 1.92, 95% CI 1.45–2.53), both of venous (OR 2.49, 95% CI 1.71–3.61) and arterial (OR 1.77, 95% CI 1.29–2.43) vessels, while its role in PMF patients is uncertain (Lussana et al. 2009).

So far, only few studies have been published addressing whether the JAK2V617F mutation may specifically affect the hemostatic system (Alvarez-Larran et al. 2008; Arellano-Rodrigo et al. 2006; Falanga et al. 2007; Robertson et al. 2007). Altogether, these studies indicate that both cellular (i.e., platelets and leukocytes) and plasma compartments of hemostasis were more activated in those patients positive for the JAK2V617F mutation. Regarding cellular components, P-selectin was found increased on platelets from JAK2V617F-positive ET patients (Arellano-Rodrigo et al. 2006), and CD14 and LAP were demonstrated to be more highly expressed on neutrophils from ET JAK2V617F mutation carriers [54], while a significantly higher expression of CD11b was observed on neutrophil and monocyte from JAK2V617F-positive PMF patients (Alvarez-Larran et al. 2008). In addition, our group could also demonstrate an elevated expression of TF in

platelets from JAK2V617F-positive ET compared to negative patients and increased levels of platelet/neutrophil aggregates (Falanga et al. 2007). The evidence that both platelets and neutrophils from JAK2V617F mutation carriers expressed increased activation features was in good agreement with the findings of increased mixed cell aggregate formation in ET patients carrying the JAK2V617F mutation (Fig. 6.3).

Among hypercoagulation parameters, plasma levels of soluble thrombomodulin were found to be elevated in JAK2V617F-positive ET patients (Falanga et al. 2007), while sP-selectin levels were significantly elevated in JAK2V617F-positive ET, PV, and PMF patients compared to negative subjects (Robertson et al. 2007). In a study by Marchetti et al. (2008), an involvement of JAK2 mutation was observed in the presence of an acquired activated protein C resistance phenotype.

There are few studies that have evaluated the molecular mechanisms by which JAK2V617F mutation can affect the prothrombotic phenotype of a cell. It has been reported that JAK2-activating mutation can cause increased red cell adhesiveness

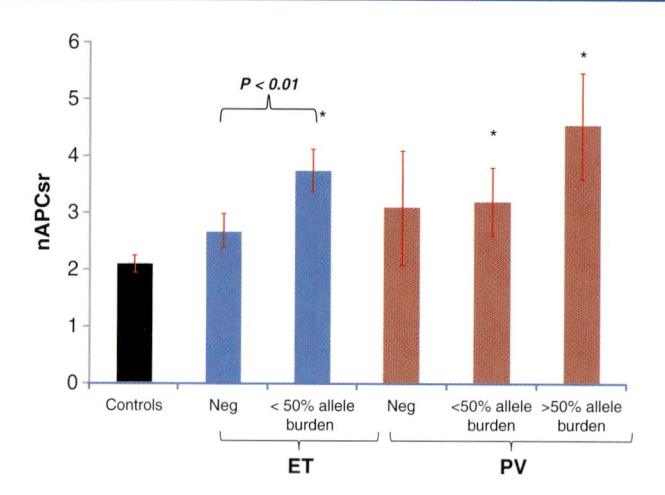

Fig. 6.4 APC resistance in ET and PV patients. APC resistance was assessed in plasma of patients with ET and PV by the thrombin generation assay in the absence and presence of APC. Data are expressed as normalized APC sensitivity ratio (*nAPCsr*). *ET* and *PV* carriers of the JAK2V617F mutation are more APC resistant than noncarriers, especially if homozygous (i.e., JAK2V617F allele burden >50%). $*p < 0.05$ versus controls (Modified from Marchetti et al. (2008))

through modification of surface adhesion molecules, facilitating thrombosis (Buss et al. 1985). In addition, JAK2 mutation may render platelet hyperresponsiveness through altered expression of cMPL signal transduction for TPO-induced platelet priming (Kubota et al. 2004). Activation of JAK2 is also involved in TF expression by neutrophil and monocyte through the MAP and PI3 kinase pathway (Rafail et al. 2008).

6.2.5 Acquired Activated Protein C (APC) Resistance

Inherited and acquired APC resistance is associated with an increased risk of thrombosis in many conditions, including pregnancy, oral contraceptive use, hormone replacement therapy, and cancer. Decreased levels of protein C and protein S can be responsible for this phenotype, and studies reported a reduction in the concentration of natural anticoagulants in this group of patients (Bucalossi et al. 1996). By using the thrombin generation assay, our group could demonstrate the occurrence of an acquired APC resistance phenotype in ET and PV patients (Marchetti et al. 2008). The results analyzed according to the presence (i.e., positivity or

negativity) and the status (i.e., heterozygosity or homozygosity) of the JAK2V617F mutation indicated that JAK2V617F mutation carriers are more APC resistant than noncarriers, especially if homozygous (i.e., JAK2V617F allele burden >50%) (Fig. 6.4). This suggests a progression in the APC-resistant phenotype determined by the JAK2V617F status and, together with previous observations, supports the hypothesis of a more hypercoagulable condition in JAK2V617F carriers. Prothrombin, factor V, free PS, and tissue factor pathway inhibitor (TFPI) levels were significantly reduced in patients, and mainly in JAK2V617F carriers. Multiple regression analysis indicated the low free PS level as a major determinant of the increased nAPCsr. Neutrophil elastase was significantly increased in all of the patients compared to controls and was significantly and inversely related to free PS plasma levels. Therefore, the increased blood cell counts, together with blood cell activation, can contribute to the chronic activation of blood coagulation and hence to the consumption of coagulation factors. A high prevalence of acquired APC resistance, in this case determined as the classical prolongation of activated partial thromboplastin time (aPTT) after addition of APC, was also reported by Arellano-Rodrigo et al. in a group of patients with ET (Arellano-Rodrigo et al. 2009). Again, decreased levels of free PS were detected and its inverse relationship with JAK2V617F allele percentage. In addition, acquired APC resistance was found to be more frequent in patients with previous history of thrombosis.

6.2.6 Plasma Microparticles

Microparticles (MPs) are membrane fragments ranging in size from 0.1 to 1 μm, released by most cell types, including blood and vascular cells, upon activation. Since microparticles are known to be elevated in thromboembolic diseases and malignancy (Zwicker et al. 2009), we hypothesized a role for microparticles in the pathogenesis of thrombosis in ET (Trappenburg et al. 2009). The levels and the cellular origin of microparticles were determined by flow cytometric analysis, while the microparticle-associated procoagulant activity was measured using a thrombin generation assay. We found a significantly higher number of circulating microparticles positive for platelet and endothelial markers and for TF in ET compared to controls. In addition, microparticle-rich plasma from patients with ET has higher thrombin generation potential, which correlated significantly with the total number of microparticles. A subsequent study by Duchemin et al. (2010) showed the occurrence of an acquired "thrombomodulin resistance" phenotype in PV and ET patients, partly determined by circulating microparticles.

Conclusions

Thrombotic complications are common in patients with ET and PV and significantly impact on morbidity and mortality in these diseases. In addition, these patients commonly present with abnormalities in laboratory coagulation tests, consistent with a hypercoagulable state.

The pathogenesis of the activation of blood coagulation in these conditions is complex and includes both abnormalities of the erythrocytes, platelets, and leukocytes, arising from the clonal proliferation of hematopoietic progenitor cells.

These abnormalities involve not only quantitative changes in the number of these cells, but also involve qualitative changes in the molecular characteristics of these cells. In patients with ET and PV, measurements of neutrophil phenotypic changes and plasma parameters of neutrophil degranulation clearly show a functional activation status of these cells. These properties, together with an increased production of procoagulant microparticles and the occurrence of an APC resistance phenotype, may contribute to the clotting activation process leading to the formation of thrombin and, ultimately, of fibrin. Clinical data indicate an association of JAK2V617F mutation with the severity of the disease. Biological data also show an association of this mutation with the expression of cellular and soluble biomarkers of clotting system activation.

Future preclinical research should focus on the pathophysiology of thrombosis in ET and PV, particularly in terms of the relationship between dysregulated JAK2 and abnormalities in blood cell count and phenotypical composition. A better understanding of the molecular events leading to the development of ET and PV may provide appropriate targets for the production of bifunctional therapies, i.e., capable to attack the malignant process, as well as to reverse the coagulopathy.

References

Adams BD et al (2010) Myeloproliferative disorders and the hyperviscosity syndrome. Hematol Oncol Clin North Am 24:585–602

Afshar-Kharghan V, Thiagarajan P (2006) Leukocyte adhesion and thrombosis. Curr Opin Hematol 13: 34–39

Alvarez-Larran A et al (2004) Increased CD11b neutrophil expression in Budd-Chiari syndrome or portal vein thrombosis secondary to polycythaemia vera. Br J Haematol 124:329–335

Alvarez-Larran A et al (2008) Increased platelet, leukocyte, and coagulation activation in primary myelofibrosis. Ann Hematol 87:269–276

Arellano-Rodrigo E et al (2006) Increased platelet and leukocyte activation as contributing mechanisms for thrombosis in essential thrombocythemia and correlation with the JAK2 mutational status. Haematologica 91:169–175

Arellano-Rodrigo E et al (2009) Platelet turnover, coagulation factors, and soluble markers of platelet and endothelial activation in essential thrombocythemia:

relationship with thrombosis occurrence and JAK2 V617F allele burden. Am J Hematol 84:102–108

Baxter EJ et al (2005) Acquired mutation of the tyrosine kinase JAK2 in human myeloproliferative disorders. Lancet 365:1054–1061

Bucalossi A et al (1996) Reduction of antithrombin III, protein C, and protein S levels and activated protein C resistance in polycythemia vera and essential thrombocythemia patients with thrombosis. Am J Hematol 52:14–20

Buss DH et al (1985) The incidence of thrombotic and hemorrhagic disorders in association with extreme thrombocytosis: an analysis of 129 cases. Am J Hematol 20:365–372

Carobbio A et al (2007) Leukocytosis is a risk factor for thrombosis in essential thrombocythemia: interaction with treatment, standard risk factors, and Jak2 mutation status. Blood 109:2310–2313

Carobbio A et al (2008) Leukocytosis and risk stratification assessment in essential thrombocythemia. J Clin Oncol 26:2732–2736

Cervantes F et al (2006) Frequency and risk factors for thrombosis in idiopathic myelofibrosis: analysis in a series of 155 patients from a single institution. Leukemia 20:55–60

Cortelazzo S et al (1995) Hydroxyurea for patients with essential thrombocythemia and a high risk of thrombosis. N Engl J Med 332:1132–1136

De Stefano V et al (2010) Leukocytosis is a risk factor for recurrent arterial thrombosis in young patients with polycythemia vera and essential thrombocythemia. Am J Hematol 85:97–100

Duchemin J et al (2010) Increased circulating procoagulant activity and thrombin generation in patients with myeloproliferative neoplasms. Thromb Res 126:238–242

Elliott MA, Tefferi A (2005) Thrombosis and haemorrhage in polycythaemia vera and essential thrombocythaemia. Br J Haematol 128:275–290

Falanga A et al (1994) Hemostatic system activation in patients with lupus anticoagulant and essential thrombocythemia. Semin Thromb Hemost 20:324–327

Falanga A et al (1999) Neutrophil activation and hemostatic changes in healthy donors receiving granulocyte colony-stimulating factor. Blood 93:2506–2514

Falanga A et al (2000) Polymorphonuclear leukocyte activation and hemostasis in patients with essential thrombocythemia and polycythemia vera. Blood 96:4261–4266

Falanga A et al (2005a) Pathogenesis of thrombosis in essential thrombocythemia and polycythemia vera: the role of neutrophils. Semin Hematol 42:239–247

Falanga A et al (2005b) Leukocyte-platelet interaction in patients with essential thrombocythemia and polycythemia vera. Exp Hematol 33:523–530

Falanga A et al (2007) V617F JAK-2 mutation in patients with essential thrombocythemia: relation to platelet, granulocyte, and plasma hemostatic and inflammatory molecules. Exp Hematol 35:702–711

Finazzi G, Barbui T (2008) Evidence and expertise in the management of polycythemia vera and essential thrombocythemia. Leukemia 22:1494–1502

Gangat N et al (2009) Leukocytosis at diagnosis and the risk of subsequent thrombosis in patients with low-risk essential thrombocythemia and polycythemia vera. Cancer 115:5740–5745

Harrison CN (2005) Platelets and thrombosis in myeloproliferative diseases. Hematology Am Soc Hematol Educ Program 1:409–415

Harrison CN et al (2005) Hydroxyurea compared with anagrelide in high-risk essential thrombocythemia. N Engl J Med 353:33–45

Huang PY, Hellums JD (1993) Aggregation and disaggregation kinetics of human blood platelets: Part I. Development and validation of a population balance method. Biophys J 65:334–343

Jensen MK et al (2000) Increased platelet activation and abnormal membrane glycoprotein content and redistribution in myeloproliferative disorders. Br J Haematol 110:116–124

Jensen MK et al (2001) Increased circulating platelet-leukocyte aggregates in myeloproliferative disorders is correlated to previous thrombosis, platelet activation and platelet count. Eur J Haematol 66:143–151

Kralovics R et al (2005) A gain-of-function mutation of JAK2 in myeloproliferative disorders. N Engl J Med 352:1779–1790

Kubota Y et al (2004) Constitutively activated phosphatidylinositol 3-kinase primes platelets from patients with chronic myelogenous leukemia for thrombopoietin-induced aggregation. Leukemia 18:1127–1137

Kwaan HC, Wang J (2003) Hyperviscosity in polycythemia vera and other red cell abnormalities. Semin Thromb Hemost 29:451–458

Landolfi R et al (1992) Increased thromboxane biosynthesis in patients with polycythemia vera: evidence for aspirin-suppressible platelet activation in vivo. Blood 80:1965–1971

Landolfi R et al (1995) Bleeding and thrombosis in myeloproliferative disorders: mechanisms and treatment. Crit Rev Oncol Hematol 20:203–222

Landolfi R et al (2004) Efficacy and safety of low-dose aspirin in polycythemia vera. N Engl J Med 350:114–124

Landolfi R et al (2006) Thrombosis and bleeding in polycythemia vera and essential thrombocythemia: pathogenetic mechanisms and prevention. Best Pract Res Clin Haematol 19:617–633

Landolfi R et al (2007) Leukocytosis as a major thrombotic risk factor in patients with polycythemia vera. Blood 109:2446–2452

Levine RL et al (2005) Activating mutation in the tyrosine kinase JAK2 in polycythemia vera, essential thrombocythemia, and myeloid metaplasia with myelofibrosis. Cancer Cell 7:387–397

Lussana F et al (2009) Association of V617F Jak2 mutation with the risk of thrombosis among patients with essential thrombocythaemia or idiopathic myelofibrosis: a systematic review. Thromb Res 124:409–417

Marchetti M, Falanga A (2008) Leukocytosis, JAK2V617F mutation, and hemostasis in myeloproliferative disorders. Pathophysiol Haemost Thromb 36:148–159

Marchetti M et al (2008) Thrombin generation and activated protein C resistance in patients with essential thrombocythemia and polycythemia vera. Blood 112:4061–4068

Michiels JJ et al (2006) Clinical and laboratory features, pathobiology of platelet-mediated thrombosis and bleeding complications, and the molecular etiology of essential thrombocythemia and polycythemia vera: therapeutic implications. Semin Thromb Hemost 32:174–207

Palandri F et al (2011) Impact of leukocytosis on thrombotic risk and survival in 532 patients with essential thrombocythemia: a retrospective study. Ann Hematol 90:933–938

Panova-Noeva M et al (2011) Platelet-induced thrombin generation by the calibrated automated thrombogram assay is increased in patients with essential thrombocythemia and polycythemia vera. Am J Hematol 86:337–342

Pearson MJ, Lipowsky HH (2000) Influence of erythrocyte aggregation on leukocyte margination in postcapillary venules of rat mesentery. Am J Physiol Heart Circ Physiol 279:H1460–H1471

Pearson TC, Wetherley-Mein G (1978) Vascular occlusive episodes and venous haematocrit in primary proliferative polycythaemia. Lancet 2:1219–1222

Posan E et al (1998) Reduced in vitro clot lysis and release of more active platelet PAI-1 in polycythemia vera and essential thrombocythemia. Thromb Res 90:51–56

Rafail S et al (2008) Leptin induces the expression of functional tissue factor in human neutrophils and peripheral blood mononuclear cells through JAK2-dependent mechanisms and TNFalpha involvement. Thromb Res 122:366–375

Robertson B et al (2007) Platelet and coagulation activation markers in myeloproliferative diseases: relationships with JAK2 V6I7 F status, clonality, and antiphospholipid antibodies. J Thromb Haemost 5:1679–1685

Schafer AI (1984) Bleeding and thrombosis in the myeloproliferative disorders. Blood 64:1–12

Schafer AI (2004) Thrombocytosis. N Engl J Med 350:1211–1219

Stuart MJ, Nagel RL (2004) Sickle-cell disease. Lancet 364:1343–1360

Tefferi A (2011) Annual Clinical Updates in Hematological Malignancies: a continuing medical education series: polycythemia vera and essential thrombocythemia: 2011 update on diagnosis, risk-stratification, and management. Am J Hematol 86:292–301

Thomas DJ et al (1977) Effect of haematocrit on cerebral blood-flow in man. Lancet 2:941–943

Trappenburg MC et al (2009) Elevated procoagulant microparticles expressing endothelial and platelet markers in essential thrombocythemia. Haematologica 94:911–918

Turitto VT, Weiss HJ (1980) Red blood cells: their dual role in thrombus formation. Science 207:541–543

Turitto VT, Weiss HJ (1983) Platelet and red cell involvement in mural thrombogenesis. Ann N Y Acad Sci 416:363–376

Villmow T et al (2002) Markers of platelet activation and platelet-leukocyte interaction in patients with myeloproliferative syndromes. Thromb Res 108:139–145

Wieczorek I et al (1995) Low proteins C and S and activation of fibrinolysis in treated essential thrombocythemia. Am J Hematol 49:277–281

Yedgar S et al (2002) The red blood cell in vascular occlusion. Pathophysiol Haemost Thromb 32:263–268

Zhao R et al (2005) Identification of an acquired JAK2 mutation in polycythemia vera. J Biol Chem 280:22788–22792

Zwicker JI et al (2009) Tumor-derived tissue factor-bearing microparticles are associated with venous thromboembolic events in malignancy. Clin Cancer Res 15:6830–6840

Part III

Specific Issues of Treatment in PV and ET

Risk Classification

7

Guido Finazzi

Contents

G. Finazzi
Department of Hematology,
Ospedali Riuniti di Bergamo, Bergamo, Italy
e-mail: gfinazzi@ospedaliriuniti.bergamo.it

7.1 Polycythemia Vera

Early studies in untreated PV patients found a high incidence of thrombotic events and a life expectancy of about 18 months after diagnosis (Chievitz and Thiede 1962). Cytoreductive treatments of blood hyperviscosity by phlebotomy or chemotherapy have dramatically reduced the number of thrombotic events, even though hematological transformations towards post-polycythemic myelofibrosis and acute leukemia still represent a major cause of death (Marchioli et al. 2005). Since there is a concern that myelosuppressive drugs given to control the proliferative phase of the disease might be implicated in the long-term complications, current treatment recommendations should be adapted on the expected risk for thrombosis of the patient (Barbui and Finazzi 2006).

7.1.1 Incidence and Type of Thrombosis and Hemorrhage

At initial presentation, the reported incidence of thrombosis and bleeding in PV patients varied from 12–39% to 1.7–20%, respectively (Barbui and Finazzi 2006). Factors that could have accounted for the relatively wide range of values include patient selection, definition of events, and accuracy in data reporting. The largest epidemiologic study (European Collaboration on Low-dose Aspirin, ECLAP) included 1,638 patients followed for a median of 2.8 years (Marchioli et al. 2005). A total of 164 deaths (10%) were recorded for an

T. Barbui and A. Tefferi (eds.), *Myeloproliferative Neoplasms*, Hematologic Malignancies,
DOI 10.1007/978-3-642-24989-1_7, © Springer-Verlag Berlin Heidelberg 2012

overall mortality rate of 3.7 per 100 persons per year. As compared with the general Italian population standardized for age and sex, the excess of mortality of PV patients was 2.1 times. Cardiovascular mortality accounted for 41% of all deaths (1.5 deaths per 100 persons per year), mainly due to large vessel arterial events, such as coronary heart disease and non-hemorrhagic stroke. The cumulative rate of non-fatal thrombosis was 3.8 events per 100 persons per year, without difference between arterial and venous thrombosis. Major and fatal bleeding were rare, accounting for only 0.8 and 0.15 events per 100 persons per year. Thus, thrombosis represents a major cause of morbidity and mortality in PV.

Particularly serious thrombotic events typically associated with PV are abdominal vein thrombosis (AVT), including Budd-Chiari syndrome and obstruction of the portal, mesenteric, and splenic system. Overall, PV and other myeloproliferative neoplasms (MPN) were reported to be the major cause of AVT, accounting for 25–65% of cases (Elliott and Tefferi 2004). Of importance, the diagnosis of MPN may be difficult in these disorders because blood cell counts and serum erythropoietin levels can be still within the normal limits or only slightly modified, and the presence of a splenomegaly is of little diagnostic value. Specialized tests, including bone marrow biopsy and endogenous erythroid colony formation, have been advocated (Chait et al. 2005), but a step forward in the diagnosis of an occult MPN in these patients has been done with the discovery of JAK2 V617F. Testing for the mutation was found positive in 40–58% of patients with Budd-Chiari syndrome and 36% of those with portal vein thrombosis (Patel et al. 2006; Primignani et al. 2006) and is now recommended in all patients presenting with AVT (Chung et al. 2006).

7.1.2 Risk Stratification According to Thrombotic Risk

7.1.2.1 Age and Previous Thrombosis

Increasing age and a history of vascular events have consistently proven to be independent predictors of thrombosis in patients with PV (Berk et al. 1986; Marchioli et al. 2005). The first to report these risk

factors were the Polycythemia Vera Study Group (PVSG) investigators in a multivariate analysis of the entire cohort of 431 patients enrolled in the seminal 01 clinical trial. Phlebotomy treatment, rate of phlebotomy, history of prior thrombosis and advanced age contributed significantly to the overall risk of thrombosis, whereas this was not found for other parameters such as sex and pre-treatment hematological indices (i.e. hematocrit, white cell, and platelet count) (Berk et al. 1986). In the ECLAP study, the incidence of cardiovascular complications was higher in patients aged more than 65 years (5.0% patient-year, hazard ratio 2.0, 95% confidence interval [CI] 1.22–3.29, $P < 0.006$) or with a history of thrombosis (4.93% patient-year, hazard ratio 1.96, 95% CI 1.29–2.97, $P=0.0017$) than in younger subjects with no history of thrombosis (2.5% patient-year, reference category) (Fig. 7.1) (Marchioli et al. 2005). At variance of the PVSG findings, performance of phlebotomy was not associated with an increased thrombotic risk (relative risk 0.89, 95% CI 0.67–1.18).

7.1.2.2 The Role of Hematocrit

The principal hemorrheologic abnormality in PV is an elevated whole blood viscosity. The blood viscosity in PV is higher than that of normal controls at all shear rates (Thomas et al. 1977). In a retrospective analysis of the records of 69 PV patients with histories of vascular thrombosis, Pearson and Wetherley-Mein (1978) demonstrated a strong correlation in univariate analysis between hematocrit level and the development of thrombotic episodes, including many cerebrovascular occlusions. Thomas and coworkers (1977) showed that cerebral blood flow is reduced in patients with PV in whom the hematocrit is 53–62%. These abnormalities were observed even in patients with hematocrits at the lower levels of normal, that is, 46–52%. Reductions in cerebral blood flow were correctable with phlebotomy. Reduction of the hematocrit by relatively small amounts frequently led to substantial improvements in whole blood viscosity and cerebral blood flow. Some PV patients apparently still maintain a higher than normal whole blood viscosity despite the normalization of the hematocrit, suggesting that an increase in hematocrit may not be the only factor responsible for increased blood viscosity.

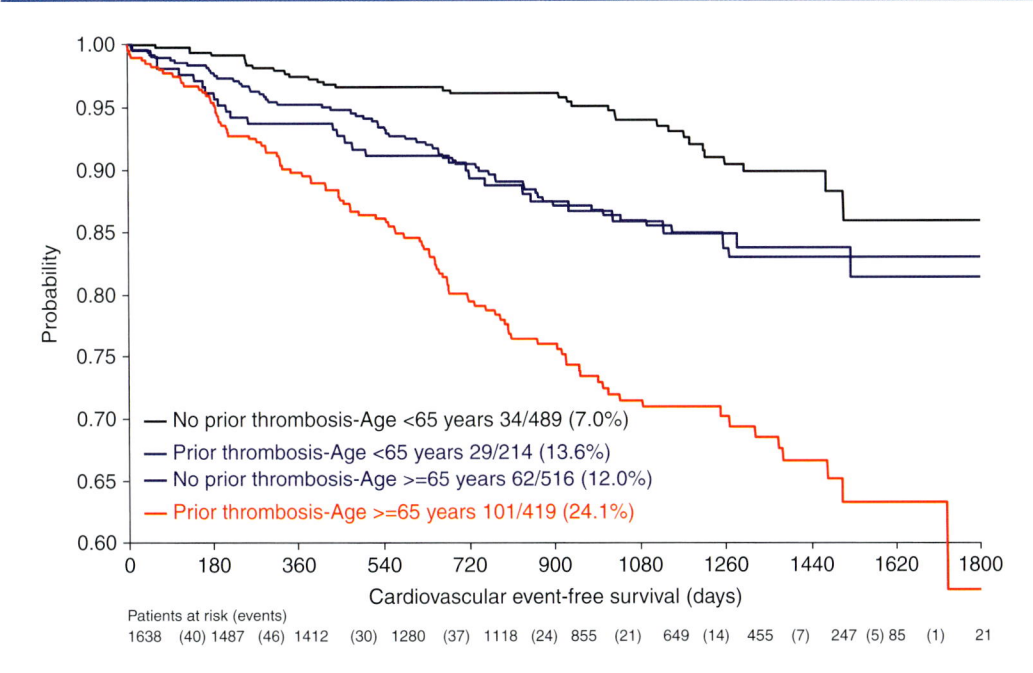

Fig. 7.1 Rate of vascular complications during follow-up in 1,638 patients with PV enrolled in the ECLAP study according to prior thrombosis and age

Almost all patients with PV are iron deficient. Decreased red cell deformability has been said to accompany iron deficiency, leading to increased blood viscosity and a decreased ability of red cells to pass through small-bore polycarbonate filters (Hutton 1979). Such abnormalities have been shown to be due to increased membrane stiffness rather than to reduced surface-volume ratio (Yip et al. 1983). Studies of patients with hemoglobinopathies due to abnormal oxygen binding who have secondary erythrocytosis provide further support to the belief that hematocrit elevations are not the sole cause of the thrombotic tendency in PV. A survey of 200 patients with these types of hemoglobinopathies has not demonstrated a higher incidence of myocardial ischemia or any other form of thrombosis, even though the red cell mass is frequently as elevated as that in patients with PV (Bunn and Forget 1986). Furthermore, Shibata and colleagues studied the risk of thrombosis in a transgenic mouse model with extreme erythrocytosis due to over-expression of EPO and did not observe an increased incidence of thrombosis (Shibata et al. 2003).

The issue of hematocrit and thrombosis in PV has been recently updated. In the ECLAP study, despite the recommendation of maintaining the hematocrit values at less than 0.45, only 48% of patients had values below this threshold, whilst 39% and 13% of patients remained between 0.45 and 0.50 and greater than 0.50, respectively (Marchioli et al. 2005). Multivariate models considering all the confounders failed to show any correlation between these hematocrit values and thrombosis (Di Nisio et al. 2006). A total of 164 deaths (10%), 145 (8.85%) major thrombosis and 226 (13.8%) total thrombosis were encountered during 4,393 person-years of follow-up (median 2.8 years). An association between relevant outcome events (thrombotic events, mortality, and hematological progression) and hematocrit in the evaluable range of 40–55% was found neither in the multivariate analysis at baseline nor in the time-dependent multivariate model (Di Nisio et al. 2006). For the time being, the recommended hematocrit target is below 45% (Barbui et al. 2011a), but the uncertainty described above prompted Italian investigators to launch a prospective, randomized clinical study (CYTO-PV) addressing the issue of the optimal target of cytoreduction in PV (EudraCT 2007-006694-91).

7.1.2.3 Platelet Number and Function

No study to date has demonstrated a significant correlation between platelet number or function and thrombosis. In the PVSG 01 clinical trial, platelet counts did not predict thrombosis, either measured at baseline or at the nearest times before the thrombotic event (Berk et al. 1986). Accordingly, an ad hoc analysis of the patients enrolled in the ECLAP study failed to show any association between platelet count and thrombotic events (Di Nisio et al. 2006). Neither the currently proposed therapeutic target of 400×10^9/L nor any other of the platelet count thresholds evaluated in this analysis predicted a higher risk of thrombosis. The concordant findings of these two major prospective studies in PV suggest that current treatment does not primarily aim at lowering the platelet count.

Qualitative platelet abnormalities occur frequently in PV patients. Increased plasma and urinary thromboxane production has been linked to increased platelet activation (Landolfi et al. 1992). A low-dose aspirin regimen selective for inhibition of platelet cyclooxygenase has been found to suppress increased thromboxane production in vivo and to clinically benefit patients with PV (GISP 1997; Landolfi et al. 2004). In addition, selected patients with PV have been afforded prompt resolution of vascular complications such as erythromelalgia or transient ischemic attacks following institution of platelet antiaggregating agents (Michiels et al. 1985). It is important to emphasize that erythromelalgia does not resolve in PV patients with phlebotomy alone or with anticoagulation but requires the use of platelet antiaggregating agents, namely aspirin. Although a variety of clinical assessments of platelet function have been used to identify patients who are potentially at a high risk of developing a life-threatening hemorrhagic or thrombotic event, the results of these studies to date have been very disappointing. It appears that the etiology of thrombosis and hemorrhage in PV is multifactorial and that the available tools are inadequate to identify those patients at highest risk.

7.1.2.4 Leukocytes

Leukocytosis was found to be an independent risk factor for thrombosis (Barbui et al. 2009). PV patients with WBC count $>15,000 \times 10^9$/L, compared to those with WBC count $<10,000 \times 10^9$/L, had a significant 70% increase of the rate of vascular complications, mainly represented by myocardial infarction (Landolfi et al. 2007). Similar findings have been reported in patients with ET (see below). Activated leukocytes may release proteases and oxygen radicals which alter endothelial cells and platelets so as to favor the development of a prothrombotic state. A series of markers of leukocyte activation, including expression of membrane CD11B and leukocyte alkaline phosphatase antigen, cellular elastase content, plasma elastase levels, and myeloperoxidase levels are elevated in patients with PV (Falanga et al. 2005). An association between these functional abnormalities and the presence of JAK2 mutation has been reported (Arellano-Rodrigo et al. 2006). Overall, these results would indicate that an increased release of neutrophil proteases may provide a mechanism by which the homeostatic pathway is activated in PV, which ultimately would contribute to the establishment of a prethrombotic state (Marchetti et al. 2008).

7.1.2.5 Other Risk Factors

Conventional risk factors for atherosclerosis, including hypertension, hyperlipidaemia, diabetes, and smoking, have been assessed in PV with variable results, possibly reflecting the size of the studies and number of patients with the risk markers of interest included. In the absence of consistent data, it seems reasonable to assume that common cardiovascular risk factors are associated in PV with the same relative risk as those estimated in the general population. According to this assumption, recent guidelines recommend that all patients should be managed aggressively for their risk condition and should be requested to stop smoking (McMullin et al. 2005; Barbui et al. 2011a). However, the use of cytotoxic drugs in otherwise low-risk patients carrying well-controlled cardiovascular risk factors is not generally indicated (McMullin et al. 2005; Barbui et al. 2011a).

Several studies have explored the contribution of inherited and acquired thrombophilic states to the occurrence of thrombotic events in PV with some conflicting results. To date, there is no convincing evidence that identification of a thrombophilic abnormality adds to the management of patients, so that routine thrombophilia screening is not currently recommended (McMullin et al. 2005; Barbui et al. 2011a).

The influence of the JAK2 V617F mutational load on the thrombotic risk has been evaluated in 173 patients with PV (Vannucchi et al. 2007). The mean mutant allele burden was 52%, with 32 patients (18%) having greater than 75% mutant allele. The burden of JAK2 V617F allele correlated with measurements of stimulated erythropoiesis (higher hematocrit, lower mean cell volume, serum ferritin, and erythropoietin levels) and myelopoiesis (higher white cell count, neutrophil count, and serum lactate dehydrogenase) and with markers of neutrophil activation (elevated leukocyte alkaline phosphatase and PRV-1 expression). As compared to those with less than 25% mutant allele, patients harboring greater than 75% JAK2 V617F allele were at higher relative risk (RR) of developing major cardiovascular events during follow-up (RR 7.1; $P = 0.003$).

7.2 Essential Thrombocythemia

A risk stratification based on thrombohemorrhagic risk is needed also for patients with ET, as for those with PV, with the purpose to focus the indication for myelosuppressive therapy on high-risk patients only and to avoid the risk of over-treatment in individuals with a low probability to develop major bleeding or thrombotic complications.

7.2.1 Incidence and Type of Thrombosis and Hemorrhage

Thrombosis and hemorrhage are the most frequent clinical complications observed in ET patients. In uncontrolled studies, reported cumulative rates for thrombosis and hemorrhage during follow-up ranged from 7% to 17% and 8% to 14%, respectively (Barbui and Finazzi 2006). In one study that also evaluated a control population (Cortelazzo et al. 1990), the incidence of thrombotic episodes

was 6.6% per patient-year in ET vs. 1.2% in control subjects, and the rate of major hemorrhagic complications was 0.33% per patient-year in ET vs. 0% in controls.

The most frequent types of major thrombosis include stroke, transient ischemic attack, myocardial infarction, peripheral arterial thrombosis, and deep venous thrombosis often occurring in unusual sites, such as hepatic (Budd-Chiari syndrome), portal, and mesenteric veins. In addition to large vessel occlusions, ET patients may suffer from microcirculatory symptoms, including vascular headaches, dizziness, visual disturbances, distal paraesthesia, and acrocyanosis cases (Elliott and Tefferi 2004). The most characteristic of these disturbances is erythromelalgia, consisting of congestion, redness, and burning pain to ischemia and gangrene of distal portions of toes and fingers (Michiels et al. 1985). The most frequent bleeding events are hemorrhages from the gastrointestinal tract followed by hematuria and other muco-cutaneous hemorrhages. Hemarthrosis and large muscle hematomas are uncommon.

7.2.2 Risk Stratification According to Thrombotic Risk

7.2.2.1 Age and Previous Thrombosis

Age over 60 and a previous thrombotic event were identified as major risk factors for thrombosis in most studies (summarized in Table 7.1). The age-related differences in the frequency of these events have been attributed to the coexistence of vascular disease in older patients (Watson and Key 1993). However, younger patients are not free of vascular thrombosis, sometimes in unusual sites, such as the portal or sagittal veins (Mitus et al. 1990). Overall, the incidence of thrombotic and hemorrhagic complications in asymptomatic patients with essential thrombocythemia less than 60 years of age who had a platelet count of less than $1,500 \times 10^9$/L has been shown to be comparable with a normal control population (Ruggeri et al. 1998). These authors have emphasized the importance of the concurrent absence of both of the formerly mentioned clinical characteristics to define a low-risk profile in young patients with essential thrombocythemia.

7.2.2.2 Platelet Count

Several large cohort studies have failed to define a relationship between the frequency of thrombotic complications and platelet number (Table 7.1). Thus, an elevated platelet count, per se, should not be considered an indication for a myelosuppressive therapy aimed at preventing thrombotic complications. Supporting this view, in a retrospective study of 99 consecutive young patients (aged <60 years) who presented with extreme thrombocytosis (platelet count $\geq 1,000 \times 10^9$/L) and without a previous history of thrombohemorrhagic complications, the incidences of major thrombosis and hemorrhage during the follow-up were similar between those who were treated with prophylactic cytoreductive therapy and those who did not receive such therapy (Tefferi et al. 2006).

The relationship between frequency of bleeding episodes and high platelet counts is much more consistent. Several studies have shown that the degree and duration of bleeding in this patient population correlate with the platelet count (Table 7.1). Bleeding events appear to occur exclusively when the platelet counts are excessively high and stop when the platelet count falls to normal. The clinical spectrum of bleeding in essential thrombocythemia patients closely resembles that observed in von Willebrand disease (Budde et al. 1993; van Genderen et al. 1996). Several groups have now shown that high platelet counts (>$1,000 \times 10^9$/L) are associated with an acquired von Willebrand syndrome and that reduction of platelet numbers is associated with correction of the von Willebrand abnormalities and cessation of bleeding episodes (Budde et al. 1993; van Genderen et al. 1996). An increase in the number of circulating platelets appears to favor the adsorption of larger von Willebrand multimers onto platelet membranes, resulting in their removal from the circulation and their subsequent degradation. The laboratory features of acquired von Willebrand syndrome in essential thrombocythemia is characteristic of a type II deficiency with a prolonged bleeding time, decreased ristocetin cofactor activity, and a decrease or absence of large von Willebrand factor multimers (Budde

et al. 1993; van Genderen et al. 1996; Elliott and Tefferi 2004).

7.2.2.3 Platelet Function

Platelets in patients with essential thrombocythemia have been known for a considerable time to be qualitatively abnormal (Landolfi et al. 2006; Finazzi et al. 2009). Although both increased and decreased platelet reactivities have been described, these findings have not been definitively associated with thrombohemorrhagic complications with two noteworthy exceptions; erythromelalgia, where the prompt relief of symptoms by cyclooxygenase inhibitors provides direct evidence that prostaglandins play a role in the development of vascular occlusion (Michiels et al. 1985), and acquired von Willebrand syndrome, which is a major cause of bleeding in patients with essential thrombocythemia (Budde et al. 1993; van Genderen et al. 1996).

Prolongation of the bleeding time has been reported in 7–19% of newly diagnosed patients with essential thrombocythemia (Finazzi et al. 2009). A close correlation between prolongation of the bleeding time and the occurrence of hemorrhage in essential thrombocythemia patients does not always exist. This is in contrast to correction of the bleeding time in those patients with essential thrombocythemia, extreme thrombocytosis, and acquired von Willebrand syndrome following reduction of platelet numbers to the normal range. It is important to emphasize that aspirin prolongs the bleeding time of patients with essential thrombocythemia to a greater degree than that of normal controls (Budde et al. 1993; van Genderen et al. 1996).

Abnormal platelet aggregation has been reported in 35–100% of patients with essential thrombocythemia. Abnormal aggregation studies are not related to prolongation of the bleeding time or to the incidence of episodes of hemorrhage or thrombosis. In essential thrombocythemia, platelet aggregation is classically defective in response to epinephrine, adenosine diphosphate (ADP), and collagen but is usually normal with arachidonic acid and ristocetin. Characteristically, in essential thrombocythemia, the first wave of aggregation is diminished, and

Table 7.1 Cohort studies of risk factors for thrombosis and bleeding in essential thrombocythemia including at least 100 patients

Study (ref)	Patients, no.	Risk factors for thrombosis (RR or P)				
		Age > 60	Previous thrombosis	Platelet count	Leukocytosis	Cardiovascular risk factors[a]
Cortelazzo et al. (1990)	100	10.3 (2.05–51.5)	13 (4.1–41.5)	NS	–	NS
Besses et al. (1999)	148	3.3 (1.5–7.4)	3.0 (1.5–6.0)	NS	–	4.7 (1.8–11.8)
Colombi et al. (1991)	103	NS	$P<0.001$	NS	–	–
Jantunen et al. (2001)	132	NS	–	NS	–	$P=0.01$
Bazzan et al. (1999)	187	NS (age >55)	–	NS	–	NS
Wolanskyi et al. (2006)	322	1.51 (1.05–2.18)	2.3 (1.25–4.24) (arterial only)	–	1.74 (1.15–2.66) (WBC $\geq 15\times10^9$/L)	NS
Carobbio et al. (2007)	439	2.3 (1.3–3.9) (age >60 and previous thrombosis evaluated together)		NS	2.3 (1.4–3.9) (WBC $\geq 8.7\times10^9$/L)	–
Passamonti et al. (2008)	605	$P<0.001$	$P=0.03$	NS	NS	–
Palandri et al. (2011)	532	2.45 (1.35–4.43)		NS	1.76 (1.95–2.97) (WBC $\geq 11\times10^9$/L)	–

Study (ref)	Patients, no.	Risk factor for bleeding
		Platelet count
van Genderen and Michiels (1994)	200 (review of published cases)	$P<0.001$ (platelets $>1,000\times10^9$/L)
Fenaux et al. (1990)	147	"Higher risk" (platelets $>2,000\times10^9$/L)
Wolanskyi et al. (2006)	322	NS
Alvarez-Larran et al. (2010)	300	$P<0.01$ (platelets $>800\times10^9$/L)

NS not significant

[a]At least one of the following: smoking, hypertension, hypercholesterolemia, diabetes

the second wave of aggregation is absent in response to epinephrine. An acquired form of platelet storage pool disease occurs frequently in essential thrombocythemia. Platelet alpha-granule content and release are abnormal, resulting in elevated plasma levels of platelet factor-4 and beta-thromboglobulin. Because the content of alpha-granule constituents has been reported to be normal in megakaryocytes isolated from essential thrombocythemia, the synthesis of these molecules is not believed to be abnormal, but rather, the release of alpha-granule constituents is believed to be a consequence of platelet activation. The finding of an acquired storage pool defect again does not correlate with platelet numbers or with the occurrence of clinical symptoms (Finazzi et al. 2009).

The survival of platelets in patients with erythromelalgia and thrombosis has been shown to be reduced to 4.2 ± 0.2 days compared with normal platelet survivals in asymptomatic essential thrombocythemia patients (6.6 ± 0.3 days) and patients with reactive thrombocytosis (8.0 ± 0.4 days) (van Genderen 1995). Thrombosis in this setting is associated with an increased platelet turnover, which can be quantitated cytometrically by measuring the number of platelets most recently released into the circulation (reticulated platelets). Treatment of erythromelalgia with aspirin increased mean platelet survival from 4.0 ± 0.3 to 6.9 ± 0.4 days and was associated with a significant elevation of platelet numbers (van Genderen 1995). These findings suggest that erythromelalgia results from platelet-mediated thrombosis of the arterial microvasculature of the extremities. Complete correction of this ischemic circulatory defect is associated with the use of platelet cyclooxygenase inhibitors, such as aspirin (van Genderen and Michiels 1994). Agents that do not inhibit platelet cyclooxygenase, such as coumadin, sodium salicylate, dipyridamole, sulfinpyrazone, and ticlopidine, are not active in the treatment of this disorder (van Genderen and Michiels 1994).

One intriguing explanation for the increased risk of thrombosis in patients with essential thrombocythemia has been proposed by Lee and Baglin (1995). These investigators demonstrated that the total amount of thrombin generated on the platelet surfaces of patients with essential thrombocythemia was markedly greater than that generated on the platelet surfaces of normal controls or patients with reactive thrombocytosis. The molecular basis of this abnormality has not been defined, but it remains possible that an abnormal membrane structure of essential thrombocythemia platelets may account for the enhanced thrombin potential that may lead to a relatively high thrombotic risk. On this ground, Trappenburg and coworkers (2009) have more recently documented increased numbers of platelet microparticles, as well as increased platelet-neutrophil and platelet-monocyte conjugates, in patients with essential thrombocythemia. Platelet microparticles support thrombin generation and leukocyte activation. Increased numbers of platelet microparticles have been associated with the development of vascular thrombosis.

7.2.2.4 Leukocyte Number and Function

A prognostic role for leukocytosis in ET, as in PV, has been advocated (Barbui et al. 2009). Two large cohort studies reported that an increased baseline leukocyte count was an independent risk factor for both thrombosis and inferior survival (Wolanskyj et al. 2006; Carobbio et al. 2007). In "low-risk" ET patients (i.e. below 60 years and without previous thrombosis), leukocytosis confers a thrombotic risk comparable to that of treated "high-risk" patients without leukocytosis (Carobbio et al. 2007). The role of WBC count in ET was mostly observed on the occurrence of myocardial infarction, as shown in Table 7.2, confirming the data reported above for PV (Carobbio et al. 2008). White blood cell (WBC) counts above 9.5×10^9/L at diagnosis were independently associated with thrombosis during follow-up (RR = 1.8, $P = 0.03$) in another study of 187 patients with ET and PV (Caramazza et al. 2009). These findings were not confirmed in a retrospective study of 407 low-risk patients with ET (Gangat et al. 2009a). Leukocytosis at the time of diagnosis, defined by a cut-off level of either 15 or 9.4×10^9/L, did not appear to be predictive of either arterial or venous thrombosis during follow-up. However, in an analysis by

Table 7.2 Sites of thrombosis according to leukocytosis at diagnosis in 657 patients with ET

	7.1 to 10×10^9/L White blood cells[a]		More than 10×10^9/L White blood cells[a]	
	HR (95% CI)	P	HR (95% CI)	P
Major thrombosis	2.21 (1.05–4.65)	0.036	3.27 (1.54–6.95)	0.002
Arterial thrombosis	2.07 (0.83–5.20)	0.121	3.12 (1.20–8.08)	0.019
Myocardial infarction	5.82 (0.64–53.2)	0.118	8.08 (1.00–65.5)	0.050
Stroke/TIA	0.88 (0.29–2.67)	0.824	1.32 (0.42–4.11)	0.631
Venous thrombosis	1.40 (0.49–4.04)	0.534	2.51 (0.86–7.29)	0.092

Multivariable models adjusted for information collected at diagnosis, including center, sex, standard risk factors, hemoglobin, hematocrit, and platelet count
[a]Reference category: WBC $\leq 7 \times 10^9$/L

Passamonti et al. (2009) of 194 low-risk ET patients, the increase in leukocyte count within 2 years of diagnosis (observed in 9% of patients), rather than leukocytosis at diagnosis, was associated with an higher risk of vascular complications during follow-up.

In ET, an in vivo leukocyte activation has been consistently documented in association with signs of activation of both platelets and endothelial cells. Interestingly, the presence of the JAK2 mutation is associated with higher platelet and leukocyte activation in these patients (Arellano-Rodrigo et al. 2006). Thus, platelet and leukocyte activation may play a role in the generation of the pre-thrombotic state that characterizes essential thrombocythemia (Falanga et al. 2005; Marchetti and Falanga, 2008). However, whether leukocytosis should be simply considered a marker for vascular disease or whether elevated WBC levels actually contribute directly to causing such disorders should be matter of prospective studies.

7.2.2.5 Other Risk Factors

The presence of the JAK2 V617F mutation in about 60% of ET patients raised the question whether mutated and non-mutated patients differ in terms of thrombotic risk. The largest prospective study on 806 patients suggested that JAK2 mutation in ET was associated with anamnestic venous but not arterial events (Campbell et al. 2005). An increased risk of thrombosis in JAK2 mutated patients was retrospectively observed by other investigators (Cheung et al. 2005; Finazzi et al. 2007). However, the rate of vascular complications was not affected by the presence of the mutation in two relatively large retrospective studies, including 150 and 130 ET patients, respectively (Antonioli et al. 2005; Wolanskyj et al. 2005). A systematic literature review was carried out to compare the frequency of thrombosis between JAK2 V617F positive and wild-type patients with essential thrombocythemia (Lussana et al. 2009). This study showed that JAK2 V617F patients have a twofold risk of developing thrombosis (odds ratio 1.92, 95% confidence interval 1.45–2.53), but a significant heterogeneity between studies should be pointed out. In addition to the prognostic role of JAK2 mutation for the first thrombotic episode, recent data would indicate that the mutation has also a role to predict recurrent thrombotic episodes in patients with ET (De Stefano et al. 2010).

Bone marrow histology is important for an accurate morphologic diagnosis of ET according to WHO criteria and for predicting survival and hematological transformations to myelofibrosis or acute leukemia (Barbui et al. 2011c). However, its role as risk factor for thrombosis is controversial. Campbell et al. (2009) have identified increased bone marrow reticulin fibrosis at diagnosis as an independent predictor of subsequent thrombotic and hemorrhagic complications. However, a recent analysis comparing 891 patients with WHO-diagnosed ET vs. 180 patients clinically presenting like ET but with an histological picture of pre-fibrotic PMF did not show any difference in the rates of arterial (1.2–1.4% patient-year, respectively) and venous (0.6% patient-year in both groups) thrombotic complications (Barbui et al. 2011c).

Table 7.3 Risk stratification in PV and ET based on thrombotic risk

Risk category	Age ≥ 60 years or history of thrombosis
Low	No
High	Yes

Extreme thrombocytosis (platelet count >1,000 × 10⁹/L) is a risk factor for bleeding, not for thrombosis

Increasing leukocyte count and JAK2 V617F mutation or allele burden have been identified as novel risk factors for thrombosis, but confirmation is required

The role of inflammation among the possible pathogenetic mechanisms of thrombosis in ET and PV has been recently highlighted by Barbui and coworkers (2011b) who correlated vascular complications with plasma levels of high-sensitivity C-reactive protein and pentraxin-3 in 244 ET and PV patients. Major thrombosis rate was higher in the highest C-reactive protein tertile ($P=0.01$) and lower at the highest pentraxin-3 levels ($P=0.045$). These associations remained significant in multivariable analysis and indicate that these inflammatory biomarkers independently and in opposite ways modulate the risk of cardiovascular events in patients with MPN.

Conclusions

By incorporating this body of knowledge in a clinically oriented scheme (Table 7.3), we have now consistent information to stratify the patients with either PV or ET in a "high-risk" or "low-risk" category according to their age and previous history of thrombosis (Barbui et al. 2011a). Putative novel variables, such as leukocytosis and JAK2 V617F mutational status and allele burden might be incorporated in the risk classification, possibly allowing better definition of the low-risk group, once more information is available and when they have been eventually validated in prospective studies.

7.3 Risk Stratification in Pregnancy

Pregnancy in MPN is an increasingly frequent and relevant problem due to improvement in diagnosis and for the trend in modern society towards delaying pregnancy until later life.

Normal pregnant women are at an increased risk of thrombosis, calculated to be approximately six times higher than in non-pregnant women, and the risk is compounded if they also have MPN. As a consequence, women with MPN may present a high incidence not only of pregnancy-related venous thromboembolism but also of other vascular complications of pregnancy involving occlusion of the placental circulation (Harrison 2005; Griesshammer et al. 2006). The paucity of published data, however, makes it difficult to obtain a clear view of the overall risk of these events.

7.3.1 Incidence and Risk Factors for Pregnancy Complications

In the Italian guidelines for the therapy of essential thrombocythemia, the outcomes of 461 pregnancies reported in retrospective and prospective cohort studies were pooled (Barbui et al. 2004). Most reports dealt with single cases or small numbers, and some suspicion of reporting bias was raised since there is a tendency to describe patients with complications rather than those with an uncomplicated pregnancy. To avoid this bias, Elliott and Tefferi (2003) restricted their review to series comprising at least six patients but, interestingly, the results were not different from those in the systematically retrieved literature that formed the basis of the ET Italian guidelines.

The mean age at pregnancy was 29 years, with a mean platelet count at the beginning of pregnancy of $1,000 × 10^9$/L. During the second trimester, a spontaneous decline was registered to a nadir of $599 × 10^9$/L. This decrease seems larger than the reduction seen in normal pregnancies, which is attributed to an increase in plasma volume. The mechanism is not known, but could involve placental or fetal production of a factor that downregulates platelet production. In the post-partum period, the platelet counts rise back up to their earlier levels, and rebound thrombocytosis may occur in some patients. This increases the probability of vascular complications at this time, which is a period of high thrombotic risk, like in other conditions of thrombophilia as well as in normal women. Overall, 50–70% of ET women had successful live births; first-trimester loss occurred in about 25–40% and late pregnancy loss in 10% of cases. This is in agreement with a Mayo Clinic study of 63 pregnancies: 60% ended in live births and 32% in first trimester miscarriages (Gangat et al. 2009b). Abruptio placentae was reported in 3.6% of cases, higher than in the general population (1%) (Barbui et al. 2004). Pre-eclampsia rates were similar to the normal population (1.7%), and intrauterine growth retardation was reported in 4–5%. Recent studies suggested that the presence of JAK2 V617F mutation may increase the risk of pregnancy loss (Passamonti et al. 2007), but adjusting management strategies on this basis is not recommended.

Maternal thrombosis or hemorrhage is uncommon. In the pooled analysis cited above, post-partum thrombotic episodes were reported in 13 patients, occurring in 5.2% of pregnancies, and minor, or major, pre- or post-partum bleeding events in other 13 cases (Barbui et al. 2004). The maternal vascular risk may be higher in women with previous venous or arterial events or hemorrhages attributed to MPN, independent of whether they occurred in a previous pregnancy or not. Similarly, severe complications in a previous pregnancy, such as ≥3 first-trimester, or ≥1 second- or third-trimester losses, birthweight <5th centile of gestation, pre-eclampsia, intrauterine death, or stillbirth, are considered to raise the risk of subsequent events for the mother and the fetus. Other vascular risk factors in pregnant women are age, obesity, immobilization, and other causes of genetic and acquired thrombophilia including antiphospholipid antibodies.

Pregnancy in polycythemia vera (PV) is rarer than in ET. A study reviewed a total of 38 pregnancies in 18 PV patients (Robinson et al. 2005); 22 successful live births were reported (57%). Similar to ET, spontaneous abortion during the first trimester was reported in 22% of cases and pre-term delivery in 13.8%.

Based on the information, consensus recommendations for risk stratification in pregnant women with MPNs have been recently developed by ELN and are summarized in Table 7.4 (Barbui et al. 2011a).

Table 7.4 Features consistent with high-risk pregnancy in Ph-neg. classical myeloproliferative neoplasms (MPN)

Previous venous or arterial thrombosis (whether pregnant or not)

Previous hemorrhage attributed to MPN (whether pregnant or not)

Previous pregnancy complication that may have been caused by MPN; e.g.

Unexplained recurrent first trimester loss (three unexplained first trimester losses)

Intrauterine growth restriction (birthweight <5th centile for gestation)

Intrauterine death or still birth (with no obvious other cause, evidence of placental dysfunction and growth restricted fetus)

Severe pre-eclampsia (necessitating pre-term delivery <34 weeks) or development of any such complication in the index pregnancy

Placental abruption

Significant ante- or post-partum hemorrhage

Marked sustained rise in platelet count rising to above $1,500 \times 10^9/L$

References

Alvarez-Larran A, Cervantes F, Pereira A et al (2010) Observation versus antiplatelet therapy as primary prophylaxis for thrombosis in low-risk essential thrombocythemia. Blood 116:1205–1210

Antonioli E, Guglielmelli P, Pancrazzi A et al (2005) Clinical implications of the JAK2 V617F mutation in essential thrombocythemia. Leukemia 19:1847–1849

Arellano-Rodrigo E, Alvarez-Larran A, Reverter JC et al (2006) Increased platelet and leukocyte activation as contributing mechanisms for thrombosis in essential thrombocythemia and correlation with the JAK2 mutational status. Haematologica 91:169–175

Barbui T, Finazzi G (2006) Evidence-based management of polycythemia vera. Best Pract Res Clin Haematol 19:483–493

Barbui T, Barosi G, Grossi A et al (2004) Practice guidelines for the therapy of essential thrombocythemia. A statement from the Italian Society of Hematology, the Italian Society of Experimental Hematology and the Italian Group for Bone Marrow Transplantation. Haematologica 89:215–222

Barbui T, Carobbio A, Rambaldi A et al (2009) Perspectives on thrombosis in essential thrombocythemia and polycythemia vera: is leukocytosis a causative factor? Blood 114:759–763

Barbui T, Thiele J, Passamonti F et al (2011c) Survival and disease progression in essential thrombocythemia are significantly influenced by accurate morphologic diagnosis: an international study. J Clin Oncol 29: 3179–3184

Barbui T, Barosi G, Birgegard G et al (2011a) Philadelphia-negative classical myeloproliferative neoplasms: critical concepts and management recommendations from European LeukemiaNet. J Clin Oncol 29:761–770

Barbui T, Carobbio A, Finazzi G et al (2011b) Inflammation and thrombosis in essential thrombocythemia and polycythemia vera: different role of C-reactive protein and pentraxin 3. Haematologica 96:315–318

Bazzan M, Tamponi G, Schinco P et al (1999) Thrombosis-free survival and life expectancy in 187 consecutive patients with essential thrombocythemia. Ann Hematol 78:539–543

Berk PD, Goldberg JD, Donovan PB et al (1986) Therapeutic recommendations in polycythemia vera based on Polycythemia Vera Study Group protocols. Semin Hematol 23:132–143

Besses C, Cervantes F, Pereira A et al (1999) Major vascular complications in essential thrombocythemia: a study of the predictive factors in a series of 148 patients. Leukemia 13:150–154

Budde A, Scharf RE, Franke P et al (1993) Elevated platelet count as a cause of abnormal von Willebrand factor multimer distribution in plasma. Blood 82:1749–1757

Bunn HF, Forget BG (1986) Hemoglobinopathy due to abnormal oxygen binding. In: Bunn HF, Forget BG (eds) Hemoglobin: molecular, genetic and clinical aspects. WB Saunders, Philadelphia

Campbell PJ, Scott LM, Buck G et al (2005) Definition of subtypes of essential thrombocythaemia and relation to polycythaemia vera based on JAK2 V617F mutation status: a prospective study. Lancet 366:1945–1953

Campbell PJ, Bareford D, Erber WN et al (2009) Reticulin accumulation in essential thrombocythemia: prognostic significance and relation to therapy. J Clin Oncol 27:2991–2999

Caramazza D, Caracciolo C, Barone R et al (2009) Correlation between leukocytosis and thrombosis in Philadelphia negative chronic myeloproliferative neoplasms. Ann Hematol 88:967–971

Carobbio A, Finazzi G, Guerini V et al (2007) Leukocytosis is a risk factor for thrombosis in essential thrombocythemia: interaction with treatment, standard risk factors and JAK2 mutation status. Blood 109:2310–2313

Carobbio A, Antonioli E, Guglielmelli P et al (2008) Leukocytosis and risk stratification assessment in essential thrombocythemia. J Clin Oncol 26:2732–2736

Chait Y, Condat B, Cazals-Hatem D et al (2005) Relevance of the criteria commonly used to diagnose myeloproliferative disorder in patients with splanchnic vein thrombosis. Br J Haematol 129:553–560

Cheung B, Radia D, Pantedelis P et al (2005) The presence of the JAK2 V617F mutation is associated with higher haemoglobin and increased risk of thrombosis in essential thrombocythaemia. Br J Haematol 132:244–250

Chievitz E, Thiede T (1962) Complications and causes of death in polycythemia vera. Acta Med Scand 172:513–523

Chung RT, Iafrate AJ, Amrein PC et al (2006) Case 15-2006: a 46-year-old woman with sudden onset of abdominal distention. N Engl J Med 354:2166–2175

Colombi M, Radaelli F, Zocchi L et al (1991) Thrombotic and hemorrhagic complications in essential thrombocythemia. A retrospective study of 103 patients. Cancer 67:2926–2930

Cortelazzo S, Viero P, Finazzi G et al (1990) Incidence and risk factors for thrombotic complications in a historical cohort of 100 patients with essential thrombocythemia. J Clin Oncol 8:556–562

De Stefano V, Za T, Rossi E et al (2010) Increased risk of recurrent thrombosis in patients with essential thrombocythemia carrying the homozygous JAK2 V617F mutation. Ann Hematol 85:97–100

Di Nisio M, Barbui T, Di Gennaro L et al (2006) The hematocrit and platelet target in polycythemia vera. Br J Haematol 136:249–259

Elliott MA, Tefferi A (2003) Thrombocythaemia and pregnancy. Best Pract Res Clin Haematol 16:227–242

Elliott MA, Tefferi A (2004) Thrombosis and haemorrhage in polycythaemia vera and essential thrombocythaemia. Br J Haematol 128:275–290

Falanga A, Marchetti M, Vignoli A et al (2005) Leukocyte-platelet interaction in patients with essential thrombocythemia and polycythemia vera. Exp Hematol 33:523–530

Fenaux P, Simon M, Caulier MT et al (1990) Clinical course of essential thrombocythemia in 147 cases. Cancer 66:549–556

Finazzi G, Rambaldi A, Guerini V et al (2007) Risk of thrombosis in patients with essential thrombocythemia and polycythemia vera according to JAK2 V617F status. Haematologica 92:135–136

Finazzi G, Hu M, Barbui T et al (2009) Essential thrombocythemia. In: Hoffman R, Benz EJ Jr, Shattil SJ, Furie B, Silberstein LE, McGlave P, Heslop H (eds) Hematology basic principles and practice, 5th edn. Churchill Livingstone, Philadelphia

Gangat N, Wolanskyj AP, Schwager SM et al (2009a) Leukocytosis at diagnosis and the risk of subsequent thrombosis in patients with low-risk essential thrombocythemia and polycythemia vera. Cancer 115:5740–5745

Gangat N, Wolanskyj AP, Schwager S et al (2009b) Predictors of pregnancy outcome in essential thrombocythemia: a single institution study of 63 pregnancies. Eur J Haematol 82:350–353

Griesshammer M, Struve S, Harrison CM (2006) Essential thrombocythemia/polycythemia vera and pregnancy: the need for an observational study in Europe. Semin Thromb Hemost 32:422–429

Gruppo Italiano Studio Policitemia (1997) Low-dose aspirin in polycythemia vera: a pilot study. Br J Haematol 97:453–456

Harrison C (2005) Pregnancy and its management in the Philadelphia negative myeloproliferative diseases. Br J Haematol 129:293–306

Hutton RD (1979) The effect of iron deficiency on whole blood viscosity in polycythaemic patients. Br J Haematol 43:191–199

Jantunen R, Juvonen E, Ikkala E et al (2001) The predictive value of vascular risk factors and gender for the development of thrombotic complications in essential thrombocythemia. Ann Hematol 80:74–78

Landolfi R, Ciabattoni G, Patrignani P et al (1992) Increased thromboxane biosynthesis in patients with polycythemia vera: evidence for aspirin-suppressible platelet activation in vivo. Blood 80:1965–1971

Landolfi R, Marchioli R, Kutti J et al (2004) Efficacy and safety of low-dose aspirin in polycythemia vera. N Engl J Med 350:114–124

Landolfi R, Cipriani MC, Novarese L (2006) Thrombosis and bleeding in polycythemia vera and essential thrombocythemia: pathogenetic mechanisms and prevention. Best Pract Res Clin Haematol 19:617–633

Landolfi R, Di Gennaro L, Barbui T et al (2007) Leukocytosis as a major thrombotic risk factor in patients with polycythemia vera. Blood 109:2446–2452

Lee LH, Baglin T (1995) Altered platelet phospholipid-dependent thrombin generation in thrombocytopenia and thrombocytosis. Br J Haematol 89:131–136

Lussana F, Caberlon S, Pagani C et al (2009) Association of V617F Jak2 mutation with the risk of thrombosis among patients with essential thrombocythemia or idiopathic myelofibrosis: a systematic review. Thromb Res 124:409–417

Marchetti M, Falanga A (2008) Leukocytosis, JAK2V617F mutation and hemostasis in myeloproliferative disorders. Pathophysiol Haemost Thromb 36:148–159

Marchetti M, Castoldi E, Spronk HM et al (2008) Thrombin generation and activated protein C resistance in patients with essential thrombocythemia and polycythemia vera. Blood 112:4061–4068

Marchioli R, Finazzi G, Landolfi R et al (2005) Vascular and neoplastic risk in a large cohort of patients with polycythemia vera. J Clin Oncol 23:2224–2232

McMullin MF, Bareford D, Campbell P et al (2005) Guidelines for the diagnosis, investigation and management of polycythaemia/erythrocytosis. Br J Haematol 130:174–195

Michiels JJ, Abels J, Steketee J et al (1985) Erythromelalgia caused by platelet mediated arteriolar inflammation and thrombosis in thrombocythemia. Ann Intern Med 102:466–471

Mitus AJ, Barbui T, Shulman LN et al (1990) Hemostatic complications in young patients with essential thrombocythemia. Am J Med 88:371–375

Palandri F, Polverelli N, Catani L et al (2011) Impact of leukocytosis on thrombotic risk and survival in 532 patients with essential thrombocythemia: a retrospective study. Ann Hematol. doi:10.1007//s00277-010-1154-3

Passamonti F, Randi ML, Rumi E et al (2007) Increased risk of pregnancy complications in patients with essential thrombocythemia carrying the JAK2 (617V>F) mutation. Blood 110:485–489

Passamonti F, Rumi E, Arcaini L et al (2008) Prognostic factors for thrombosis, myelofibrosis and leukemia in essential thrombocythemia: a study of 605 patients. Haematologica 93:1645–1651

Passamonti F, Rumi E, Pascutto C et al (2009) Increase in leukocyte count over time predicts thrombosis in patients with low-risk essential thrombocythemia. J Thromb Haemost 7:1587–1589

Patel RK, Lea N, Heneghan A et al (2006) Prevalence of the activating JAK2 tyrosine kinase mutation V617F in the Budd-Chiari syndrome. Gastroenterology 130:2031–2038

Pearson TC, Wetherley-Mein G (1978) Vascular occlusive episodes and venous haematocrit in primary proliferative polycythemia. Lancet 2:1219–1222

Primignani M, Barosi G, Bergamaschi G et al (2006) Role of the JAK2 mutation in the diagnosis of chronic myeloproliferative disorders in splanchnic vein thrombosis. Hepatology 44:1528–1534

Robinson S, Bewley S, Hunt BJ et al (2005) The management and outcome of 18 pregnancies in women with polycythaemia vera. Haematologica 90:1477–1483

Ruggeri M, Finazzi G, Tosetto A et al (1998) No treatment for low-risk thrombocythaemia: results from a prospective study. Br J Haematol 103:772–777

Shibata J, Hasegawa J, Siemens HJ et al (2003) Hemostasis and coagulation at a hematocrit level of 0.85: functional consequences of erythrocytosis. Blood 101:4416–4422

Tefferi A, Gangat N, Wolanskyj AP (2006) Management of extreme thrombocytosis in otherwise low-risk essential thrombocythemia: does number matter? Blood 108:2493–2494

Thomas DJ, du Boulay GH, Marshall J et al (1977) Cerebral blood flow in polycythemia. Lancet 2:161–163

Trappenburg MC, van Schilfgaarde M, Marchetti M et al (2009) Elevated procoagulant microparticles expressing endothelial and platelet markers in essential thrombocythemia. Haematologica 94:911–918

van Genderen PJJ (1995) Platelet consumption in thrombocythemia complicated by erythromelalgia: reversal by aspirin. Thromb Haemost 73:210–214

van Genderen PJJ, Michiels JJ (1994) Erythromelalgic, thrombotic and hemorrhagic manifestations of thrombocythaemia. Presse Med 23:73–77

van Genderen PJJ, Budde A, Michiels JJ et al (1996) The reduction of large von Willebrand factor multimers in plasma in essential thrombocythemia is related to the platelet count. Br J Haematol 93:962–965

Vannucchi AM, Antonioli E, Guglielmelli P et al (2007) Prospective identification of high-risk polycythemia vera patients based on JAK2 (V617F) allele burden. Leukemia 21:1952–1959

Watson KV, Key N (1993) Vascular complications of essential thrombocythemia: a link to cardiovascular risk factors. Br J Haematol 83:198–203

Wolanskyj AP, Lasho TL, Schwager SM et al (2005) JAK2 V617F mutation in essential thrombocythaemia:

clinical associations and long-term prognostic relevance. Br J Haematol 131:208–213

Wolanskyj AP, Schwager SM, McClure RF et al (2006) Essential thrombocythemia beyond the first decade: life expectancy, long-term complication rates, and prognostic factors. Mayo Clin Proc 81:159–166

Yip R, Mohandas N, Clark MR et al (1983) Red cell membrane stiffness in iron deficiency. Blood 62:99–106

Goal of Therapy and Monitoring the Response in Polycythemia Vera and Essential Thrombocythemia

8

Jean-Jacques Kiladjian

Contents

8.1 Introduction

Polycythemia vera (PV) and essential thrombocythemia (ET) are the most indolent Philadelphia-negative myeloproliferative neoplasms (MPN). In fact, several studies have shown that life expectancy in ET is almost similar to that of the general age- and sex-matched population, but life expectancy of PV patients is however significantly altered, especially after the first decade of follow-up (Passamonti et al. 2004; Cervantes et al. 2008). Evolution of PV and ET is characterized by a short-term risk of vascular complications (thrombosis and hemorrhages) and a longer-term risk of evolution to myelofibrosis (MF), myelodysplastic syndromes (MDS), or acute myeloid leukemia (AML). However, in a recent retrospective study from the Swedish Cancer Registry that included 4,389 and 2,559 patients with a diagnosis of PV and ET, respectively, a significant overall excess mortality compared to reference population was found (Bjorkholm et al. 2011). Contrary to high-risk MF where treatment aims to prolong survival that may require therapies with high risks of complications, current therapeutic strategies in PV and ET are based on the risk of thrombosis, aiming to reduce mortality and morbidity due to vascular events (Barbui et al. 2011a).

8.2 *Primum Non Nocere*

In diseases with a low impact on overall survival such as PV and especially ET, the main goal of therapy should be to first do no harm, i.e., do not

J.-J. Kiladjian
Clinical Investigations Center,
Saint-Louis Hospital and Paris Diderot University,
Paris, France
e-mail: jean-jacques.kiladjian@sls.aphp.fr

T. Barbui and A. Tefferi (eds.), *Myeloproliferative Neoplasms*, Hematologic Malignancies,
DOI 10.1007/978-3-642-24989-1_8, © Springer-Verlag Berlin Heidelberg 2012

Table 8.1 Goals of therapy in polycythemia vera (PV) and essential thrombocythemia (ET), possible actions, and monitoring tools

Goal	Action	Monitoring tools
Avoid thrombosis	Treat generic cardiovascular risk factors	Hematocrit in PV
	Antiplatelet therapy (low-dose aspirin)	*Leukocytes?*
	Cytoreductive therapy in high-risk patients	*JAKV617F burden?*
Avoid hemorrhage	Cytoreductive therapy in high-risk patients	Platelet count
Avoid evolution to MF/MDS/AML	Avoid clearly leukemogenic therapies	Spleen size
		CBC
	IFNa (or anagrelide) if <40 years old	Bone marrow
		LDH?
Control of symptoms	IFNa for pruritus	MPN-SAF
	JAK-inhibitors?	

Investigational items (not validated in prospective trials) are in italics followed by a question mark
MF myelofibrosis, *MDS* myelodysplastic syndrome, *AML* acute myeloid leukemia, *IFNa* interferon alpha, *CBC* complete blood count, *LDH* serum lactate dehydrogenase, *MPN-SAF* myeloproliferative neoplasm symptom assessment form

overtreat patients who are at very low risk of developing disease-related complications (Spivak 2002). In MPN, a proper diagnosis and classification, in particular accurate diagnosis of early stages of MF that mimic ET (Barbui et al. 2011b) or identification of early stages of PV that can present with apparently isolated thrombocytosis (Cassinat et al. 2008; Kiladjian et al. 2008b), is crucial to guide management and therapy. For example, when the diagnosis of ET is made according to the 2008 World Health Organization (WHO) guidelines (Tefferi et al. 2007), including a strict analysis of bone marrow biopsy findings, a large retrospective study showed a normal life expectancy and a very low rate of disease complication in those WHO-defined ET patients (Barbui et al. 2011b). In such patients, the usefulness of cytoreductive therapy is highly debatable, and the first goal of therapy should be aggressive management of other cardiovascular risk factors, such as diabetes, hypertension, hypercholesterolemia, and smoking (Table 8.1).

8.3 Risk of Vascular Complications

The major goal of PV and ET management is currently the reduction of the risk of vascular complication and mainly the risk of thrombosis (Table 8.1) (Finazzi and Barbui 2007; Beer et al. 2011). Accordingly, the European Leukemia Net (ELN) recently published management guidelines in MPN underscoring that a major goal of

therapy in PV and ET patients is "to avoid first occurrence and/or recurrence of thrombotic and/or hemorrhagic complications" (Barbui et al. 2011a). Several parameters, discussed in another chapter of this book, allow accurate assessment of this vascular risk, the most important being the age of the patient (above 60 years) and a history of vascular event. Obviously, no therapeutic strategy can modify such parameters, which, when present, are sufficient to trigger a cytoreductive therapy. However, blood counts have also been shown to influence the risk of vascular events.

8.3.1 Erythrocytosis and Blood Viscosity

The hallmark of PV is erythrocytosis, i.e., an excess of red blood cells in the circulation, historically measured by isotopic red cell mass determination and usually estimated by the hematocrit or the hemoglobin level. Diagnosis of PV according to WHO therefore requires as first major criterion an elevation of either hemoglobin, or hematocrit, or red cell mass (Tefferi et al. 2007). A major consequence of this increased red cell mass is an increase in blood viscosity and therefore an increased risk of clotting (especially in large vessels) with a direct and exponential relationship between hematocrit and blood viscosity (Pearson and Wetherley-Mein 1978). Accordingly, the primary objective in the treatment of PV (Finazzi and Barbui 2007) has always been to reduce the hematocrit within the normal range (or even lower) since the earliest clinical trials conducted by the Polycythemia Vera Study Group (PVSG) (Berk et al. 1986). The target hematocrit required to reduce the risk of thrombosis due to hyperviscosity is currently considered to be 0.45 (Barbui et al. 2011a). This threshold, however, is somehow arbitrary, and one could consider different hematocrit targets in men and women (0.45 and 0.42, respectively) (Spivak 2002), or that higher values (up to 0.55) could be safe targets in PV (Di Nisio et al. 2007).

8.3.2 Platelet Count and Vascular Risk

In ET, although the degree of thrombocytosis is not a reliable indicator of thrombotic risk, a very high platelet count may predict for hemorrhagic complications (Fenaux et al. 1990; Besses et al. 1999; Carobbio et al. 2008a, b). In addition, the two seminal randomized clinical trials performed in ET and published to date have both shown a reduction in the vascular complications of high-risk patients receiving cytoreductive therapy (Cortelazzo et al. 1995; Harrison et al. 2005). In the Cortelazzo et al. study, ET patients treated with hydroxyurea had significantly lower incidence of vascular complications compared to untreated patients (Cortelazzo et al. 1995). In the PT-1 trial, hydroxyurea showed superiority compared to anagrelide, a selective platelet-reducing agent, in the primary composite end point chosen for this study (time from randomization until the patient died from thrombosis or hemorrhage or had an arterial or a venous thrombotic event or a serious hemorrhage). However, the incidence of vascular complications in anagrelide-treated patients was clearly much lower than in untreated patients from the Bergamo trial, suggesting that lowering the platelet count may be beneficial in terms of vascular complications in high-risk ET (Harrison et al. 2005).

In contrast, thrombocytosis has never been shown to influence the risk of thrombosis in PV (Elliott and Tefferi 2005; Schafer 2006). In the PVSG-01 clinical trial, platelet count did not predict thrombosis, and analysis of the patients enrolled in the large European "ECLAP" study failed to show any association between platelet count and thrombotic events (Berk et al. 1986; Di Nisio et al. 2007). Therefore, platelet count is not a target for therapy in PV, at least regarding the aim to reduce the risk of thrombosis.

8.3.3 Leukocytosis and JAK2V617F Mutation

More recently, two other parameters were shown in retrospective studies to influence the risk of thrombosis: leukocytosis and JAK2V617F mutation (either its presence versus absence, or the proportion of cells carrying the mutation in JAKV617F-positive patients) (Vannucchi et al. 2007; Barbui et al. 2009; Gangat et al. 2009). Their value as potential prognostic markers is discussed in another chapter, but to date, the experts of the ELN considered that leukocytosis and JAK2V617F allele burden should not be considered as targets for therapy in PV and ET, until they are validated in prospective studies (Barbui et al. 2011a).

8.3.4 In Summary

A major goal of therapy in PV and ET is to avoid vascular complications. Widely validated disease-related targets to reach this objective are: erythrocytosis in PV (correlated with a risk of thrombosis) and extreme thrombocytosis in ET (correlated with a risk of bleeding). Leukocytosis and JAK2V617F allele burden are interesting candidates but should not be used per se as reasons to initiate cytoreductive therapy (Table 8.1).

8.4 Minimize the Risk of Evolution to Myelofibrosis, Myelodysplastic Syndromes, and Acute Myeloid Leukemia

Hematological evolutions to MF, MDS, or AML are recognized long-term complications of Ph-negative MPN (Schafer 2004; Campbell and Green 2006). Such evolution is indeed a matter of concern in PV and ET patients who are expected to live for several decades, although the exact incidence of such transitions is still debated (Finazzi et al. 2005; Kiladjian et al. 2006). They can occur spontaneously as long-term sequelae of the chronic phase or be favored by the use of leukemogenic therapies such as radioactive phosphorus or alkylating agents (Kiladjian et al. 2003; Bjorkholm et al. 2011).

8.4.1 Avoid the Use of Drugs with Recognized Leukemogenic Potential

Several therapies have been shown in clinical trials to be clearly associated with an increased risk of hematological evolution. PVSG-01 study in PV showed that ^{32}P and chlorambucil therapies were associated with much higher risks of leukemia and nonhematological malignancy compared to phlebotomy (Berk et al. 1995). The French Polycythemia Study Group (FPSG) conducted a randomized clinical trial comparing hydroxyurea to pipobroman as first-line therapy in PV patients younger than 65 years. There were no differences between the two groups in vascular end points or rates of leukemia or nonhematological malignancy at first analyses of this study (Najean and Rain 1997). However, long-term analyses after a median follow-up of 16.3 years showed that pipobroman is clearly leukemogenic, the cumulative incidence of AML/MDS being 6.6%, 16.5%, and 24% in the HU arm and 13%, 34%, and 52% in the pipobroman arm at 10, 15, and 20 years, respectively (Kiladjian et al. 2011b). Such drugs being associated with a clearly demonstrated risk of leukemia in randomized trials must not be used as first-line therapy and are second-line therapies reserved for patients with short life expectancy (Barbui et al. 2011a).

8.4.2 Careful Use of Cytotoxic Agents in Younger Patients

In patients diagnosed with PV or ET at younger age (<40 years), the use of cytotoxic agents should be carefully examined. Lifelong exposition to cytotoxic drugs could be harmful, especially if resistance or intolerance to first-line therapy occurs leading to treatment change, considering that the sequential use of more than one cytoreductive agent may enhance the risk of AML (Finazzi et al. 2005). Therefore, interferon alpha is often proposed as first-line therapy in patients younger than the age of 40 years, assuming that it is not leukemogenic (Finazzi and Barbui 2007; Barbui et al. 2011a; Beer et al. 2011). Anagrelide is not cytotoxic and likely not mutagenic and can also be an alternative to conventional therapies for selected younger ET patients (Birgegard 2006; Beer et al. 2011).

8.5 Control of Disease-Related Symptoms

Neglected for a long time, self-reported symptoms are now recognized as an important part of the management of MPN patients. Indeed, quality of life of PV and ET patients is not only burdened by vascular events, but also by a series of symptoms including pruritus, fatigue, and constitutional symptoms, resulting in restricted participation in both social functions and physical activity (Mesa et al. 2007). These symptoms are widely observed regardless of cultural background and can be measured using the Myeloproliferative Neoplasm Symptom Assessment Form (MPN-SAF), a comprehensive and reliable instrument that is validated in multiple languages (Scherber et al. 2011). Of note, besides the difficulty to capture those symptoms, their management is often difficult. For example, intractable pruritus can represent a disabling condition in some PV patients, and symptomatic therapies (including antihistamines, selective serotonin uptake inhibitor, and photochemotherapy) often fail to control this symptom. Interferon alpha has been reported to be effective in this situation, but it is difficult to propose in patients with otherwise low-risk disease.

The new class of JAK kinase inhibitors could bring an important improvement regarding the issue of disease-related symptoms control. The first reported clinical trial results with one of these new drugs, INCB018424 or ruxolitinib, showed rapid and durable improvement of debilitating symptoms in PMF patients, associated with a marked diminution of levels of circulating inflammatory cytokines (Verstovsek et al. 2010). Preliminary reports with other JAK-inhibitors suggest that this rapid and until now unachievable efficacy to reduce a large array of symptoms in MPN is a shared characteristic of members of this new class of drugs (Pardanani et al. 2011). However, it is too early to anticipate their usefulness in PV and ET patients in the absence of clinical studies' results, although they should rapidly be part of the therapeutic arsenal to treat symptomatic PMF patients.

8.6 Special Situations

Goals of therapy in PV and ET patients also include the management of a series of special clinical situations, which will not de described here since they are discussed in details in another chapter. These issues are comprised of pregnancy, thrombotic or hemorrhagic events, management of MPN in children, and surgery.

8.7 Monitoring Therapy Efficacy

To achieve the goals of therapy listed above in PV and ET, a series of actions are necessary, including (but not restricted to) the prescription of drugs (Table 8.1). Thus, measuring the efficacy of these therapies to achieve their objective is mandatory in clinical practice, to detect failures requiring a rapid switch to second-line options.

As discussed in paragraph 1 of this section, erythrocytosis and thrombocytosis are relevant targets to reduce the risks of thrombosis and bleeding, respectively. Once safe thresholds have been determined, it is theoretically easy to assess treatment efficacy. The ELN has proposed two sets of criteria to define on the one hand the response (Barosi et al. 2009) and on the other hand the resistance and intolerance to hydroxyurea (Barosi et al. 2010). Of note, these definitions were primarily developed for use in clinical trials. Indeed, comparisons or meta-analyses of clinical studies in MPN have been hampered due to the use of heterogeneous definitions of response or resistance/intolerance to therapies. The general use of unified definitions will hopefully help in assessing the efficacy of new therapies. The ELN definition of response is split in three sets of categories, namely clinical-hematological, molecular, and histological response (Barosi et al. 2009).

8.7.1 Clinical-Hematological Response

At present, only clinical-hematological criteria can be employed for monitoring the response to conventional cytoreductive therapy, since no drug has produced yet relevant effects on mutated allele burden or bone marrow histopathology, with the exception of interferon alpha discussed below (and allogeneic bone marrow transplantation (BMT) discussed in a special chapter of this book).

In clinical practice, criteria for clinical resistance and intolerance to hydroxyurea can be used for decision-making when assessing the opportunity to move patients to second-line therapies and/or for identifying those suitable for enrollment in clinical trials with novel drugs (Barosi et al. 2010). The relevance of criteria defining response to hydroxyurea in daily practice is less evident. Although this clinical-hematological definition of response will prove a usefulness to analyze clinical trials, its relevance in clinical practice has been questioned in a study showing the absence of association between the ELN response category and the risk of thrombosis in ET (Carobbio et al. 2010). One should keep in mind that MPN "response" to a therapy does not necessarily mean "efficacy." For example, reduction of the platelet count within the normal range evidences the "response" of ET to an active drug, but does not necessarily protect against the occurrence of a thrombotic event which demonstrates lack of efficacy, as shown in the aforementioned study (Carobbio et al. 2010). Besides the uncertainties about the relevant thresholds and definitions, monitoring of clinical-hematological response should focus on regular assessment of disease-related symptoms, splenomegaly, and evolution of blood cell counts. Common sense suggests that resolution of symptoms and normalization of abnormal parameters should indicate a favorable clinical-hematological response!

8.7.2 Molecular and Histological Response

At the exclusion of allogeneic BMT, current therapies have not been shown to consistently induce molecular or histological responses, and these levels of response must not be routinely assessed in clinical practice.

A possible exception to this rule could be interferon alpha therapy. With respect to molecular response, two independent phase 2 clinical studies of pegylated interferon alpha-2a have shown a major reduction in the JAK2V617F allele burden during therapy (Kiladjian et al. 2008a; Quintas-Cardama et al. 2009), including significant numbers of complete molecular responses. It is important to emphasize that the elimination of JAK2V617F in this setting is not necessarily indicative of cure of the MPN and that clinical implications of these molecular responses remain uncertain and require validation. Still, major reduction or eradication of JAK2V617F shows at least that interferon alpha has a specific effect on the clone bearing this mutation and raises the hope that this therapy will result in a favorable change in the natural history of patients with MPNs (Kiladjian et al. 2011a). In addition to such molecular response, two studies have reported a normalization of bone marrow morphology after interferon alpha therapy in few patients (Larsen et al. 2009; Silver and Vandris 2009). Such promising results have yet to be confirmed in larger prospective studies, along with a clear demonstration of good tolerance to establish interferon alpha as a new standard of care in PV and ET.

JAK-inhibitors are also candidates for inducing molecular or histological responses, at the image of tyrosine kinase–inhibitor targeted therapy in chronic myelogenous leukemia (CML). Some differences between CML and MPN on the one hand, and between bcr-abl inhibitors and JAK-inhibitors currently available on the other hand, may however explain disappointing molecular and histological responses observed to date in JAK-inhibitors' trials in MPN (Verstovsek et al. 2010; Pardanani et al. 2011). In Philadelphia-negative MPN, JAK2V617F is not the unique molecular target responsible of disease development and progression in a significant number of patients, and several investigators have shown that PV and ET are often oligoclonal rather than monoclonal diseases (Kiladjian et al. 2010; Klampfl et al. 2011). In addition, although JAK-inhibitors may display certain degree of selectivity toward members of the JAK family, none of the drugs currently developed are specific of the V617F mutation (Agrawal et al. 2011). However, at the time of this publication, median follow-up of patients treated with such drugs is still short, and definitive conclusion regarding their ability to reduce the JAK-mutated burden or reverse bone marrow abnormalities cannot be firmly drawn.

Conclusion

The main goal of therapy in PV and ET is currently to reduce the risk of vascular events, which remain the most frequent short-term complications leading to significant mortality and morbidity. Several tools have been developed to help clinicians to decide how to treat those patients: risk factors predicting the risk of vascular events are well defined; consensual international guidelines about the choice between therapeutic agents are available; resistance and intolerance to hydroxyurea can be objectively detected; the response to therapies can be monitored. Of note, overall survival of PV and ET patients constantly improved over the last decades, mainly due to better assessment and management of the vascular risk.

Still, one should keep in mind that those very efficient therapies are only palliative, and that our ultimate goal that should be cure of the disease is not yet achievable for PV and ET patients. Living with a malignant disease, even indolent, may have an impact in many aspects (social, professional, familial, etc.) of patient's daily life, an aspect of PV and ET still underestimated by physicians. Results obtained with pegylated interferon alpha-2a in few patients, including clinical-hematological, molecular, and histological complete responses, are encouraging, showing that a curative approach could be achievable in selected patients. New therapeutic agents (JAK-inhibitors, chromatin-modifying agents, inhibitors of antiapoptotic proteins, etc.) and strategies combining several of these new agents will hopefully open new avenues in the therapy of PV and ET patients in the near future.

References

Agrawal M, Garg RJ et al (2011) Experimental therapeutics for patients with myeloproliferative neoplasias. Cancer 117(4):662–676

Barbui T, Carobbio A et al (2009) Perspectives on thrombosis in essential thrombocythemia and polycythemia vera: is leukocytosis a causative factor? Blood 114(4):759–763

Barbui T, Barosi G et al (2011a) Philadelphia-negative classical myeloproliferative neoplasms: critical concepts and management recommendations from European LeukemiaNet. J Clin Oncol 29(6):761–770

Barbui T, Thiele J et al (2011b) Survival and disease progression in essential thrombocythemia are significantly influenced by accurate morphologic diagnosis: an international study. J Clin Oncol 29:3179–3184

Barosi G, Birgegard G et al (2009) Response criteria for essential thrombocythemia and polycythemia vera: result of a European LeukemiaNet consensus conference. Blood 113(20):4829–4833

Barosi G, Birgegard G et al (2010) A unified definition of clinical resistance and intolerance to hydroxycarbamide in polycythaemia vera and primary myelofibrosis: results of a European LeukemiaNet (ELN) consensus process. Br J Haematol 148(6):961–963

Beer PA, Erber WN et al (2011) How I treat essential thrombocythemia. Blood 117(5):1472–1482

Berk PD, Goldberg JD et al (1986) Therapeutic recommendations in polycythemia vera based on Polycythemia Vera Study Group protocols. Semin Hematol 23(2):132–143

Berk PD, Wasserman L et al (1995) Treatment of polycythaemia vera, a summary of clinical trends conducted by the polycythaemia vera sub-group. In: Wasserman L, Berk PD (eds) Treatment of polycythaemia vera, a summary of clinical trends conducted by the Polycythaemia Vera Study Group. W.B. Saunders, Philadelphia, pp 166–194

Besses C, Cervantes F et al (1999) Major vascular complications in essential thrombocythemia: a study of the predictive factors in a series of 148 patients. Leukemia 13(2):150–154

Birgegard G (2006) Anagrelide treatment in myeloproliferative disorders. Semin Thromb Hemost 32(3):260–266

Bjorkholm M, Derolf AR et al (2011) Treatment-related risk factors for transformation to acute myeloid leukemia and myelodysplastic syndromes in myeloproliferative neoplasms. J Clin Oncol 29(17):2410–2415

Campbell PJ, Green AR (2006) The myeloproliferative disorders. N Engl J Med 355(23):2452–2466

Carobbio A, Antonioli E et al (2008a) Leukocytosis and risk stratification assessment in essential thrombocythemia. J Clin Oncol 26(16):2732–2736

Carobbio A, Finazzi G et al (2008b) Thrombocytosis and leukocytosis interaction in vascular complications of essential thrombocythemia. Blood 112(8):3135–3137

Carobbio A, Finazzi G et al (2010) Hydroxyurea in essential thrombocythemia: rate and clinical relevance of responses by European LeukemiaNet criteria. Blood 116(7):1051–1055

Cassinat B, Laguillier C et al (2008) Classification of myeloproliferative disorders in the JAK2 era: is there a role for red cell mass? Leukemia 22(2):452–453

Cervantes F, Passamonti F et al (2008) Life expectancy and prognostic factors in the classic BCR/ABL-negative myeloproliferative disorders. Leukemia 22(5):905–914

Cortelazzo S, Finazzi G et al (1995) Hydroxyurea for patients with essential thrombocythemia and a high risk of thrombosis. N Engl J Med 332(17):1132–1136

Di Nisio M, Barbui T et al (2007) The haematocrit and platelet target in polycythemia vera. Br J Haematol 136(2):249–259

Elliott MA, Tefferi A (2005) Thrombosis and haemorrhage in polycythaemia vera and essential thrombocythaemia. Br J Haematol 128(3):275–290

Fenaux P, Simon M et al (1990) Clinical course of essential thrombocythemia in 147 cases. Cancer 66(3):549–556

Finazzi G, Barbui T (2007) How I treat patients with polycythemia vera. Blood 109(12):5104–5111

Finazzi G, Caruso V et al (2005) Acute leukemia in polycythemia vera: an analysis of 1638 patients enrolled in a prospective observational study. Blood 105(7):2664–2670

Gangat N, Wolanskyj AP et al (2009) Leukocytosis at diagnosis and the risk of subsequent thrombosis in patients with low-risk essential thrombocythemia and polycythemia vera. Cancer 115(24):5740–5745

Harrison CN, Campbell PJ et al (2005) Hydroxyurea compared with anagrelide in high-risk essential thrombocythemia. N Engl J Med 353(1):33–45

Kiladjian JJ, Gardin C et al (2003) Long-term outcomes of polycythemia vera patients treated with pipobroman as initial therapy. Hematol 4(3):198–207

Kiladjian JJ, Rain JD et al (2006) Long-term incidence of hematological evolution in three French prospective studies of hydroxyurea and pipobroman in polycythemia vera and essential thrombocythemia. Semin Thromb Hemost 32(4 Pt 2):417–421

Kiladjian JJ, Cassinat B et al (2008a) Pegylated interferon-alfa-2a induces complete hematologic and molecular responses with low toxicity in polycythemia vera. Blood 112(8):3065–3072

Kiladjian JJ, Cervantes F et al (2008b) The impact of JAK2 and MPL mutations on diagnosis and prognosis of splanchnic vein thrombosis: a report on 241 cases. Blood 111(10):4922–4929

Kiladjian JJ, Masse A et al (2010) Clonal analysis of erythroid progenitors suggests that pegylated interferon alpha-2a treatment targets JAK2V617F clones without affecting TET2 mutant cells. Leukemia 24(8): 1519–1523

Kiladjian JJ, Mesa RA et al (2011a) The renaissance of interferon therapy for the treatment of myeloid malignancies. Blood 117(18):4706–4715

Kiladjian JJ et al (2011b) Treatment of polycythemia vera with hydroxyurea and pipobroman: final results of a randomized trial initiated in 1980. J Clin Oncol 29(29):3907–3913

Klampfl T, Harutyunyan A et al (2011) Genome integrity of myeloproliferative neoplasms in chronic phase and during disease progression. Blood 118(1):167–176

Larsen TS, Moller MB et al (2009) Minimal residual disease and normalization of the bone marrow after long-term treatment with alpha-interferon2b in polycythemia vera. A report on molecular response patterns in seven patients in sustained complete hematological remission. Hematology 14(6):331–334

Mesa RA, Niblack J et al (2007) The burden of fatigue and quality of life in myeloproliferative disorders (MPDs): an international Internet-based survey of 1179 MPD patients. Cancer 109(1):68–76

Najean Y, Rain JD (1997) Treatment of polycythemia vera: the use of hydroxyurea and pipobroman in 292 patients under the age of 65 years. Blood 90(9):3370–3377

Pardanani A, Vannucchi AM et al (2011) JAK inhibitor therapy for myelofibrosis: critical assessment of value and limitations. Leukemia 25(2):218–225

Passamonti F, Rumi E et al (2004) Life expectancy and prognostic factors for survival in patients with polycythemia vera and essential thrombocythemia. Am J Med 117(10):755–761

Pearson TC, Wetherley-Mein G (1978) Vascular occlusive episodes and venous haematocrit in primary proliferative polycythaemia. Lancet 2(8102):1219–1222

Quintas-Cardama A, Kantarjian H et al (2009) Pegylated interferon alfa-2a yields high rates of hematologic and molecular response in patients with advanced essential thrombocythemia and polycythemia vera. J Clin Oncol 27(32):5418–5424

Schafer AI (2004) Thrombocytosis. N Engl J Med 350(12):1211–1219

Schafer AI (2006) Molecular basis of the diagnosis and treatment of polycythemia vera and essential thrombocythemia. Blood 107(11):4214–4222

Scherber R, Dueck AC et al (2011) The Myeloproliferative Neoplasm Symptom Assessment Form (MPN-SAF): International Prospective Validation and Reliability Trial in 402 patients. Blood 118(2):401–408

Silver RT, Vandris K (2009) Recombinant interferon alpha (rIFN alpha-2b) may retard progression of early primary myelofibrosis. Leukemia 23(7):1366–1369

Spivak JL (2002) Polycythemia vera: myths, mechanisms, and management. Blood 100(13):4272–4290

Tefferi A, Thiele J et al (2007) Proposals and rationale for revision of the World Health Organization diagnostic criteria for polycythemia vera, essential thrombocythemia, and primary myelofibrosis: recommendations from an ad hoc international expert panel. Blood 110(4):1092–1097

Vannucchi AM, Antonioli E et al (2007) Clinical profile of homozygous JAK2 617V>F mutation in patients with polycythemia vera or essential thrombocythemia. Blood 110(3):840–846

Verstovsek S, Kantarjian H et al (2010) Safety and efficacy of INCB018424, a JAK1 and JAK2 inhibitor, in myelofibrosis. N Engl J Med 363(12):1117–1127

First-Line Therapy and Special Issues Management in Polycythemia Vera and Essential Thrombocythemia

9

Tiziano Barbui

Contents

9.1 Introduction

Polycythemia vera (PV) and essential thrombocythemia (ET) are chronic myeloproliferative neoplasms (MPN) characterized by clonal expansion of an abnormal hematopoietic stem/progenitor cell. Natural history of these chronic myeloproliferative neoplasms (MPN) is marked by thrombohemorrhagic complications and a propensity to transform into myelofibrosis and acute leukemia. Recommendations for management are based on a limited number of randomized clinical trials conducted within national or international collaborative groups and on several observational studies describing the clinical course of the diseases and indirectly evaluating the role of different treatments. Thus, sound methodological evidence is limited, and clinical expertise consensus still plays a major role to guide therapy. In practice, the first step to approach an individual patient with PV or ET is to identify the potential risk to develop major thrombotic or hemorrhagic complications (see Chap. 7). Then, treatment should be stratified with the aim to focus cytotoxic chemotherapy on high-risk patients. In this chapter, the current evidence on the optimal first-line treatment of patients with PV and ET is reviewed and discussed.

9.2 Low-Risk Patients

9.2.1 Phlebotomy

The clonal proliferation of hematopoietic precursors leading to progressive expansion of myeloid cells with a predominant increase of red cells characterizes the PV hematological phenotype. The consequent blood hyperviscosity is a major cause of vascular disturbances which severely impact on morbidity and mortality.

T. Barbui
Research Foundation Ospedale Maggiore
(FROM) and Hematology Department,
Ospedali Riuniti, Bergamo, Italy
e-mail: tbarbui@ospedaliriuniti.bergamo.it

Blood viscosity has been proved to be an exponential function of the hematocrit (Hct), leading to increments of red cell aggregation and creating the potential for vascular stasis. The resulting resistance to blood flow, the interplay between platelet, leukocytes, and vessel wall are the major determinants of the risk of thrombosis (Spivak 2004). The immediate goal of therapy is to reach and maintain a target Hct level with phlebotomy, and long-term objective to induce a condition of iron deficiency that will impose a constrain to erythropoiesis.

On the basis of old uncontrolled studies showing increased incidence of vascular occlusive events as well as suboptimal cerebral blood flow in ranges of Hct values between 46% and 52% (Pearson and Wetherley-Mein 1978), the use of aggressive target of Hct lower than 45% in males and 42% in females has been advised. The only randomized study comparing phlebotomy with myelosuppressive therapy was performed by the Polycythemia Vera Study Group (PVSG) more than 20 years ago (Berk et al. 1986). In this trial, patients treated in the phlebotomy arm with Hct target set at 45% had a better overall median survival at 13.9 years than the other two arms (chlorambucil 8.9 years, radiophosphorus 11.8 years) due to a reduced incidence of acute leukemia and other malignancies, albeit an excess of thrombosis was observed during the first 3 years of phlebotomy treatment. In the large prospective observation study by European investigators (ECLAP, *European Collaboration on Low-dose Aspirin in Polycythemia*) (Di Nisio et al. 2007) despite the recommendation of maintaining the Hct values at less than 0.45, only 48% of patients had values below this threshold, while 39% and 13% remained between 0.45 and 0.50 and greater than 0.50, respectively. Multivariate analysis considering all the confounders failed to show any correlation between Hct values in the range between less than 45% and 50% and incidence of thrombosis. These findings prompted Italian investigators to launch a national-based multicenter, randomized controlled trial aimed to assessing the benefit/risk profile of cytoreductive therapy with phlebotomy and/or hydroxyurea aimed at maintaining Hct <45% (control arm) vs. at maintaining

Hct in the range of 45–50%(experimental arm). The primary end point of this trial is cardiovascular death plus thrombotic events (stroke, acute coronary syndrome, transient ischemic attack, pulmonary embolism, abdominal thrombosis, deep vein thrombosis, and peripheral arterial thrombosis). Results of this trial will be available in 2013.

In clinical practice, phlebotomy should be started withdrawing 250–500 cc of blood daily or every other day until a hematocrit between 40% and 45% is obtained. In the elderly or those with a cardiovascular disease, smaller amount of blood (200–300 cc) should be withdrawn twice weekly. Once normalization of the hematocrit has been obtained, blood counts at regular intervals (every 4–8 weeks) will establish the frequency of future phlebotomies. Sufficient blood should be removed to maintain the hematocrit below 45%. Supplemental iron therapy should not be given.

9.2.2 Low-Dose Aspirin (ASA)

For patients without hematological disease, low-dose aspirin is both of definite and substantial benefit for secondary prevention of occlusive vascular disease, but evidence of its benefit in primary prevention of vascular occlusive disease is controversial with the risks of hemorrhage outweighing any benefit in several studies (Patrono et al. 2008). In the past, the potential risk of bleeding limited the use of aspirin in PV. The only randomized clinical trial evaluating efficacy and safety of aspirin in PV has been conducted by investigators of ECLAP (Landolfi et al. 2004). This placebo-controlled, double-blind study randomized 532 PV subjects to receive 100 mg ASA or placebo. After a follow-up of about 3 years, there was a statistically significant 59% reduction of major thromboses (both arterial and venous) without a significant increase of hemorrhagic complications in the ASA group. In absolute terms, out of 1,000 people treated with aspirin, three people had a fatal thrombotic event, compared with 22 people treated with placebo (risk difference 1.9%, 95% CI 0–4%).

Thus, the utility of low-dose aspirin as first-line therapy in PV is generally accepted since the net risk/benefit ratio is favorable in all risk categories.

Because of the possible increase of the bleeding risk, combination of ASA plus other antiaggregating agents such as clopidogrel may be considered with caution in PV patients at high risk of thrombotic events and at low to moderate bleeding risk.

In ET, some conflicting opinions reflected in national guidance or consensus documents (Barbui et al. 2004; Harrison et al. 2010) exist regarding the use of aspirin for patients with "low-risk" essential thrombocythemia since no clinical trials are available. A recent publication from Spain (Alvarez-Larran et al. 2010) questions the benefit of low-dose aspirin in low-risk ET, and the conclusion was that antiplatelet therapy reduces the incidence of venous thrombosis in *JAK2*-positive patients and the rate of arterial thrombosis only in patients with associated cardiovascular risk factors. While these results are provocative, the data is limited by its retrospective nature, the potential bias in that it is unclear why certain patients were allocated "antiplatelet" agents or not, and that the "antiplatelet" agents used were not uniformly low-dose aspirin. However, until additional data become available, the routine use of long-term aspirin in ET asymptomatic cases should be indicated with great caution, particularly in patients with a high bleeding risk (e.g., gastric ulcers or esophageal varices secondary to splanchnic vein thrombosis and portal hypertension), and perhaps in extreme thrombocytosis (Harrison and Barbui 2011).

Moreover, combining aspirin with some cytoreductive drugs may enhance the risk of bleeding. In the PT-1 randomized study comparing hydroxyurea vs. anagrelide in high-risk patients with ET (discussed in section 9.3), low-dose aspirin was given to both groups. An increased rate of major bleeding was registered in the anagrelide plus aspirin arm, and this may be due to a synergistic effect of the two drugs on platelet function inhibition (Harrison et al. 2005).

9.3 High-Risk Patients

The most commonly used first-line therapy drugs for the treatment of high-risk PV and ET patients include hydroxyurea (HU) and interferon alpha (IFN-alpha).

9.3.1 Hydroxyurea

HU is an antimetabolite that prevents DNA synthesis and was introduced in the therapy of PV and ET by PVSG. These investigators assumed this drug to be not leukemogenic, and in a paper summarizing their long-term experience in 51 PV patients followed for a median of 8.6 years, they reported an incidence of leukemia of 9.8% (vs. 3.7% in the historical phlebotomized controls) but less myelofibrosis (7.8% vs. 12.7%), fewer total deaths (39.2% vs. 55.2%), and less thrombotic events in comparison with historical phlebotomy arm (Fruchtman et al. 1997).

In the ECLAP study, HU alone was not found to enhance the risk of leukemia in comparison with patients treated with phlebotomy only (hazard ratio 0.86, 95% CI 0.26–2.88; $p=0.8$); however, the risk was significantly increased by exposure to radiophosphorus, busulfan, or pipobroman (hazard ratio 5.46, 95% CI 1.84–16.25; $p=0.002$). In addition, the use of HU in patients already treated with alkylating agents or radiophosphorus also enhanced the leukemic risk (hazard ratio 7.58, 95% CI 1.85–31; $p=0.0048$) (Finazzi et al. 2005). A randomized clinical trial did not find significant differences in the rate of leukemic transformation in PV patients treated with HU or pipobroman, an alkylating agent with a mechanism of action that also involves metabolic competition with pyrimidine basis (Najean and Rain 1997). However, different results were observed by prolonging the observation time. In a recent long-term analysis of the above mentioned study comparing HU to Pipobroman in 292 PV patients (median follow-up 16.3 years), median survival was 20.3 years in HU arm and 15.4% in Pipobroman arm. Cumulative incidence of AML/MDS at 10, 15, and 20 years was 6.6%, 16.5%, and 24% in the HU arm and 13%, 34% and 52% in the pipobroman arm (Kiladjian et al. 2011b). A similar trend was observed by Gangat et al. (2007) who reported a rate of AML of 2.4%, 4%, 11.6%, and 16.7% in PV patients given no chemotherapy, HU only, other single cytotoxic drugs only.

Very recently, in a nationwide cohort of 11,039 MPN patients, a nested case–control study including 162 AML and MDS patients and 242 matched controls was conducted in Sweden (Bjorkholm et al. 2011). Results indicate that the risk of AML/MDS was not significantly enhanced by HU given as a sole therapy. Of note, 25% of patients who developed leukemia were never exposed to cytotoxic therapy supporting the notion of a major role for intrinsic MPN related factors in leukemogenesis of MPN.

HU has also emerged as first-line therapy in high-risk patients with ET because of its efficacy and only rare acute toxicity. The efficacy of HU in preventing thrombosis in high-risk ET patients was demonstrated in a seminal randomized clinical trial (Cortelazzo et al. 1995). One hundred and fourteen patients were randomized to long-term treatment with HU ($n=56$) or to no cytoreductive treatment ($n=58$). During a median follow-up of 27 months, 2 thromboses were recorded in the HU-treated group (1.6% pt-yr) compared with 14 in the control group (10.7% pt-yr; $p=0.003$). Some long-term follow-up studies revealed that a proportion of ET patients treated with HU developed acute leukemia, particularly when given before or after alkylating agents or radiophosphorus (Sterkers et al. 1998; Finazzi et al. 2000). In other studies, however, the use of this drug as the only cytotoxic treatment was rarely associated with secondary malignancies. In an analysis of 25 ET patients younger than 50 years and treated with HU alone for high risk of thrombosis, no case of leukemic or neoplastic transformation occurred after a median follow-up of 8 years (range 5–14 years) (Finazzi et al. 2003). HU plus aspirin has been compared head to head to anagrelide plus aspirin in a randomized clinical trial (PT-1) including 809 ET patients (Harrison et al. 2005). Patients in the anagrelide arm showed an increased rate of arterial thrombosis (OR 2.16, 95% CI 1.04–2.37; $p=0.03$), major bleeding (OR 2.61, CI 1.27–5.33; $p=0.008$), and myelofibrotic transformation (OR 2.92, CI 1.24–6.86, $p=0.01$) but a decreased incidence of venous thrombosis (OR 0.27, CI 0.11–0.71, $p=0.006$) compared to HU. In addition, anagrelide was more poorly tolerated than HU and presented significantly greater rates of cardiovascular ($p<0.0001$), gastrointestinal ($p<0.02$),

neurological ($p<0001$), and constitutional ($p<0.001$) complications. Transformation to acute leukemia was comparable between the two arms (4 anagrelide vs. 6 HU) although the small number of transformations and short follow-up prevent firm conclusions about leukemogenicity of the two drugs. Responses to treatment in the PT-1 trial was influenced by JAK2 status (Campbell et al. 2005). Patients who were V617F positive randomized to anagrelide had higher rates of arterial thrombosis than those randomized to hydroxyurea (19 vs. 5 patients; $p=0.003$), whereas for V617F-negative patients, there were equal numbers of arterial thromboses in the two groups (ten patients in each group; $p=0.9$). In addition, V617F-positive patients required substantially lower doses of hydroxyurea and yet had greater reductions in platelet counts, white cell counts, and hemoglobin concentration than did V617F-negative patients. No such effect was seen in patients receiving anagrelide. These findings suggest that V617F-positive patients gain particular benefit from hydroxyurea compared with anagrelide. Therapy with anagrelide, but not with hydroxyurea, was also associated with progressive anemia and an increase in bone marrow fibrosis (Campbell et al. 2009).

The increased fibrosis was reversible in a small number of patients upon withdrawal of anagrelide, and follow-up trephine biopsies are therefore recommended for patients receiving this agent, perhaps every 2–3 years. It is important to note that the diagnosis of ET in the PT1-trial was made according to the PVSG classification, and it remains questionable if these recommendations can be applied to ET patients diagnosed according to the World Health Organization (WHO) classification. In a recent study (Barbui et al. 2011a), representatives from seven international centers of excellence for myeloproliferative neoplasms convened to create a clinicopathologic database of patients ($n=1,104$) previously diagnosed as having ET. Study eligibility criteria included availability of treatment-naïve bone marrow specimens obtained within 1 year of diagnosis. All bone marrows subsequently underwent a central re-review by a WHO author. Diagnosis was confirmed as

ET in 891 patients (81%) and revised to early/prefibrotic PMF in 180 (16%); 33 were not evaluable or represented reactive cases. Ten/fifteen-year survival, leukemic transformation, fibrotic progression rates, and survival were significantly worse in early/prefibrotic PMF vs. ET. However, thrombosis rates were similar between the two groups. These results validate the clinical relevance of strict adherence to WHO criteria in the diagnosis of ET.

In this connection, useful information is expected from the Anahydret trial (Gisslinger et al. 2007). Anahydret is a randomized single-blind international multicenter phase III study designed to evaluate the noninferiority of anagrelide vs. hydroxyurea in 258 high-risk ET patients diagnosed according to the 2008 WHO diagnostic criteria. This classification, at variance of PVSG criteria required in the PT-1 trial, included a more homogenous category of patients excluding those with early myelofibrosis who, at diagnosis, present different hematological and clinical features in comparison with WHO-ET. Moreover, contrary to PT-1 enrolling criteria that included all comers with ET, these were de novo diagnosed and cytotoxic naïve patients. During the whole study period, 11 major ET-related complications occurred in the anagrelide group (five arterial events, two venous thrombotic complications, and four bleedings) and 12 major events were seen in the hydroxyurea arm (five arterial events, five venous thrombotic events, and two bleedings). Transformations to myelofibrosis were not reported. This study provides preliminary evidence for noninferiority of anagrelide compared to hydroxyurea in the first-line treatment of ET diagnosed according to the WHO classification. However, compared to PT-1, the number of patients enrolled was small, duration of follow-up relatively short, and considerably fewer end-point events were recorded. It is therefore questionable whether this study has the statistical power to detect the differences observed in the PT-1 study. Therefore, anagrelide does appear to provide partial protection from thrombosis, particularly in JAK2 V617F–negative ET

patients, and may be suitable as second-line therapy for patients in whom hydroxyurea is inadequate or not tolerated, according with the criteria described above (Harrison et al. 2005; Barbui and Finazzi 2005).

Concerning side effects of hydroxyurea, Antonioli et al. (2011) reported a rate of 5% strengthening the good tolerability of this drug.

In clinical practice, the starting dose of HU is 15–20 mg/kg/day until response is obtained (for response criteria, see chapter). Thereafter, a maintenance dose should be administered to keep the response without reducing WBC count values below $2,500 \times 109/L$. Supplemental phlebotomy should be performed if needed in PV patients. Complete hemogram should be recorded every 2 weeks during the first 2 months, then every month, and, in steady state in responding patients, every 3 months.

9.3.2 Interferon Alpha as First-Line Therapy

IFN-alpha was considered for the treatment of patients with MPN since this agent suppresses the proliferation of hematopoietic progenitors, has a direct inhibiting effect on bone marrow fibroblast progenitor cells, and antagonizes the action of platelet-derived growth factor, transforming growth factor beta, and other cytokines, which may be involved in the development of myelofibrosis. Published reports concern small consecutive series of patients in whom hematological response and side effects were evaluated. One review analyzed the cumulative experience with IFN-alpha in 279 patients with PV from 16 studies (Lengfelder et al. 1996). Overall responses were 50% for reduction of Hct to less than 0.45% without concomitant phlebotomies, 77% for reduction in spleen size, and 75% for reduction of pruritus. In a review article, Silver (2006) updated his experience on the long-term use (median 13 years) of IFN-alpha in 55 patients with PV. Complete responses, defined by phlebotomy free, Hct less than 45%, and platelet number below $600 \times 10^9/L$, were reached in the great majority of cases after 1–2 years of treatment, and the maintenance dose could be decreased in half of the patients. Noteworthy is the absence of thrombo-hemorrhagic events during this long follow-up.

IFN-alpha has been also used in ET patients. The results of several cohort studies, reviewed in Lengfelder et al. (1996), indicate that reduction of platelet count below 600×10^9/L can be obtained in about 90% of cases after about 3 months with an average dose of 3 million IU daily. IFN-alpha is not known to be teratogenic and does not cross the placenta. Thus, it has been used successfully throughout pregnancy in some ET patients with no adverse fetal or maternal outcome. The main problem with IFN-alpha therapy, apart from its costs and parental route of administration, is the incidence of side effects. Fever and flu-like symptoms are experienced by most patients and usually require treatment with paracetamol. Signs of chronic IFN-alpha toxicity, such as weakness, myalgia, weight and hair loss, and severe depression, limit its long-term use. Pegylated forms of IFN-alpha allow weekly administration, potentially improving compliance and possibly providing more effective therapy. A phase II study has shown that following pegylated interferon alpha-2a therapy, the malignant clone as quantitated by the percentage of the mutated allele JAK2 V617F was reduced (Kiladjian et al. 2006). More limited effects on JAK2 mutational status have been reported after therapy with pegylated interferon alpha-2b in a small group of patients with PV and ET (Samuelsson et al. 2006). Kiladjian et al. (2008b) performed a prospective sequential quantitative evaluation of the percentage of mutated JAK2 allele (percentage of V617F) by real-time polymerase chain reaction (PCR) in patients treated with pegylated interferon alpha-2a. The percentage of JAK2 V617F was decreased in 26 (89.6%) of 29 treated patients, from a mean of 45% to a mean of 22.5% after 12 months of treatment (median decrease of 50%; $p < .001$), with no evidence for a plateau being achieved. In two patients, JAK2 V617F was no longer detectable after 12 months, such complete molecular response being observed in a total of seven patients (24%) at time of last analysis after a median follow-up of 31.4 months. These impressive results have been confirmed by the M.D. Anderson Cancer Center investigators (Quintas-Cardama et al. 2009). In a phase II study of pegylated interferon alpha-2a in 79 patients with PV and ET, an overall hematologic response rate was observed in 80% of PV and 81% of ET (complete in 70% and 76% of patients, respectively). The molecular response rate was 38% in ET and 54% in PV, being complete (undetectable JAK2 V617F) in 6% and 14%, respectively. The JAK2 V617F mutant allele burden continued to decrease with no clear evidence for a plateau. Contrary to these findings, no significant JAK2 V617F changes were obtained by recombinant interferon alpha-2b; whether this finding represents a qualitative difference between two agents remains to be determined (Silver et al. 2009). The tolerability of PEG-IFN, gastrointestinal and cardiovascular symptoms, makes it necessary to discontinue the drug in about one third of patients. Thus, this agent may have an important role in the treatment of PV and other clonal MPN.

According to European LeukemiaNet (ELN) recommendations (Barbui et al. 2011b):

First line therapy (Table 9.1) in all patients with PV should be phlebotomy to maintain the hematocrit less than 45%, and low-dose aspirin (75–100 mg). Cytoreduction is strongly indicated in high risk cases defined by age and previous major vascular events. Poor tolerance to or high need of phlebotomy, symptomatic or progressive splenomegaly, severe disease related symptoms, platelet counts greater than 1.5×109/L or progressive leukocytosis are other indications to cytoreduction. Either HU or IFN alpha are the first-line therapy at any age. Intermittent busulfan may be considered in elderly patients. No cytoreductive drugs in otherwise low-risk patients carrying well-controlled cardiovascular risk factors is recommended. All patients with ET (Table 9.2) presenting microvascular disturbances should be managed with low-dose aspirin (75–100 mg). Cytoreduction with HU is the first-line therapy in high risk patients at any age. The use of cytoreductive drugs in otherwise low-risk patients carrying well-controlled cardiovascular risk factors is not generally indicated.

Table 9.1 Flow-chart recommended first-line treatment for patients with PV

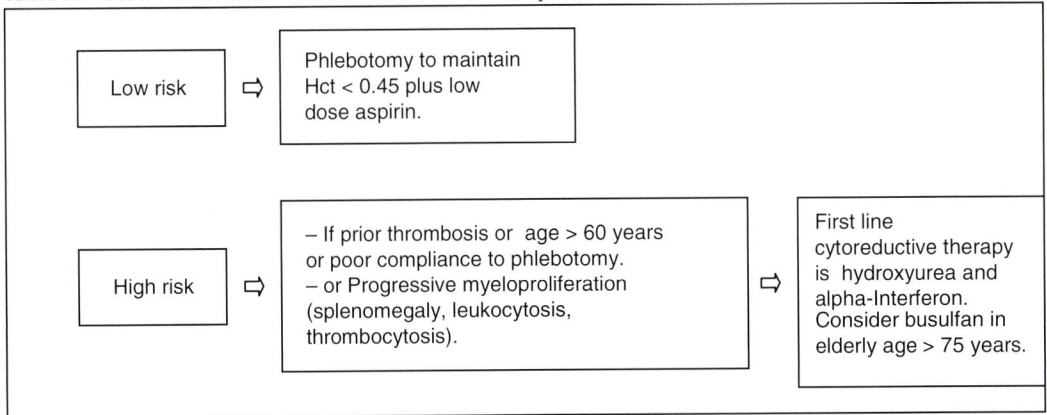

Table 9.2 Flow-chart recommended first line treatment for patients with ET

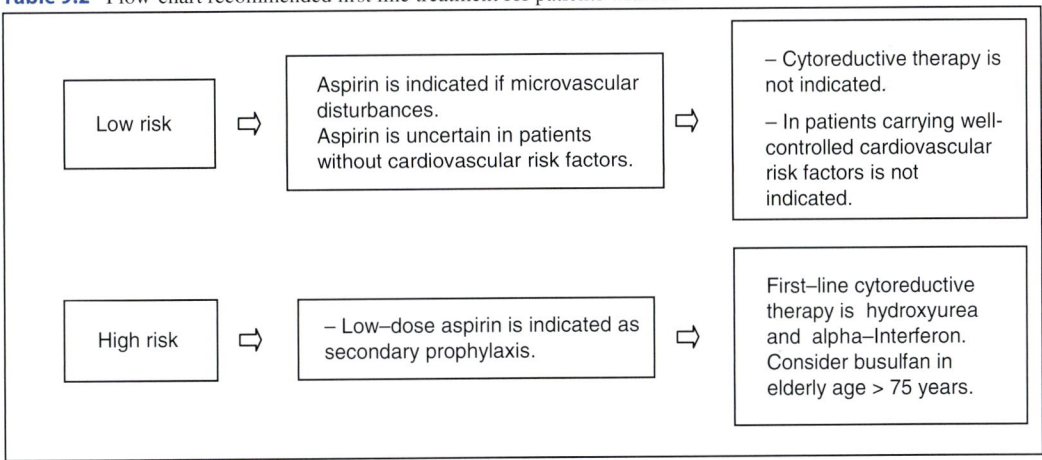

9.4 First-Line Therapy in Special Clinical Situations

Special issues in myeloproliferative neoplasms (MPN) comprise clinical conditions with high relevance for the duration and quality of the patient's life, but with limited evidence to support sound diagnostic and therapeutic recommendations. These issues include MPN in pregnancy, in children, abdominal vein thrombosis, bleeding complications, surgery, and pruritus. Practical suggestions to guide clinical decisions in these settings remain largely empirical, but recently developed guidelines based on ELN experts' consensus may help to tackle these problems (Barbui et al. 2011a, b).

9.4.1 Pregnancy

As outlined by the recent English guidelines (Harrison et al. 2010), patients should be managed

Table 9.3 Risk-adapted management of pregnancy in ET

1. Risk stratification

    At least one of the following defines high-risk pregnancy:

        Previous major thrombotic or bleeding complication

        Previous severe pregnancy complications[a]

        Platelet count $>1,500 \times 10^9/L$

2. Therapy

    (a) Low-risk pregnancy:

        Aspirin 100 mg/day

        LMWH 4,000 U/day after delivery until 6 weeks postpartum

    (b) High-risk pregnancy

        As above, plus:

        If previous major thrombosis or severe pregnancy complications: LMWH throughout pregnancy (stop aspirin if bleeding complications)

        If platelet count $>1,500 \times 10^9/L$: consider IFN-α

        If previous major bleeding: avoid aspirin and consider IFN-α to reduce thrombocytosis

[a]Severe pregnancy complications: >3 first-trimester or >1 second- or third-trimester losses, birth weight <5th centile of gestation, pre-eclampsia, intrauterine death or stillbirth

by a multidisciplinary team, and a detailed personal and family history should be taken. It is recommended that the patient should stop any possible teratogenic drug at least 3 months before conception. Depending on the risk of maternal vascular events and pregnancy morbidity, the various treatment options range from no therapy through aspirin alone or low molecular weight heparin (LMWH) to cytoreductive therapy.

According to ELN recommendations (Table 9.3), in the absence of clear contraindications, all patients with ET and PV should be given aspirin (75 or 100 mg daily) throughout pregnancy and for at least 6 weeks after delivery. Low-dose aspirin is considered safe in pregnancy and should preferably be started before conception to facilitate placental and fetal development. Bleeding complications are rare, but particular attention should be paid to patients with a platelet count above 1,000 to $1,500 \times 10^9/L$, as the risk of bleeding may increase significantly.

LMWH is indicated for prophylaxis and treatment of deep venous thrombosis and to reduce fetal morbidity in high-risk pregnant women with ET (Table 9.3). The suggested dose of enoxaparin is 4,000 U (40 mg) once daily, increasing to 4,000 U twice daily from 16 weeks and dropping to 4,000 U daily for 6 weeks postpartum. To increase the antithrombotic efficacy in very high-risk situations, LMWH was used in combination with low-dose aspirin.

Cytoreductive therapy in pregnancy is a very controversial area. During pregnancy, hematocrit and platelet count may undergo a natural fall, and this could reduce the need for phlebotomy or cytoreductive drugs. According to the Italian guidelines and expert judgment (Barbui et al. 2004; Harrison et al. 2010), candidates for platelet-lowering drugs are women with a previous history of major thrombosis or major bleeding, or when platelet count is greater than 1,000 to $1,500 \times 10^9/L$, or when familial thrombophilia or cardiovascular risk factors are documented. If cytoreduction must be given, interferon alpha is probably the safest option. Other cytotoxic drugs like hydroxyurea, busulfan, and anagrelide should be avoided, particularly during organogenesis in the first trimester.

9.4.2 Children

MPN are rare in children. The most frequent is ET (Dame and Sutor 2005). Diagnostic criteria for MPN in children are the same as in adults, but family screening is recommended to differentiate JAK2 V617F–negative ET from rare familial disorders due to mutations of TPO or MPL other than W515, particularly MPL S505N. Also, in case of JAK2 V617F–negative or exon 12–negative erythrocytosis with normal or slightly reduced erythropoietin levels, a familial history should prompt a search for rare mutations in *EPO-R*. Screening for inherited thrombophilia is recommended for children with a familial or personal history of thrombosis.

By definition, children with ET are at low vascular risk unless a major thrombotic or hemorrhagic event has occurred. Thus, cytoreductive therapy should be used only as a last resort. In the rare cases that need treatment, the English guidelines underline that the selection of a cytotoxic or cytoreductive agent is best made after discussion with the child and parents, and that hydroxyurea (HU) is well tolerated and efficacious in controlling symptoms (Harrison et al. 2010). Anagrelide and IFN-alpha are other options, but all these drugs have limitations. Adverse effects of interferon alpha such as flu-like syndrome, neuropsychiatric symptoms, and autoimmune phenomena can be particularly dangerous for children. Anagrelide is not licensed as first-line therapy for ET in Europe. The long-term leukemogenicity of HU may be a special concern for children, although none of the pediatric patients treated with this agent have yet undergone malignant transformation.

> According to ELN experts, cytoreductive drugs should be used only as a last resort. There are insufficient data to recommend a specific agent, and the choice should be tailored on individual basis. Use of aspirin in children <12 years should be considered with caution because of risk of Reye syndrome (Belay et al. 1997).

9.4.3 Treatment of Thrombosis

According to ELN experts (Barbui et al. 2011a, b), patients with spontaneous venous thromboembolism should be given low molecular weight heparin at therapeutic dose, followed by warfarin or acenocumarol with the aim of keeping PT INR in the conventional therapeutic range (2.0–3.0). The anticoagulant duration should follow the national guidelines for the treatment of thrombosis in malignancy. Low-dose aspirin therapy is recommended for patients with a recent major arterial vascular event (ischemic stroke, transient ischemic attack, peripheral arterial occlusion, myocardial infarction, unstable angina).

Patients presenting with erythromelalgia should be treated with low-dose aspirin. This dose is effective in the majority of the patients. If no relief within 24–48 h, a larger dose should be given. Appropriate cytoreduction, with the goal to optimize the control of the blood cell counts, is recommended in all patients with major vascular events, as described above.

9.4.4 Splanchnic Vein Thrombosis

Abdominal vein thrombosis, including extrahepatic portal vein occlusion, Budd-Chiari syndrome, and mesenteric vein thrombosis, is characteristically encountered in MPNs (Chung et al. 2006). Diagnosis may be difficult because symptoms (abdominal pain, hepatomegaly, ascites) are not specific. Doppler ultrasonography, CT scanning, and MRI are usually required to achieve a diagnosis (Chait et al. 2005). In these thromboses, MPN may not be clinically obvious because concurrent hypersplenism, occult gastrointestinal bleeding, or hemodilution can mask blood count abnormality. Of significant diagnostic help is the determination of JAK2 V617F mutation, which is found in about 45% of patients with Budd-Chiari syndrome and 34% with portal vein thrombosis (Patel et al. 2006; Kiladjian et al. 2008c).

Splanchnic vein thrombosis should be managed according to current guidelines (Martinelli et al. 2008). Full-dose heparinization is recommended, despite the high risk of gastrointestinal bleeding, followed by lifelong oral anticoagulation with a PT INR range of 2.0–3.0. In a survey of the current outcome of portal vein thrombosis in 136 patients, 42 (31%) of whom had a myeloproliferative disorder, anticoagulant therapy reduced the risk of recurrence or extension of thrombosis by two thirds without any real increase in the incidence or severity of bleeding (Condat et al. 2001). In the Budd-Chiari syndrome, intensive medical management including anticoagulation is mandatory, and more aggressive procedures should be considered in the most severe cases. Examples of such procedures include transjugular intrahepatic portosystemic shunt, angioplasty (with or without stenting), surgical shunts, and even liver transplantation (Narayanan Menon et al. 2004). Joint management with a liver team, follow-up of varices, and warning about pregnancy are recommended by ELN experts (Barbui et al. 2011b). For those patients with thrombocytosis, HU should be used to restore platelet counts to 400×10^9/L or less as soon as possible.

> According to ELN, treatment of splanchnic vein thrombosis includes LMWH followed by long-life oral anticoagulation with PT INR range 2.0–3.0. Invasive procedures should be limited only if needed, liver transplantation if needed. Joint management with a liver team, follow-up of varices and warning about pregnancy are recommended in this context. For those patients with thrombocytosis, hydroxyurea should be used to restore counts to 400×10^9/L or less as soon as possible.

9.4.5 Bleeding

Hemorrhage is both a less frequent and generally less severe clinical complication than thrombosis in patients with MPN. Hemorrhagic symptoms are more frequent in patients with platelet counts in excess of 1,000 to $1,500 \times 10^9$/L; these symptoms may be related to acquired von Willebrand syndrome (AvWS), a deficiency of von Willebrand factor (Elliott and Tefferi 2003). Normalization of the platelet count was accompanied by regression of the hemorrhagic tendency so that a practical consequence is to consider cytoreductive therapy for ET patients whose platelet count is over $1,500 \times 10^9$/L (Barbui et al. 2004). Serious bleeding may be triggered by simultaneous antithrombotic therapy with anticoagulants or antiplatelet agents. These drugs should be avoided in patients with previous hemorrhagic events such as gastric ulcers or esophageal varices secondary to abdominal vein thrombosis and portal hypertension. If anagrelide is used, concurrent aspirin therapy should be prescribed with caution.

Treatment of bleeding events in MPN should start with withdrawal of any concomitant anti-thrombotic therapy and correction of extreme thrombocytosis, if it is associated with AvWS. This situation is usually treated with HU, but platelet pheresis may be indicated in an emergency. Platelet transfusions have been rarely used, although the defective platelet function in MPNs may represent a rationale for their indication. Recombinant factor VII has been reported to be useful in MPN patients with uncontrolled, life-threatening bleeding (Cervera et al. 2005), but further study is needed. Occasional patients may present with simultaneous bleeding and thrombosis; treatment of these difficult cases should be individually tailored and based on the prevalent clinical symptoms.

9.4.6 Surgery

Patients with MPN have an increased risk of morbidity and mortality when they require surgical procedures (Ruggeri et al. 2008). The optimal management of MPN during surgery is uncertain because prospective studies are lacking. The appropriate control of erythrocytosis and thrombocytosis with phlebotomy and/or myelosuppression has been recommended (Barbui et al. 2011a, b). The platelet count should be kept below 400×10^9/L, particularly when splenectomy is planned, because of the potential for postoperative extreme thrombocytosis, which may lead to the development of AvWS and associated hemorrhagic diathesis. Aspirin should be withheld for at least 1 week before elective surgery involving a high risk of bleeding, surgery (e.g., neurosurgery) in which even minor bleeding could result in life-threatening complications, or surgery requiring heparin prophylaxis. LMWH at a prophylactic dose (4,000 U subcutaneously, starting 12 h before surgery) is indicated for all patients with MPN because of the high thrombotic risk, although there are no prospective studies in this setting. Surgical patients with MPN must be followed carefully for the paradoxical predisposition to both bleeding and thrombotic perioperative complications. In cases of splenectomy, echoscan of the abdominal veins is recommended, typically within 1–2 weeks after surgery, to exclude asymptomatic splanchnic vein thrombosis.

9.4.7 Pruritus

Intractable pruritus (typically aquagenic) can be a disabling condition in some patients with MPN, particularly PV. The pathogenesis is unknown, although JAK2 V617F–induced constitutive activation and agonist hypersensitivity in basophils of these patients have been recently demonstrated (Pieri et al. 2009). A number of small studies have tried to address this clinical problem (reviewed in Saini et al. 2010). Antihistamines, such as cyproheptadine (4–16 mg/day), may be beneficial. If unsuccessful, interferon alpha (3.0×10^6 units subcutaneously three times a week) or pegylated interferon (0.5–1.0 μg/kg/week) was reported to be effective in most patients. Other treatment options include paroxetine, a selective serotonin uptake inhibitor, at a dosage of 20 mg/day, and photochemotherapy using psoralen and ultraviolet A light. Novel targeted therapies with inhibitors of JAK2 V617F were found to be useful in controlling this symptomin phase I, II and III clinical trial (see chapter Verstovsek).

References

Alvarez-Larran A, Cervantes F, Pereira A et al (2010) Observation versus antiplatelet therapy as primary prophylaxis for thrombosis in low-risk essential thrombocythemia. Blood 116:1205–1210

Antonioli E, Guglielmelli P, Pieri L et al (2011) Side effects of hydroxyurea in classic chronic myeloproliferative neoplasms. A retrospective study of 3,411 patients. 16th Congress EHA, London (abstract)

Barbui T, Finazzi G (2005) When and how to treat essential thrombocythemia. N Engl J Med 353:85–86

Barbui T, Barosi G, Grossi A et al (2004) Practice guidelines for the therapy of essential thrombocythemia. A statement from the Italian Society of Hematology, the Italian Society of Experimental Hematology and the Italian Group for Bone Marrow Transplantation. Haematologica 89:215–232

Barbui T, Thiele J, Passamonti F et al (2011a) Survival and risk of leukemic transformation in essential thrombocythemia are significantly influenced by accurate morphologic diagnosis: an international study on 1,104 patients. J Clin Oncol 29:3179–3184

Barbui T, Barosi G, Birgegard G et al (2011b) Philadelphia-negative classical myeloproliferative neoplasms: criti-cal concepts and management recommendations from European LeukemiaNet. J Clin Oncol 29:761–770

Belay ED, Bresee JS, Holman RC et al (1997) Reye's syndrome in the United States from 1981 through 1997. N Engl J Med 340:1377–1382

Berk PD, Goldberg JD, Donovan PB et al (1986) Therapeutic recommendations in polycythemia vera based on Polycythemia Vera Study Group protocols. Semin Hematol 23:132–143

Bjorkholm M, Derolf AR, Hultcranz M et al (2011) Treatment related risk factors for transformation to acute myeloid leukemia and myelodysplastic syndromes in myeloproliferative neoplasms. J Clin Oncol. doi:10.1200/JCO.2011.34.7542

Campbell PJ, Scott LM, Buck G et al (2005) Definition of subtypes of essential thrombocythaemia and relation to polycythemia vera based on JAK2 V617F mutation status: a prospective study. Lancet 366:1945–1953

Campbell PJ, Bareford D, Erber WN et al (2009) Reticulin accumulation in essential thrombocythemia: prognostic significance and relation to therapy. J Clin Oncol 27:2991–2999

Cervera JS, Mena-Duran AV, Piqueras CS (2005) The use of recombinant factor VIIa in a patient with essential thrombocythemia with uncontrolled surgical bleeding. Thromb Haemost 93:383–384

Chait Y, Condat B, Cazals-Hatem D et al (2005) Relevance of the criteria commonly used to diagnose myeloproliferative disorder in patients with splanchnic vein thrombosis. Br J Haematol 129:553–560

Chung RT, Iafrate AJ, Amrein PC et al (2006) Case 15–2006: a 46-year-old woman with sudden onset of abdominal distention. N Engl J Med 354:2166–2175

Condat B, Pessione F, Hillaire S et al (2001) Current outcome of portal vein thrombosis in adults: risk and benefit of anticoagulant therapy. Gastroenterology 120:490–497

Cortelazzo S, Finazzi G, Ruggeri M et al (1995) Hydroxyurea in the treatment of patients with essential thrombocythemia at high risk of thrombosis: a prospective randomized trial. N Engl J Med 332:1132–1136

Dame C, Sutor AH (2005) Primary and secondary thrombocytosis in childhood. Br J Haematol 129:165–177

Di Nisio M, Barbui T, Gennaro D et al (2007) The hematocrit and platelet target in polycythemia vera. Br J Haematol 136:249–259

Elliott MA, Tefferi A (2003) Thrombocythaemia and pregnancy. Best Pract Res Clin Hematol 16:227–242

Finazzi G, Ruggeri M, Rodeghiero F et al (2000) Second malignancies in patients with essential thrombocythemia treated with busulphan and hydroxyurea: long-term follow-up of a randomized clinical trial. Br J Haematol 110:577–583

Finazzi G, Ruggeri M, Rodeghiero F et al (2003) Efficacy and safety of long-term use of hydroxyurea in young patients with essential thrombocythemia and a high risk of thrombosis. Blood 101:3749

Finazzi G, Caruso V, Marchioli R et al (2005) Acute leukemia in polycythemia vera. An analysis of 1,638 patients enrolled in a prospective observational study. Blood 105:2664–2670

Fruchtman SM, Mack K, Kaplan ME et al (1997) From efficacy to safety: a polycythemia vera study group report on hydroxyurea in patients with polycythemia vera. Semin Hematol 34:17–23

Gangat N, Strand J, Li CY et al (2007) Leucocytosis in polycythemia vera predicts both inferior survival and leukaemic transformation. Br J Haematol 138:354–358

Gisslinger H, Kralovics R, Gotic M et al (2007) Non-inferiority of anagrelide compared to hydroxyurea in newly diagnosed patients with essential thrombocythemia. The ANAHYDRET-Study. Blood 110:3547 (abstract)

Harrison C, Barbui T (2011) Aspirin in low-risk essential thrombocythemia, not so simple after all? Leuk Res 35:286–289

Harrison CN, Campbell PJ, Buck G et al (2005) Hydroxyurea compared with anagrelide in high-risk essential thrombocythemia. N Engl J Med 353:33–45

Harrison CN, Bareford D, Butt N et al (2010) Guideline for investigation and management of adults and children presenting with a thrombocytosis. Br J Haematol 149:352–375

Kiladjian JJ, Cassinat B, Turlure P et al (2006) High molecular response rate of polycythemia vera patients treated with pegylated interferon alpha-2a. Blood 108:2037–2040

Kiladjian JJ, Chevret S, Dosquet C et al (2008a) Long-term outcome in polycythemia vera: final analysis of a randomized trial comparing hydroxyurea (HU) to pipobroman (Pi). Blood 112: abstract 1746

Kiladjian JJ, Cassinat B, Chevret S et al (2008b) Pegylated interferon alpha-2a induces complete hematologic and molecular responses with low toxicity in polycythemia vera. Blood 112:3065–3072

Kiladjian JJ, Cervantes F, Leebek FWG et al (2008c) The impact of JAK2 and MPL mutations on diagnosis and prognosis of splanchnic vein thrombosis: a report on 241 cases. Blood 111:4922–4929

Landolfi R, Marchioli R, Kutti J et al (2004) Efficacy and safety of low-dose aspirin in polycythemia vera. N Engl J Med 350:114–124

Lengfelder E, Griesshammer M, Hehlmann R (1996) Interferon-alpha in the treatment of essential thrombocythemia. Leuk Lymphoma 22(suppl 1):135–142

Martinelli I, Franchini M, Mannucci PM (2008) How I treat rare venous thrombosis. Blood 112:4818–4823

Najean Y, Rain JD for the French Polycythemia Study Group (1997) Treatment of polycythemia vera: the use of hydroxyurea and pipobroman in 292 patients under the age of 65 years. Blood 90:3370–3377

Narayanan Menon KV, Shah V, Kamath PS (2004) The Budd-Chiari syndrome. N Engl J Med 350:578–585

Patel RK, Lea N, Heneghan A et al (2006) Prevalence of the activating JAK2 tyrosine kinase mutation V617F in the Budd-Chiari syndrome. Gastroenterology 130:2031–2038

Patrono C, Baigent C, Hirsh J et al (2008) Antiplatelet drugs: American College of Chest Physicians Evidence-Based Clinical Practice Guidelines (8th edition). Chest 133:234S–256S

Pearson TC, Wetherley-Mein G (1978) Vascular occlusive episodes and venous haematocrit in primary proliferative polycythaemia. Lancet 2:1219–1222

Pieri L, Bogani C, Guglielmelli P et al (2009) The JAK2V617F mutation induces constitutive activation and agonist hypersensitivity in basophils from patients with polycythemia vera. Haematologica 94:1484–1488

Quintas-Cardama A, Kantarjian H, Manshouri T et al (2009) Pegylated interferon alpha-2a yields high rates of hematologic and molecular response in patients with advanced essential thrombocythemia and polycythemia vera. J Clin Oncol 27:5418–5424

Ruggeri M, Rodeghiero F, Tosetto A et al (2008) Postsurgery outcomes in patients with polycythemia vera and essential thrombocythemia: a retrospective survey. Blood 111:666–671

Saini KS, Patnaik MM, Tefferi A (2010) Polycythemia vera-associated pruritus and its management. Eur J Clin Invest 40:828–834

Samuelsson J, Mutschler M, Birgegard G et al (2006) Limited effects on JAK2 mutational status after pegylated interferon alpha-2b therapy in polycythemia vera and essential thrombocythemia. Haematologica 91:1281–1282

Silver RT (2006) Long-term effects of the treatment of polycythemia vera with recombinant interferon-alpha. Cancer 107:451–458

Silver RT, Vandris K, Goldman JJ et al (2009) Decrease in JAK2V617F allele burden is not a prerequisite to clinical response in patients with polycythemia vera. Blood 114:1908 (abstract)

Spivak J (2004) Daily aspirin. Only half the answer. N Engl J Med 350:99–101

Sterkers Y, Preudhomme C, Lai J-L et al (1998) Acute myeloid leukemia and myelodysplastic syndromes following essential thrombocythemia treated with hydroxyurea: high proportion of cases with 17p deletion. Blood 91:616–622

Primary and Secondary Antithrombotic Prophylaxis

10

Leonardo Di Gennaro and Raffaele Landolfi

Contents

L. Di Gennaro • R. Landolfi (✉)
Haemostasis Research Center,
Catholic University School of Medicine,
Institute of Internal Medicine and Geriatrics,
Rome, Italy
e-mail: rlandolfi@rm.unicatt.it

10.1 Introduction

Polycythemia vera (PV) and essential thrombocythemia (ET) are relatively benign myeloproliferative neoplasms (MPNs) and require a treatment strategy mainly aimed at preventing thrombotic complications (Landolfi and Di Gennaro 2011). Over the last three decades, much effort has been devoted at elucidating the pathogenesis of thrombophilia, at describing their clinical manifestations, as well as at providing effective and safe antithrombotic options. The availability of safer cytoreductive drugs and the wider use of aspirin have contributed to reduce the incidence of both neoplastic and vascular complications and to improve life expectancy of these patients (Cervantes et al. 2008).

However, the pathogenesis of thrombosis in MPNs remains elusive. The controversial role of several disease-related abnormalities and of other individual and environmental factors accounts for some heterogeneity in treatment decisions, especially in patients with intermediate vascular risk. Age and vascular history are to date the two main risk factors for thrombosis in PV or ET subjects and still guide clinicians in the stratification of individual risk and in therapeutic decisions (Marchioli et al. 2005; Passamonti et al. 2004; Tefferi et al. 2011; Barbui et al. 2011a, b). The role of classical risk factors is, however, likely to be important, and in addition recent data draw attention toward the possible association of thrombotic risk with the inflammation and with old and novel MPNs-related mutations. These factors can be taken into consideration in conditions of intermediate/uncertain vascular risk and will be discussed here in order to propose an approach to antithrombotic prophylaxis patients which integrates novel findings with well-established information and also takes into consideration evidence coming from vascular prevention in the general population.

10.2 Thrombotic Diathesis in Polycythemia Vera and Essential Thrombocythemia: Incidence and Clinical Characteristics

Thrombophilia of PV and ET patients is characterized by an increased incidence of arterial and venous thromboses and by microcirculatory disturbances which often manifest at diagnosis or in the preclinical phase of the disease.

Arterial thromboses represent 60–70% of all cardiovascular events and include acute myocardial infarction, cerebral and peripheral arterial occlusion. Also venous thromboses, such as deep venous thrombosis and pulmonary embolism, are frequent manifestations in MPNs. Splanchnic thromboses, which include portal vein thrombosis, mesenteric thrombosis and thrombosis of the hepatic veins, have an unusually high prevalence among young female subjects (Chait et al. 2005; Briere 2006). Fatal cardiovascular events and disease transformation to myelofibrosis or leukemia account for most of the deaths in PV and ET. The mortality rate is increased in PV patients in an age-dependent manner, while life expectancy may be normal in the majority of patients with ET (Cervantes et al. 2008). Microcirculatory disturbances are represented by erythromelalgia, headache, dizziness, hearing and visual disturbances, Raynaud-like phenomena and superficial thrombophlebitis (Landolfi et al. 2006; Michiels et al. 2006a). Also miscarriages in women with latent or manifest MPNs are attributed to an impaired microcirculation (Griesshammer et al. 2006). Erythromelalgia is the best characterized manifestation and can affect more than 5% of patients,

particularly in the early phases of the disease, generally characterized by an active proliferating activity (Michiels 1997). The inhibition of platelet prostaglandin production by aspirin is dramatically effective in reversing the attack. Microcirculatory disturbances are quite characteristic of PV and ET patients and, when observed in otherwise healthy subjects, should lead to consider a latent myeloproliferative disorder (Michiels et al. 2006). Whether patient with past history of these disturbances should be considered at high thrombotic risk is currently unclear. In addition, diagnosis of many of these manifestations may be somewhat uncertain due to the transient and often vague nature of symptoms. A careful evaluation of history and the demonstration of rapid and complete reversal of symptoms after aspirin are considered important for diagnostic confirmation.

10.3 Antithrombotic Strategy: General Interventions for All Patients

Since thrombosis can be an early complication of MPNs, an effective antithrombotic strategy has to be adopted as soon as the disease is diagnosed. This strategy shall include treatment of blood hyperviscosity in patients with PV, interventions on lifestyle and cardiovascular risk factors, as well as aspirin use in the majority of subjects. An accurate evaluation of the vascular risk is then used for appropriately tailoring the cytoreductive intervention in each patient.

10.3.1 Treatment of Blood Hyperviscosity in PV Patients

At the time of diagnosis, PV patients often have red cell mass values between 36 and 66 mL/kg and haematocrit values between 0.50 and 0.75. These haematocrit levels are associated with a high risk of major arterial and venous thrombosis at the time of PV diagnosis (Berk et al. 1995). In a PVSG study, the incidence of major vascular episodes was correlated with haematocrit levels

Table 10.1 Treatment options in PV and ET patients according to risk stratification

| Risk level | Suggested treatment | | Score |
	Polycythemia vera	Essential thrombocythemia	
Low	Phlebotomy low-dose aspirin	Low-dose aspirin	<1.5
Low with platelet count >1,000×109/L	Phlebotomy low-dose aspirin provided ristocetin cofactor activity >30%	Low-dose aspirin provided ristocetin cofactor activity >30%	<1.5
Intermediate	Phlebotomy low-dose aspirin	Low-dose aspirin IFN or HU	1.5–3
High	Phlebotomy low-dose aspirin HU	Low-dose aspirin HU	3.1–6
Very high	Phlebotomy low-dose aspirin HU Consider more aggressive treatment	Low-dose aspirin HU Consider more aggressive treatment	>6

| Scoring system | | | |
Risk factor	Score	Risk factor	Score
Age <40	0	Dyslipidemia	0.5
40–55	1	Hypertension	0.5
56–65	2.5	Smoke	1.5
>65	3.5	Diabetes	1.5
Leukocyte count (>12×10⁹/L)	1	Past history of thrombosis	3.5

HU Hydroxyurea, *IFN* Interferon-α

(Messinezy et al. 1985). The vascular risk was highest at haematocrits above 0.50 (risk from 35% to 50%) and moderately increased at haematocrits between 0.45 and 0.50. For reducing the risk of vascular events, the treatment of hyperviscosity is an essential and urgent need after PV diagnosis. Thus, phlebotomy is recommended to bring and maintain the haematocrit below 45% in males and below 42% in females (Pearson and Wetherley-Mein 1978; Pearson 1997). As reported in Table 10.1, treatment of blood hyperviscosity applies to all PV subjects, although the best strategy to maintain the target haematocrit value is different in patients with different vascular risk. A recent analysis of the ECLAP data failed to show a clear effect on thrombotic risk of haematocrit values in the range of 0.45–0.50 (Marchioli et al. 2005). Thus, it is not clear whether phlebotomy should be performed with the aim of reducing the haematocrit to less than 0.45, as classically recommended, or whether it could be adequate to decrease the haematocrit below 0.50. Future prospective studies are needed to answer this question in PV patients with different vascular risk. Waiting for these studies, it seems prudent to maintain haematocrit values lower than 0.48 also in low-risk PV subjects (Barbui et al. 2004; Di Nisio et al. 2007; Crisa et al. 2010).

10.3.2 Interventions on Lifestyle and Cardiovascular Risk Factors

The identification and appropriate management of cardiovascular risk factors and the promotion of a healthy lifestyle are in MPNs, as in the general population, a cornerstone of vascular prevention. On the contrary, the importance of a healthy lifestyle is frequently scotomized in MPNs due to the tendency to consider the thrombosis as "caused" by the disease rather than by the interplay of various factors, as summarized in Fig. 10.1. In this view, the presence of MPN disorder should raise further attention toward the need for adequately recognizing and treating any modifiable risk factor and for encouraging the patient toward a healthy lifestyle. A successful intervention on lifestyle and all modifiable risk factor requires full patient adherence, and this underlines the importance of sharing with him treatment decisions and goals.

Interventions on lifestyle are aimed at achieving healthy eating habit, appropriate physical activity and abstinence from smoking. Several epidemiological studies performed in the general population indicate that nutrition and physical activity are predictors of age-specific mortality and cardiovascular event.

Fig. 10.1 Thrombosis in myeloproliferative neoplasms: pathogenetic mechanisms and prophylaxis

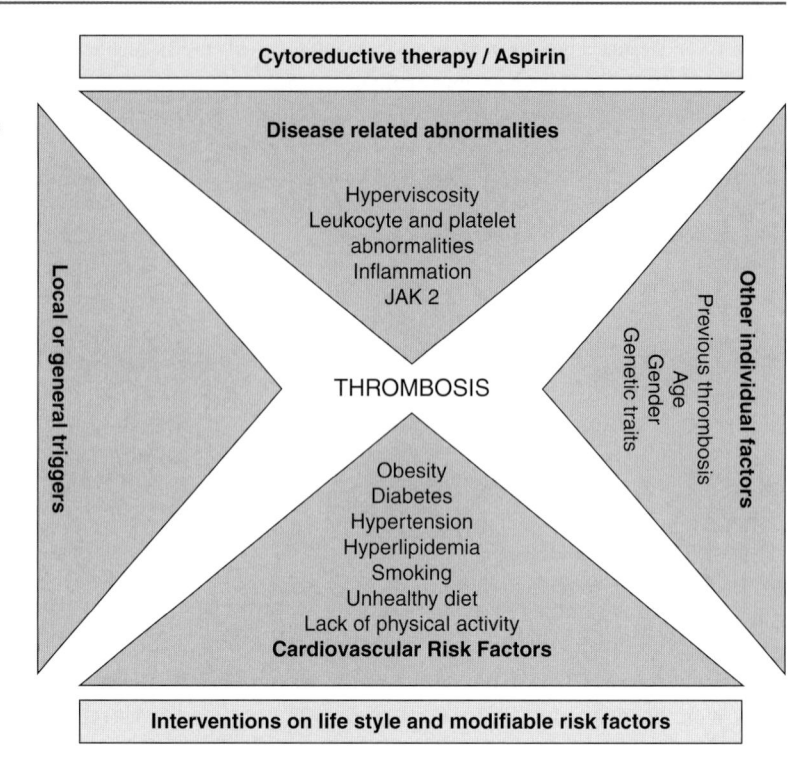

All patients should achieve a normal body weight, increase physical activity, reduce alcohol and sodium intake and increase consumption of fresh fruits, vegetables and low-fat dairy products. Body mass index and waist circumference should be routinely measured in all subjects with the aim of maintaining a body mass index between 18.5 and 24.9 and a waist circumference of <80 cm in women and <95 cm in men.

Clinicians should encourage 30–60 min of moderate-intensity exercise for 3 days a week, supplemented by an increase in daily physical activities. Particular attention has to be given to smoking habit which has an important effect on vascular risk and which was found to be surprisingly common among PV patients recruited in the ECLAP observational study (Landolfi et al. 2007). In a multivariate analysis of data from the same study, smoke was associated with a significant risk of arterial thrombotic events (HR 1.90; 95% confidence interval 1.15–3.14; $P=0.0120$) (Landolfi et al. 2007). A similar finding had been reported also in ET subjects (Besses et al. 1999;

Jantunen et al. 2001). Therefore, smoking cessation is absolutely recommended and can be achieved with the help of techniques which may include counselling, nicotine replacement and oral smoking cessation medications.

Arterial hypertension, hypercholesterolemia, obesity and metabolic syndrome are major risk factors for the development of cardiovascular disease in general population (McTigue et al. 2003) but have not been convincingly shown to be independent predictors of thrombosis in MPNs patients. Only one multivariate analysis on ET patients demonstrated the independent contribution of hypercholesterolemia in predicting thrombosis (Besses et al. 1999). We recommend an appropriate treatment of all these risk factors and the fully adoption of the seventh report of the Joint National Committee on Prevention, Detection, Evaluation, and Treatment of High Blood Pressure. This recommends 140 and 90 mmHg as upper limits for systolic and diastolic blood pressure in subjects without chronic kidney disease or diabetes while, in the presence of these conditions, achieving the target level of 130/80 mmHg is considered mandatory (Smith et al. 2006, Chobanian et al. 2003). Physicians should prefer, as initial anti-hypertensive drugs, ß-blockers and/or angiotensin-converting enzyme (ACE) inhibitors and subsequently add other drugs such as thiazides to achieve target blood pressure levels (Smith et al. 2006, Chobanian et al. 2003).

Indeed, in the particular setting of myeloproliferative disorders, there are only short reports on the use of these drugs (Nomura et al. 1996; Marusic-Vrsalovic et al. 2003), but there are no reasons to question their efficacy.

Generally, management of dyslipidemia is initially approached by reducing the intake of saturated fats (to <7% of total calories), trans-fatty acids and cholesterol (to <200 mg/day). For risk reduction, it should also be encouraged an increased dietary intake of omega-3 fatty acids and/or their supplementation (1 g/die) (Smith et al. 2006). Generally, hypercholesterolemia resistant to diet and physical activity is rare in MPNs, but when present, it should be adequately treated. Statins have antiproliferative, antiangiogenic and antithrombotic effects, which may be helpful in MPNs subjects (Hasselbalch and Riley 2006). The efficacy of statins in MPNs has yet to be tested in prospective studies, but their possible use in MPNs deserves clinical and scientific attention. As regard to diabetes, there is a clear increase risk of developing cardiovascular disease and stroke in both type 1 and type 2 diabetes mellitus (Greenland et al. 2010). The ECLAP observational study showed that diabetes was a possible predictor of survival and cardiovascular mortality in MPNs patients (Finazzi and Barbui 2005; Marchioli 2005). Although the evidence is limited, diabetes has to be considered an important risk factor also in MPNs and should be adequately managed (Table 10.1). In addition to interventions on lifestyle, hypoglycemic drugs should be used for achieving glycemic control as assessed by near-normal HbA_{1c} level. In diabetic subjects, an aggressive treatment of hypertension with an ACE inhibitor or an angiotensin receptor blocking (ARB) agent is mandatory.

10.3.3 Aspirin and Other Antiplatelet Agents: Mechanism of Action and Use in MPNs

Aspirin is a salicylic acid derivative having anti-inflammatory, analgesic, antipyretic, anti-rheumatic and antithrombotic activity. It is rapidly absorbed in the stomach and upper small intestine and hydrolyzed primarily in the liver to salicylic acid. This is then conjugated with glycine and glucuronic acid and excreted in the urine. The aspirin half-life is approximately 20 min, but its antiplatelet effect lasts for the all lifespan of circulating platelets due to the permanent inactivation of prostaglandin PGH-synthase, also referred to as COX-1 (Patrono 1994). This isozyme catalyzes, as prostaglandin PGH-synthase 2 or COX-2, the conversion of arachidonate to prostaglandin $(PG)H_2$, which is a substrate for several downstream isomerases that generate different bioactive prostanoids, including thromboxane (TX) A_2 and prostacyclin (PGI_2) (Vane 1971).

Thromboxane (TX) A_2 is the main platelet prostanoid and is capable to induce irreversible platelet aggregation, vasoconstriction, vascular smooth muscle cell proliferation and atherogenic process (Patrono et al. 1985). The clinical pharmacology of platelet COX inhibition by aspirin has been investigated through measurements of serum and urinary excretion of TXB_2 metabolites (Patrono et al. 1986). Single oral doses of 5–100 mg of aspirin result in dose-dependent inhibition of platelet COX activity, with 100 mg almost completely suppressing the biosynthesis of TXA_2 in normal subjects and in patients with atherosclerotic vascular disease as well as in PV and ET subjects with very high platelet count (Landolfi et al. 1992; Patrono et al. 1994; Rocca et al. 1995). Biochemical, pharmacological and clinical observations support the concept that the inactivation of platelet prostaglandin G/H synthase and, overall, ability to irreversibly suppress the synthesis of TXA_2 platelet largely account for the antithrombotic effect of aspirin (Patrono et al. 2005). The pathways of platelet activation targeted by aspirin and other antiplatelet drugs are shown in Fig. 10.2.

In the general population, the efficacy of aspirin in reducing myocardial infarction, stroke and

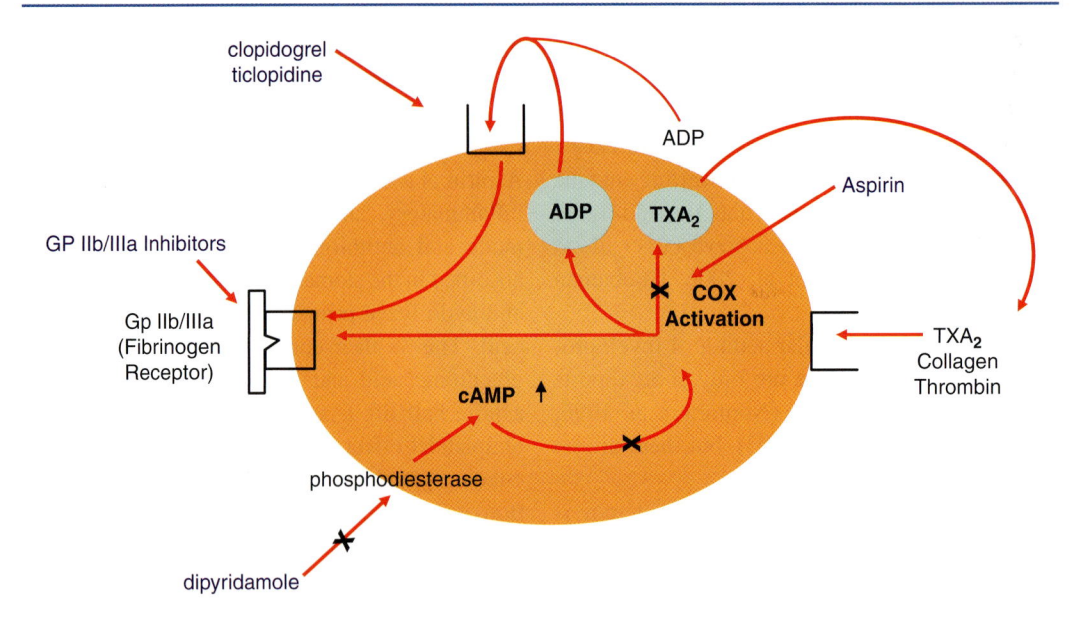

Fig. 10.2 Mechanism of action of main antiplatelet agents (Modified from Schafer (1996)). *ADP* adenosine diphosphate, *cAMP* cyclic adenosine monophosphate, *COX* cyclooxygenase, *TXA*$_2$ thromboxane A$_2$

vascular disease death in men and women with established cardiovascular disease is well known so that life-long aspirin administration is recommended in the majority of these subjects. The benefit risk ratio of aspirin use as primary prevention in subjects with no vascular risk is less clear.

A recent meta-analysis of primary prevention studies found a significant 12% relative risk reduction of vascular events by aspirin, with no significant difference among different risk categories (Baigent et al. 2009). The risk of myocardial infarction was reduced, as in secondary prevention, by approximately 30% while there was no significant effect on stroke.

However, aspirin significantly increased also the risk of bleeding, mostly gastrointestinal, in both men and women so that up to a certain vascular risk (2% per annum), benefits were offset by the harms. Particularly in patients with history of gastrointestinal disease or symptoms, physicians should weigh the potential harms of aspirin being aware that available evidence indicates that the use of an alternative antiplatelet agent such as clopidogrel is associated with a hemorrhagic risk similar to that of low-dose aspirin (Chan et al. 2005; Patrono et al. 2005).

Several findings indicate that in MPNs, the benefit/risk profile of aspirin use may have a favourable benefit/risk ratio also in subjects at low vascular risk.

First, one should consider that the so-called low-risk PV and ET subjects have a vascular risk of approximately 2% per annum (Marchioli et al. 2005; Tefferi 2011) which, in the general population, is a widely accepted threshold for aspirin use. In addition, the hypothesis of a high aspirin efficacy in MPNs subjects is supported by both clinical and pharmacological studies. All microvascular disturbances in PV and ET have been also attributed to platelet aggregate formation and have been shown to be selectively sensitive to low dose of aspirin. This evidence allowed to attribute the pathogenesis of these disturbances to a TXA$_2$-dependent mechanism (Van Genderen et al. 1997; Michiels 1997). On the other hand, TXA$_2$ biosynthesis in vivo is markedly increased in the majority of PV and ET patients, as shown by the stable increase in the urinary excretion of the major TXA$_2$ metabolites 11-dehydro-TXB$_2$ and 2,3-dinor-TXB$_2$ found in asymptomatic subjects (Landolfi et al. 1992; Rocca et al. 1995; Patrono et al. 1994). Thromboxane hyperproduction, for being abolished by very low aspirin dose, reflects an increased platelet production in response to physiological stimuli. TX biosynthesis is relatively independent from haematocrit, platelet count, treatment and clinical history, thus suggesting an abnormal in vivo platelet activation selectively sensitive to aspirin.

In PV patients, aspirin administration was first evaluated in a small size trial performed by the Polycythemia Vera Study Group. In this study, 163 PV patients were randomized to be treated with radiophosphorus or phlebotomy plus an antiplatelet therapy constituted by a combination of high-dose aspirin (900 mg/day) and dipyridamole. After a follow-up of about 17 months, the trial was stopped due to an excess of major gastrointestinal bleedings in the aspirin arm (Tartaglia et al. 1986).

Risks and benefits of a much lower aspirin dose were more recently reassessed by the ECLAP study which can be considered a primary prophylaxis trial (Landolfi et al. 2004). This trial randomized 532 PV subjects to receive 100 mg aspirin or placebo. After a follow-up of about 3 years, data analysis showed a significant reduction (RR 0.41) of major thromboses (both arterial and venous) without a significant increase of hemorrhagic complications in the aspirin group. The high aspirin efficacy and the uniform sensitivity of all events to this agent support the hypothesis of a key role of platelet thromboxane in the pathogenesis of PV thrombophilia.

In low-risk ET patients, low-dose aspirin has never been tested in prospective randomized clinical trial. Recently, the benefit of low-dose aspirin was retrospectively investigated in a low-risk ET population (Alvarez-Larran et al. 2010). The authors compared the incidence rates of arterial and venous thrombosis in low-risk ET patients treated with antiplatelet drugs with that of patients who did not receive this treatment. While the overall rate of thrombotic events was not significantly different between the two patient groups, aspirin seemed to protect from venous thrombosis JAK2V617F-positive subjects and from arterial thrombosis patients with cardiovascular risk factors (IRR: 2.5; 95% CI: 1.02–6.1; $p = 0.047$).

These data seem to support the current attitude to extend to the vast majority of PV and ET subjects the use of aspirin at low doses (50–100 mg/day), provided there are no contraindications (Landolfi et al. 2004; Tefferi 2011). In this regard, defining aspirin contraindication may be controversial. While allergy to aspirin constitutes a true contraindication to its use (Touraine et al. 2005), history of gastrointestinal disease or symptoms should only lead to more carefully weigh the potential harms of aspirin use against its benefits (Chan et al. 2005; Patrono et al. 2005).

As in general population, another antiplatelet agent can be recommended for patients who are unable to take aspirin because of an aspirin allergy (Baigent et al. 2009). The mechanism of action of thienopyridine antiplatelet agents (ticlopidine and clopidogrel) and dipyridamole is showed in Fig. 10.2.

Thienopyridines (ticlopidine and clopidogrel), also known as ADP receptor antagonist, have been shown to have an important role in the management of atherosclerotic (cerebral, cardiac and peripheral) vascular disease in the general population (Patrono and Rocca 2010).

Dipyridamole, by inhibiting phosphodiesterase, increases the levels of c-AMP which serves as an intracellular signal to suppress platelet activation and subsequent aggregation. Therefore, this agent, when used in conjunction with aspirin, has been demonstrated to have a role particularly in the secondary prevention of stroke (Halkes et al. 2006).

As shown in Fig. 10.2, we have also considered GP IIb/IIIa antagonists (abciximab, tirofiban and eptifibatide), which block the final common pathway for platelet aggregation and represent potent antiplatelet drugs. These drugs are, however, particularly indicated as adjunctive therapy during percutaneous coronary intervention.

As discussed below, an aggressive antithrombotic strategy based on the combination of aspirin with another antiplatelet drug, such as ticlopidine or clopidogrel in patients with previous myocardial infarction or with dipyridamole in patients with previous stroke, might be most beneficial in avoiding a recurrence of thrombotic event. Interestingly, clopidogrel has been reported to reduce parameters of leukocyte activation (Evangelista et al. 2005), and thus its use may be more appropriate in MPNs patients in whom the thrombophilic state is increasingly attributed to platelet and leukocyte activation and to platelet-leukocyte interaction. However, no data are available as to a different efficacy or safety of clopidogrel in this specific setting. This is an important issue since, as reported above, several findings indicate that the thrombotic diathesis of PV and ET patients may have, in comparison to that of general population, peculiar features which include an increased of sensitivity to aspirin. Certainly many of MPNs patients are being given clopidogrel after an acute coronary syndrome or a percutaneous revascularization, but at the moment, there is a paucity of data on the use of thienopyridines in prevention or therapy of thrombosis in myeloproliferative disorders. In the next future, a more aggressive antiplatelet regimen, such as that based on the combined antiplatelet therapy, might be proposed and tested in subjects with very high risk of thrombosis and low bleeding risk as it has been suggested in particular cases, such as recurrence of thrombosis in aspirin-treated patients (Tefferi 2011). This issue is further discussed in the primary prevention section.

10.4 Cytoreductive Strategies in Patients with Different Vascular Risk

The most appropriate cytoreductive strategy in the individual patient has to be chosen on the basis of the vascular risk. Most young patients with no vascular history have a low or intermediate vascular risk. Patient older than 65 years with three traditional cardiovascular risk factors and patient with previous vascular event should be considered at the same risk (see Table 10.1).

In the chart reported in Table 10.1, patient assignment to a certain risk level is made by the use of a scoring system. This system has the advantage of considering the impact of age in a more progressive manner than that based on a single threshold level and considers several other cardiovascular risk factors (Marchioli et al. 2005; Carobbio et al. 2007; Landolfi et al. 2007; Gangat et al. 2009; Tefferi 2011). Also some laboratory

disease-related parameters are considered. For example, a high white blood cell count might contribute to change the patient's risk stratification (Landolfi et al. 2007; Carobbio et al. 2007; Alvarez-Larrán et al. 2007). Multivariate analysis of data from the ECLAP observational study arm in PV patients showed that the risk of arterial thrombosis, particularly of myocardial infarction, was increased in patients with white blood cell count higher than $>10 \times 10^9$/L. This increase was statistically significant when WBC was higher than 15×10^9/L (hazard ratio 1.71; 95% confidence interval 1.10–2.65; $P=0.0171$) (Landolfi et al. 2007). Leukocytosis was found a risk factor for thrombosis also confirmed in ET subjects (Carobbio et al. 2007; Gangat et al. 2007).

There is currently no evidence that cytoreductive treatment other than phlebotomy is needed for low- and intermediate-risk PV patients with PV. Cytoreductive therapy for both PV and ET is not curative, and there is little evidence to suggest a favourable effect on thrombosis-free survival. However, this is based on studies of relatively small size, and additional data from large clinical trials are needed. Avoiding cytoreduction is generally recommended also for low-risk ET patients. Thrombotic deaths seem very rare in low-risk ET patients, and there are no data indicating that fatalities can be prevented by starting cytoreductive drugs early. Treatment of intermediate ET risk subjects is quite controversial since the thrombotic risk may not be high enough to justify the use of potentially mutagenic or toxic drugs. The safety of hydroxyurea is still debated while anagrelide is associated with several side effects which include palpitations, congestive heart failure, headache and depression, and its long-term effects are unknown. Also IFN therapy has well-known side effects. Thus, treatment of intermediate-risk subjects must be individualized, with frank discussion with the patient regarding the potential risks and side effects of cytoreductive therapy. An indication to cytoreductive treatment is extreme thrombocytosis (i.e., platelet count $>1,500 \times 10^9$/L) or the presence of bleeding symptoms since aspirin use may cause major bleeding in these subjects. Interferon-α is preferred to HU in high-risk women of child-bearing potential.

Interferon is also the first choice in all the subjects intolerant or resistant to HU (Kiladjian et al. 2008). Anagrelide has a potent platelet-reducing activity devoid of leukemogenic potential and may be an alternative to HU in younger patients. Risks and benefits of this drug were evaluated in large retrospective analysis (Fruchtman et al. 2005) and by a randomized clinical trial comparing anagrelide and HU (Harrison et al. 2005) in aspirin-treated ET subjects. This trial showed the superior efficacy of HU, thus indicating that in high-risk patients, anagrelide should be used in subjects resistant or intolerant to HU or in young subjects with intermediate vascular risk.

10.5   Secondary Prevention

A large retrospective study by De Stefano et al. analysed a cohort of 494 high-risk patients (235 PV and 259 ET subjects) who had suffered from at least one major thrombotic event (De Stefano et al. 2008). In this study, arterial thromboses accounted for 69% of thrombotic events, and cerebrovascular accidents were about 39% of these events. The re-thrombosis preferentially occurred in the same district of the first event as observed also in PV subjects followed in the ECLAP observational study (Landolfi et al. 2007). Hereditary thrombophilic states and high leukocyte were found to be associated with a higher risk of recurrence, thrombotic risk being higher in the 2 years after the first thrombotic event and slowly declining thereafter (De Stefano et al. 2008). In patients with first arterial thrombosis, aspirin use was associated with about a quarter of reduction in the risk of recurrence, thus showing a benefit similar to that observed in the general population of patients with previous myocardial infarction or previous cerebrovascular event (Baigent et al. 2009). In fact, in patients with vascular history, aspirin reduces the risk of a vascular event (non-fatal myocardial infarction, non-fatal stroke or vascular death) by approximately one-quarter, this resulting from one-third reduction in non-fatal myocardial infarction, one-quarter reduction in non-fatal stroke and one-sixth reduction in death from a vascular or unknown cause (Baigent et al. 2009). As reported in Table 10.1, all patients with vascular history should receive HU in addition to aspirin. In patients with very high thrombotic risk or having a recurrence while receiving aspirin, a different and more aggressive antithrombotic treatment may be considered, according to the type of event. Below, we discuss the antithrombotic strategy to be chosen in the secondary prevention of cerebrovascular and cardiovascular events as well as after venous thromboembolism.

10.5.1   Secondary Prevention of Cerebrovascular Events

In this paragraph, we will not discuss the use of thrombolytic therapy in acute stroke. We have no data about these treatments in MPNs subjects. However, in selected cases, according to current guidelines, the use of thrombolytic drugs such as recombinant tissue plasminogen activator (r-TPA), streptokinase, or urokinase might be safe also in these patients.

In acute ischemic stroke, in the absence of contraindications, clinicians should administer aspirin therapy (initial dose of 150–325 mg followed by 75–100 mg/die) (Albers et al. 2008). The use of aspirin within 48 h of stroke onset can reduce both stroke recurrence risk and mortality (Sandercock et al. 1997; Chen et al. 1997), while there is no evidence that early treatment with anticoagulants decreases mortality.

Moreover, it is reasonable that PV or ET patients with stroke should also begin HU in order to minimize their risk (starting dose 500 mg twice per day). The dose of HU is aimed to keep platelet count lower than 400×10^9/L and leukocyte count higher than 2×10^9/L (Tefferi and Vainchenker 2011). As in general population, also in MPNs, subjects with stroke, oral anticoagulation can be suggested only in case of concomitant atrial fibrillation with rheumatic heart disease, prosthetic heart valves, or intracardiac thrombus, documented intraluminal thrombus, or arterial dissections (Albers et al. 2008). Aspirin may be used safely in combination with low-dose heparin also for deep venous thrombosis prophylaxis. In fact, venous thrombosis is a frequent complication of stroke, with about 5% of early deaths attributed to pulmonary embolism (Collins et al. 1994).

In general population, the combination of aspirin 25 mg and extended-release dipyridamole 200 mg twice daily, and clopidogrel 75 mg/die are all acceptable options for secondary prevention stroke or TIA. However, in MPNs, aspirin use seems to have an efficacy on cerebral ischemic events not found in other clinical conditions, and this may be related to the suggested role of thromboxane hyperproduction in the thrombotic tendency of these patients. In PV and ET patients with history of cerebrovascular disease, aspirin use was found associated with a 67% reduction in the risk of recurrence (De Stefano et al. 2008). However, in patients having a stroke recurrence under aspirin treatment, the combination of aspirin with dipyridamole or the use of clopidogrel can be considered.

10.5.2 Secondary Prevention in Acute Coronary Syndromes

Antithrombotic therapy is a mainstay in the management of patients with acute coronary artery disease. As in general population, PV and ET patients with acute coronary syndrome should be treated with aspirin initially at a dose 160–200 mg and then indefinitely at a dose of 75–100 mg/die in the absence of contraindication. In all patients, aspirin should be associated with clopidogrel at a daily dose of 75 mg, and this dual treatment should be continued for at least 12 months (Becker et al. 2008). In case of allergy to aspirin, only clopidogrel can be prescribed. Moreover, ACE inhibitors and beta-blockers have to be continued indefinitely in all patients, and clinicians have to assess fasting lipid profile within 24 h of hospitalization and initiate lipid-lowering medication to maintain low-density lipoprotein cholesterol lower than 100 mg/dL. For patients with a large anterior myocardial infarction, significant heart failure, intracardiac thrombus shown by transthoracic echocardiography, atrial fibrillation, and with a history of a thromboembolic event, we suggest the combined use of moderate-intensity

(INR, 2.0–3.0) oral VKA plus low-dose aspirin (<100 mg/day) for at least 3 months after acute coronary event. All these recommendations are based on studies performed in the general population. In MPNs, patients with coronary syndromes, an aggressive pharmacological cytoreduction is also recommended since several findings indicate that hydroxyurea is very effective in secondary prevention of coronary syndromes (Harrison et al. 2005; De Stefano et al. 2008).

For all MPN patients with previous acute coronary syndromes, the use of HU and low-dose aspirin (75–100 mg/die) is mandatory. Although there is no convincing evidence of a differential efficacy of aspirin and hydroxyurea in the various arterial districts, patients with previous myocardial infarction should be treated with these two agents with a possible indication to a more aggressive use of hydroxyurea in subjects with previous myocardial infarction and persistent leukocytosis. In fact, in a prospective study performed from GIMEMA-MPD Group (De Stefano et al. 2008), a multivariate analysis showed that cytoreduction was independently effective in preventing recurrence of thrombosis and reduced the risk by 47%. This efficacy resulted more pronounced in patients with a first coronary syndrome, in which there was a 70% reduction in the risk of a recurrence of coronary event (De Stefano et al. 2008). In addition, leukocytosis was found associated with a high risk of MI recurrence (Landolfi et al. 2007).

For patients with previous large anterior MI, significant heart failure and atrial fibrillation, the combined use of moderate-intensity (INR, 2.0–3.0) oral VKA plus low-dose aspirin (<100 mg/day) for at least 3 months after the MI can be suggested.

Finally, one should consider the possibility that in patients at very high vascular risk, the association of aspirin with clopidogrel might be continued for more than the recommended 12 months.

10.5.3 Secondary Prevention of Venous Thromboembolism

Treatment of venous thrombosis in PV and ET patients should not differ from that recommended in the general population (Hirsh et al. 2008;

Geerts et al. 2008) where unfractionated heparin, low molecular weight heparins, or fondaparinux are used whenever a rapid anticoagulation is needed, and oral anticoagulants are the treatment of choice beyond the acute phase.

Low molecular weight heparins, in comparison to unfractionated heparin, have a more predictable anticoagulant activity since a variable resistance to unfractionated heparin may arise from increased heparin clearance, elevations in fibrinogen or factor VIII levels and elevations of heparin-binding proteins in plasma. Among these proteins, one has to consider the role of platelet factor 4, which is likely to be more abundantly released in patients with thrombocytosis and/or increased platelet activation (Gayoso 1999). This might support the preferential use of low molecular weight heparins in MPN subjects (Landolfi et al. 2008).

Unfractionated heparin is preferred in patients with renal failure or in case of low molecular weight heparins unavailability. Acute treatment with heparins has to be initiated as soon as possible with oral anticoagulant and continued until INR is ≥2.0 for at least 24 h.

In the general population, oral anticoagulation is continued for at least 3 months. Longer treatment durations are recommended in cases of recurrence or in presence severe of a major thrombophilic condition. Myeloproliferative neoplasms are one of such states, but decisions on optimal treatment duration have to consider additional variables such as the treatment of underlying disease as well as the location of thrombosis. Deep vein thrombosis of lower limbs in patients with unrecognized disease or in subjects not receiving chemotherapy can be treated by cytoreduction and a short-term anticoagulation (3–6 months) followed by low-dose aspirin. In fact, differently from general population, in patients with MPNs, aspirin seems efficacious also in venous thromboembolism (Landolfi et al. 2004; De Stefano et al. 2008). Therefore, in case of a first venous thrombosis, an indefinite use of aspirin could be acceptable as an alternative strategy after a limited period of oral anticoagulant therapy.

Long-term treatment of VTE manifesting in patients receiving chemotherapy and aspirin may be more controversial.

Cytoreduction in patients with first venous thrombosis resulted associated with about a 30% reduction in the risk of recurrence (De Stefano et al. 2008). In PT-1 trial HU, aspirin-treated patients seemed to show a lower efficacy in preventing venous thromboembolism compared to anagrelide (Harrison et al. 2005).

10.6 Concluding Remarks

The search for new antithrombotic strategies for PV and ET subjects has undoubtedly become a priority for future research. Early recognition of the myeloproliferative disorder and wider use of aspirin and cytoreduction have likely contributed to lower the incidence of thrombotic events. However, thrombotic recurrences in patients with thrombotic history remain unacceptably high. Physicians' awareness of such a high risk needs to be increased in order to avoid an overestimation of the neoplastic risk of hydroxyurea in high-risk young subjects and/or of the bleeding risk of patients with gastrointestinal symptoms. In addition, in very high-risk patients, the association of hydroxyurea and aspirin, which is currently viewed as an aggressive treatment, does not seem well suited to the patients' risk level. This calls for the adoption of more aggressive antithrombotic or cytoreductive strategies or for the search for novel treatment approaches.

References

Albers GW, Amarenco P, Easton JD et al (2008) Antithrombotic and thrombolytic therapy for ischemic stroke: American College of Chest Physicians Evidence-Based Clinical Practice Guidelines (8th Edition). Chest 133:630S–669S

Alvarez-Larrán A, Cervantes F, Bellosillo B et al (2007) Essential thrombocythemia in young individuals: frequency and risk factors for vascular events and evolution to myelofibrosis in 126 patients. Leukemia 21: 1218–1223

Alvarez-Larrán A, Cervantes F, Pereira A et al (2010) Observation versus antiplatelet therapy as primary prophylaxis for thrombosis in low-risk essential thrombocythemia. Blood 116:1205–1210

Baigent C, Blackwell L, Collins R, Antithrombotic Trialists' (ATT) Collaboration et al (2009) Aspirin in the primary and secondary prevention of vascular disease: collaborative meta-analysis of individual participant data from randomised trials. Lancet 373: 1849–1860

Barbui T, Barosi G, Grossi A et al (2004) Practice guidelines for the therapy of essential thrombocythemia. A statement from the Italian Society of Hematology, the Italian Society of Experimental Hematology and the Italian Group for Bone Marrow Transplantation. Haematologica 89:215–232

Barbui T, Barosi G, Birgegard G et al (2011a) Philadelphia-negative classical myeloproliferative neoplasms: critical concepts and management recommendations from European LeukemiaNet. J Clin Oncol 29:761–770

Barbui T, Carobbio A, Finazzi G et al (2011b) Inflammation and thrombosis in essential thrombocythemia and polycythemia vera: different role of C-reactive protein and Pentraxin 3. Haematologica 96:315–318

Becker RC, Meade TW, Berger PB, American College of Chest Physicians et al (2008) The primary and secondary prevention of coronary artery disease: American College of Chest Physicians Evidence-Based Clinical Practice Guidelines (8th Edition). Chest 133:776S–814S

Berk P, Wasserman LR, Fruchtman SM et al (1995) Treatment of polycythemia vera: a summary of clinical trials conducted by the Polycythemia Vera study Group. In: Wasserman LR, Berk PD, Berlin NI (eds) Polycythemia vera and the myeloproliferative disorders. Saunders, Philadelphia

Besses C, Cervantes F, Pereira A et al (1999) Major vascular complications in essential thrombocythemia: a study of the predictive factors in a series of 148 patients. Leukemia 13:150–154

Briere JB (2006) Budd-Chiari syndrome and portal vein thrombosis associated with myeloproliferative disorders: diagnosis and management. Semin Thromb Haemost 32:208–218

Carobbio A, Finazzi G, Guerini V et al (2007) Leukocytosis is a risk factor for thrombosis in essential thrombocythemia: interaction with treatment, standard risk factors and Jak2 mutation status. Blood 109:2310–2313

Cervantes F, Passamonti F, Barosi G (2008) Life expectancy and prognostic factors in the classic BCR/ABL-negative myeloproliferative disorders. Leukemia 22:905–914

Chait Y, Condat B, Casalz-Hatem D et al (2005) Relevance of the criteria commonly used to diagnose myeloproliferative disorder in patients with splanchnic thrombosis. Br J Haematol 129:553–560

Chan FK, Ching JY, Hung LC et al (2005) Clopidogrel versus aspirin and esomeprazole to prevent recurrent ulcer bleeding. N Engl J Med 352:238–244

Chen ZM, Collins R, Liu LS et al (1997) CAST (Chinese Acute Stroke Trial) Collaborative Group. Randomised placebo-controlled trial of early aspirin use in 20,000 patients with acute ischaemic stroke. Lancet 349: 1641–1649

Chobanian AV, Bakris GL, Black HR et al (2003) Seventh report of the Joint National Committee on Prevention, Detection, Evaluation, and Treatment of High Blood Pressure. Hypertension 42:1206–1252

Collins R, Peto R, Baigent C et al (1994) Antiplatelet Trialists' Collaboration. Collaborative overview of randomised trials of antiplatelet therapy: III. Reduction in venous thrombosis and pulmonary embolism by antiplatelet prophylaxis among surgical and medical patients. BMJ 308:235–246

Crisa E, Venturino E, Passera R et al (2010) A retrospective study on 226 polycythemia vera patients: impact of median hematocrit value on clinical outcomes and survival improvement with anti-thrombotic prophylaxis and non-alkylating drugs. Ann Hematol 89:691–699

De Stefano V, Za T, Rossi E et al (2008) Recurrent thrombosis in patients with polycythemia vera and essential thrombocythemia: incidence, risk factors, and effect of treatments. Haematologica 93:372–380

Di Nisio M, Barbui T, Di Gennaro L et al (2007) The haematocrit and platelet target in polycythemia vera. Br J Haematol 136:249–259

Evangelista V, Manarini S, Dell'Elba G et al (2005) Clopidogrel inhibits platelet-leukocyte adhesion and platelet-dependent leukocyte activation. Thromb Haemost 94:568

Finazzi G, Barbui T (2005) Risk-adapted therapy in essential thrombocythemia and polycythemia vera. Blood Rev 19:243–252

Fruchtman SM, Petitt RM, Gilbert HS et al (2005) Anagrelide: analysis of long term efficacy, safety and leukemogenic potential in myeloproliferative diseases. Leuk Res 29:481–491

Gangat N, Wolanskyj AP, McClure RF et al (2007) Risk stratification for survival and leukemic transformation in essential thrombocythemia: a single institutional study of 605 patients. Leukemia 21:271–276

Gangat N, Wolanskyj AP, Schwager SM et al (2009) Leukocytosis at diagnosis and the risk of subsequent thrombosis in patients with low-risk essential thrombocythemia and polycythemia vera. Cancer 115: 5740–5745

Gayoso JM (1999) 5-year incidence of thrombocytosis and the effect on heparin dose response and heparin requirements. J Extra Corpor Technol 31:184–190

Geerts WH, Bergqvist D, Pineo GF, American College of Chest Physicians et al (2008) Prevention of venous thromboembolism: American College of Chest Physicians Evidence-Based Clinical Practice Guidelines (8th Edition). Chest 133:381S–453S

Greenland P, Alpert JS, Beller GA et al (2010) ACCF/AHA guideline for assessment of cardiovascular risk in asymptomatic adults: a report of the American College of Cardiology Foundation/American Heart Association Task Force on Practice Guidelines. J Am Coll Cardiol 56:e50–e103

Griesshammer M, Struve S, Harrison CM (2006) Essential thrombocythemia/polycythemia vera and pregnancy: the need for an observational study in Europe. Semin Thromb Hemost 32:422–429

Halkes PH, van Gijn J, Kappelle LJ et al (2006) Aspirin plus dipyridamole versus aspirin alone after cerebral ischaemia of arterial origin (ESPRIT): randomised controlled trial. Lancet 367:1665–1673

Harrison CN, Campbell PJ, Buck G et al (2005) A randomized comparison of hydroxyurea with anagrelide in high-risk essential thrombocythemia. N Engl J Med 353:33–45

Hasselbalch HC, Riley CH (2006) Statins in the treatment of polycythaemia vera and allied disorders: an antithrombotic and cytoreductive potential? Leuk Res 30:1217–1225

Hirsh J, Guyatt G, Albers GW et al (2008) Antithrombotic and thrombolytic therapy: American College of Chest Physicians Evidence-Based Clinical Practice Guidelines (8th Edition). Chest 133:110–112

Jantunen R, Juvonen E, Ikkala E et al (2001) The predictive value of vascular risk factors and gender for the development of thrombotic complications in essential thrombocythemia. Ann Hematol 80:74–78

Kiladjian JJ, Cassinat B, Chevret S et al (2008) Pegylated interferon-alfa-2a induces complete hematological and molecular responses with low toxicity in polycythemia vera. Blood 112:3065–3072

Landolfi R, Di Gennaro L (2011) Pathophysiology of thrombosis in myeloproliferative neoplasms. Haematologica 96:183–186

Landolfi R, Ciabattoni G, Patrignani P et al (1992) Increased thromboxane biosynthesis in patients with polycythemia vera: evidence for aspirin-suppressible platelet activation in vivo. Blood 80:1965–1971

Landolfi R, Marchioli R, Kutti J et al (2004) Efficacy and safety of low-dose aspirin in polycythemia vera. N Engl J Med 350:114–124

Landolfi R, Cipriani MC, Novarese L (2006) Thrombosis and bleeding in polycythemia vera and essential thrombocythemia: pathogenetic mechanisms and prevention. Best Pract Res Clin Haematol 19:617–633

Landolfi R, Di Gennaro L, Barbui T et al (2007) Leukocytosis as a major thrombotic risk factor in patients with polycythemia vera. Blood 109:2446–2452

Landolfi R, Di Gennaro L, Falanga A (2008) Thrombosis in myeloproliferative disorders: pathogenetic facts and speculation. Leukemia 22:2020–2028

Marchioli R, Finazzi G, Landolfi R et al (2005) Vascular and neoplastic risk in a large cohort of patients with polycythemia vera. J Clin Oncol 23:2224–2232

Marusic-Vrsalovic M, Dominis M, Jaksic B, Kusec R (2003) Angiotensin I-converting enzyme is expressed by erythropoietic cells of normal and myeloproliferative bone marrow. Br J Haematol 123:539–541

McTigue KM, Harris R, Hemphill B et al (2003) Screening and interventions for obesity in adults: summary of the evidence for the U.S. Preventive Services Task Force. Ann Intern Med 139:933–949

Messinezy M, Pearson TC, Pochazka A et al (1985) Treatment of primary proliferative polycythemia by venesection and low dose busulphan. Retrospective study from one centre. Br J Haematol 61:657–666

Michiels JJ (1997) Erythromelalgia and thrombocythemia: a disease of platelet prostaglandin metabolism. Semin Thromb Hemost 23:335–338

Michiels JJ, Berneman Z, Bockstaele DV et al (2006a) Clinical and laboratory features, pathology of platelet-mediated thrombosis and bleeding complications and the molecular etiology of essential thrombocythemia and polycythemia vera: therapeutic implications. Semin Thromb Hemost 32:174–207

Michiels JJ, Berneman Z, Schroyens W et al (2006b) The paradox of platelet activation and impaired function: Platelet-von Willebrand factor interactions, and the etiology of thrombotic and hemorrhagic manifestations in essential thrombocythemia and polycythemia vera. Semin Thromb Hemost 32:589–604

Nomura S, Sugihara T, Tomiyama T et al (1996) Polycythaemia vera: response to treatment with angiotensin-converting enzyme inhibitor. Eur J Haematol 57:117–119

Passamonti F, Rumi E, Pungolino E et al (2004) Life expectancy and prognostic factors for survival in patients with polycythemia vera and essential thrombocythemia. Am J Med 117:755–761

Patrono C (1994) Aspirin as an antiplatelet drug. N Engl J Med 330:1287–1294

Patrono C, Rocca B (2010) The future of antiplatelet therapy in cardiovascular disease. Annu Rev Med 61:49–61

Patrono C, Ciabattoni G, Patrignani P et al (1985) Clinical pharmacology of platelet cyclooxygenase inhibition. Circulation 72:1177–1184

Patrono C, Ciabattoni G, Pugliese F et al (1986) Estimated rate of thromboxane secretion into the circulation of normal humans. J Clin Invest 77:590–594

Patrono C, Ciabattoni G, Patrignani P et al (1994) Eicosanoid biosynthesis and metabolism in myeloproliferative disorders. Ann N Y Acad Sci 744:229–236

Patrono C, García Rodríguez LA, Landolfi R, Baigent C (2005) Low-dose aspirin for the prevention of atherothrombosis. N Engl J Med 353:2373–2383

Pearson TC (1997) Hemorheologic considerations in the pathogenesis of vascular occlusive events in polycythemia vera. Semin Thromb Hemost 23:433–439

Pearson TC, Wetherley-Mein G (1978) Vascular occlusive episodes and venous haematocrit in primary proliferative polycythaemia. Lancet 2:1219–1222

Rocca B, Ciabattoni G, Tartaglione R et al (1995) Increased thromboxane biosynthesis in essential thrombocythemia. Thromb Haemost 74:1225–1230

Sandercock P, Collins R, Counsell C et al (1997) International Stroke Trial (IST). A randomised trial of aspirin, subcutaneous heparin, both, or neither among 19435 patients with acute ischaemic stroke: International Stroke Trial Collaborative Group. Lancet 349:1569–1581

Schafer AI (1996) Antiplatelet therapy. Am J Med 101: 199–209

Smith SC, Allen J, Blair S et al (2006) AHA/ACC guidelines for secondary prevention for patients with coronary and other atherosclerotic vascular disease: 2006 update. J Am Coll Cardiol 47:2130–2139

Tartaglia AP, Goldberg JD, Berk PD et al (1986) Adverse effects of antiaggregating platelet therapy in the treatment of polycythemia vera. Semin Hematol 23:172–176

Tefferi A (2011) Annual clinical updates in hematological malignancies: a continuing medical education series:

polycythemia vera and essential thrombocythemia: 2011 update on diagnosis, risk-stratification, and management. Am J Hematol 86:292–301

Tefferi A, Vainchenker W (2011) Myeloproliferative neoplasms: molecular pathophysiology, essential clinical understanding, and treatment strategies. J Clin Oncol 29:573–582

Touraine F, Moldovan D, Touraine P et al (2005) Aspirin and non steroidal anti-inflammatory drugs hypersensitivity review (2002–2004). Allerg Immunol 37:279–282

van Genderen PJ, Mulder PG, Waleboer M et al (1997) Prevention and treatment of thrombotic complications in essential thrombocythemia: efficacy and safety of aspirin. Br J Haematol 97:179–184

Vane JR (1971) Inhibition of prostaglandin synthesis as a mechanism of action for aspirin-like drugs. Nat New Biol 231:232–235

Polycythemia Vera and Essential Thrombocythemia: When to Change Therapy – Second-Line Options

11

Alessandro M. Vannucchi

Contents

11.1 Introduction

The management of a patient with polycythemia vera (PV) or essential thrombocythemia (ET) who fails, or develops intolerance to, first-line therapy is an "orphan" field in terms of evidence-based experience as well as number and characteristics of available conventional drugs. On the contrary, it is becoming an "ever-changing" field as concerns novel drugs since, in the last couple of years, trials with JAK1 and JAK2 inhibitors or histone deacetylase inhibitors have included only the category of patients refractory or intolerant to hydroxyurea, who are the most obvious candidates to second-line therapy. In this chapter, we will discuss only about conventional drugs that are currently employed for second-line treatment, while novel drugs are the topic of Chap. 18.

11.2 When to Consider Shifting a Patient to Second-Line Therapy

Two different situations could be envisaged for considering "second-line" therapy for PV or ET (Barbui et al. 2011) (Table 11.1).

The first case is that of a low-risk patient (young age, no thrombotic history, no overwhelming cardiovascular risk factors) who has been managed for some time with phlebotomies plus low-dose aspirin (in case of PV) or observation only plus/minus aspirin (in case of ET) and

A.M. Vannucchi
Section of Hematology,
University of Florence,
Florence, Italy
e-mail: amvannucchi@unifi.it

Table 11.1 ELN criteria for patient shifting to second-line therapy in case of "low-risk" and "high-risk" patients with PV or ET

Polycythemia vera	Essential thrombocythemia
Low-risk	
Shift to high-risk category	Shift to high-risk category
Uncontrolled leuko-/thrombocytosis	Increase of platelet count >1,500×10⁹/L
Significant spleen enlargement	
Intolerance/too many phlebotomies	
High-risk	
Intolerant to first-line therapy	Intolerant to first-line therapy
Resistant to first-line therapy	Resistant to first-line therapy

is currently in need of treatment with cytotoxic drugs. Reasons for becoming "in need of a treatment" might be represented by a shift in risk category (i.e., the patient becomes "high risk" because of aging or the development of major cardiovascular event(s)) or the worsening of the illness as manifested by: uncontrolled myeloproliferation (progressive leukocytosis; thrombocytosis greater than $1,500 \times 10^9$/L, known to be associated with an increased risk of hemorrhages); poor tolerance to, or a too high rate of, phlebotomies (in case of PV); progressive enlargement of the spleen that eventually becomes symptomatic; and occurrence of severe systemic manifestations. In these instances, the therapeutic attitude is the same as for first-treated high-risk subjects (Barbui et al. 2011; Barbui and Finazzi 2005; Finazzi and Barbui 2007; Vannucchi and Guglielmelli 2010; Vannucchi et al. 2009): hydroxyurea and/or interferon-alpha is the drug of choice, considering that interferon availability is regulated by country-specific laws and provided it is not otherwise contraindicated.

The second case is that of a "high-risk" patient who has already been managed for a while with first-line therapy based on hydroxyurea or interferon-alpha, plus low-dose aspirin, and currently develops intolerance or refractoriness to this treatment.

11.3 Intolerance or Refractoriness to Hydroxyurea

Most patients on hydroxyurea respond to, and tolerate quite well, adequate doses of the drug that result in the achievement of a satisfactory hematological and symptomatic control of the disease (Barosi et al. 2009). However, some subjects show since the very beginning, or develop with time, refractoriness or intolerance to hydroxyurea. Specific criteria for defining intolerance or refractoriness to hydroxyurea have been developed as consensus statement from the ELN experts (Barosi et al. 2007, 2010); they are listed in Table 11.2.

Refractoriness can be defined as the inability of the patient to reach specific treatment goals with maximized doses of the drug that are otherwise tolerated in terms of hematological and/or extra-hematological toxicity. It is suggested that a dose of at least 2 g daily of hydroxyurea, or 2.5 g daily if the body weight is greater than 80 kg, should be tried before defining refractoriness; however, most patients do not tolerate well such high doses for long periods, and in clinical practice, it happens quite frequently that definition of refractoriness in one individual is actually set at a suboptimal dose of hydroxyurea. Factors that limit an increase of the daily dose of hydroxyurea to maximized level, or prevent its steady maintenance, are usually represented by hematological toxicity (neutropenia, thrombocytopenia, or anemia, especially in ET) and gastrointestinal disturbances.

On the other hand, patients can develop *intolerance* to hydroxyurea independent of the dose. Intolerance might present as gastrointestinal complains (nausea, intestinal cramping, diarrhea), cutaneous toxicity, fever, or lung involvement (Randi et al. 2005).

Cutaneous side effects related to hydroxyurea are quite common and range in severity from diffuse alopecia, skin atrophy, and diffuse or local hyperpigmentation to uncommon painful leg ulcers, dermatomyositis-like eruption, hydroxyurea-associated nonmelanoma skin cancers, or squamous dysplasia (Ruzzon et al. 2006).

Table 11.2 European LeukemiaNet criteria of resistance or intolerance to hydroxyurea in patients with PV and ET

PV:

1. Need for phlebotomy to keep hematocrit <45% after 3 months of at least 2 g/day of hydroxyurea

2. Uncontrolled myeloproliferation, i.e., platelet count >400×10^9/L *and* white blood cell count >10×10^9/L after 3 months of at least 2 g/day of hydroxyurea

3. Failure to reduce massive splenomegaly by more than 50% as measured by palpation, *or* failure to completely relieve symptoms related to splenomegaly, after 3 months of at least 2 g/day of hydroxyurea

4. Absolute neutrophil count <1.0×10^9/L *or* platelet count <100×10^9/L or hemoglobin <100 g/L at the lowest dose of hydroxyurea required to achieve a complete or partial clinico-hematological response

5. Presence of leg ulcers or other unacceptable hydroxyurea-related nonhematological toxicities, such as mucocutaneous manifestations, gastrointestinal symptoms, pneumonitis, or fever at any dose of hydroxyurea

ET:

1. Platelets >600,000/μL after 3 months of at least 2 g/day of hydroxyurea (2.5 g/day in patients with a body weight >80 kg)

2. Platelets >400,000/μL and WBC less than 2,500/μL at any dose of hydroxyurea

3. Platelets >400,000/μL and Hb less than 10 g/dL at any dose of hydroxyurea

4. Presence of leg ulcers or other unacceptable mucocutaneous manifestations at any dose of hydroxyurea

5. Hydroxyurea-related fever

Cutaneous ulcers are typically, but not exclusively, located in the lower extremities in the perimalleolar or pretibial region or in the back of the foot; they display round shape and a diameter of up to several centimeters and are often delimited by erythematous and atrophic epidermis (Best et al. 1998). Several patients present multiple lesions and describe them as extremely painful. No histopathologic criteria contribute to diagnosis, and no consistent correlation has been found between the appearance of ulcers and either the daily dose, cumulative dose, or the duration of hydroxyurea therapy (Bader et al. 2000). These cutaneous lesions should be carefully searched by the physician, since patients often disqualify them, attributing to trivial local causes, and do not refer to the hematologist unless they are very painful, as it happens in the most advanced cases. Thus, it is important to alert the patient, at the time of first prescribing hydroxyurea, about the possibility of such side effects and to stress the appropriateness of a prompt referral in case they develop. Local (poor hygiene, peripheral vein insufficiency, use of noncomfortable shoes) and systemic factors (diabetes, hypertension, poor nutrition, among the others) likely contribute to ulcer development and maintenance. No specific treatment has been shown to have a significant impact on ulcer sealing, that indeed is

a long process that can take months; topical drugs including antibiotics, wound surgical toilette, patches, activated platelet-rich plasma preparations, or hyperbaric oxygen therapy have all been variably used and with variable, most often unsatisfactory, results. Ideally, the patient should be referred to colleagues and nurses experienced in ulcer management. Local infections are common and can lead to septic complications. Hydroxyurea assumption should be stopped, whenever possible; however, there is not enough information to say whether hydroxyurea continues to be contraindicated after complete sealing of an ulcer. In my experience, some patients assumed again hydroxyurea for a long period without developing novel ulcers, but in others, ulcerations reappeared soon.

Dysplastic precarcinomatous lesions, called actinic keratosis, as well squamous cell carcinoma (basalioma), have been reported at apparently increased rate in patients with PV or ET during treatment with hydroxyurea, but a precise estimate is lacking (Best and Petitt 1998). Actinic keratosis develops as multiple lesions in sun-exposed area, with burning sensation, pruritus, and pain. Interruption or reduction of HU treatment is often accompanied by an improvement of the lesions but usually does not lead to a complete resolution (Salmon-Ehr et al. 1998).

Avoiding prolonged sun exposure should be recommended. Other adverse cutaneous manifestations attributed to hydroxyurea, mainly dyschromic lesions and dermatitis, can localize on the face, the hands, and feet. Nail hyperpigmentation develops as single or multiple brown or black vertical streaks as well as diffuse hyperpigmentation; they have only aesthetic relevance and are not an indication for halting the treatment.

Mucosal lesions attributed to hydroxyurea are mostly represented by painful and burning mouth ulcers, that in most severe cases can reduce food assumption and cause weight loss or teeth decay (Paleri and Lindsey 2000); other regions such as the female external genitals or the perianal region can be involved as well (Karincaoglu et al. 2003). There is usually a clear cause–effect relationship with the assumption of the drug, as shown by the usually rapid resolution of the lesions once the drug has been interrupted and, conversely, their rapid reappearance after drug reassumption in most subjects. There is no specific rule for management, and treatment should be stopped in case of multiple, painful, and refractory manifestations.

Pulmonary toxicity attributable to hydroxyurea has been reported very rarely. It manifests as rapid-onset breathlessness without fever; a chest radiograph might demonstrate diffuse heterogeneous opacities, while traction bronchiectasis without honeycombing or ground-glass infiltrates has been described using high-resolution lung CT (Sandhu et al. 2000). Histological analysis of lung biopsy in a few cases showed areas of interstitial fibrosis with reactive alveolar macrophages (Loo et al. 2009). Immediate interruption of the drug is required, and in the few reported cases, it was usually followed by resolution of illness.

Hydroxyurea-related *fever* is a relatively uncommon manifestation that usually appears a few days or weeks after starting therapy (Lannemyr and Kutti 1999). High body temperature (>38.5–39°C) develops within hours of drug assumption, with chills, cramping, illness, and sometimes back or bone pain; it recedes after a few hours spontaneously or with paracetamol. Subsequent assumptions of hydroxyurea, even after a while, challenge again these symptoms, thus preventing further use of the drug in all instances (Lossos and Matzner 1995).

However, while a number of anecdotal cases of hydroxyurea toxicity have been reported in the literature, epidemiologic data from large series of patients are not yet available. To collect information on the rate and characteristics of HU-related side effects, Italian investigators examined 3,411 MPN patients, of whom 963 were PV; 1,912 ET; 357 primary myelofibrosis (PMF); 93 post-polycythemia vera (PV-); and 86 post-essential thrombocythemia (PET-) myelofibrosis. A total of 184 patients (5%) who developed HU-related side effects were identified: 16 of them developed fever, 167 mucocutaneous lesions, and 1 pneumonitis. Pulmonary toxicity attributed to HU was diagnosed in a 68-year-old male with JAK2V617F-negative PMF who was under 1 g daily of hydroxyurea since 10 years. High-degree (>39°C) fever associated with hydroxyurea intake developed in 16 patients, 8 males and 8 females, with a median age of 64 years (range, 50–79 years). The appearance of hydroxyurea-related fever was reported after a median period of 31 days (range, 1–109) of treatment at a median dosage of 0.5 g daily (range, 0.15–1 g) and a median cumulative dose of 15 g (range, 0.5–52.5 g) per patient. Mucocutaneous lesions were referred by 167 patients; 28 patients developed mucosal lesions, 118 patients presented cutaneous ulcers, while other cutaneous manifestations including keratosis, dyschromia, basalioma, and dermatitis developed in 21 patients. Two patients reported both mucosal and cutaneous lesions. With the intrinsic limitations of the retrospective design, this study has provided an estimate of the rate of hydroxyurea-related side effects (5%) overall confirming the good tolerability of the drug (personal communication).

According to the ELN criteria (Table 11.2), patients who show refractoriness or develop intolerance to first-line hydroxyurea are candidates to second-line therapeutic options (Barosi et al. 2007, 2010).

11.4 Intolerance/Refractoriness to Other First-Line Drugs

11.4.1 Interferon

Fever and flu-like symptoms develop in most patients treated with conventional interferon-alpha; these can be usually managed with prophylactic assumption of paracetamol (Kiladjian et al. 2008). These manifestations, together with other more severe toxicities represented by myalgia, weight loss, new appearance or worsening of autoimmune diseases, and severe depression, caused discontinuation of the treatment in 14–42% and 10–35% of PV and ET patients, respectively, according to a number of small trials (reviewed in, Kiladjian et al. 2011). In the largest series reported by R.T. Silver, that included 55 PV patients treated with conventional forms of interferon-alpha, only 8 (15%) discontinued the treatment (Silver 2006).

Pegylated forms of interferon-alpha might have better tolerance in both PV and ET, according to recent studies (Kiladjian et al. 2006a; Quintas-Cardama et al. 2009). In the largest of these, that enrolled 40 PV and 39 ET patients and used PEG-IFN-alpha-2a (Quintas-Cardama et al. 2009), 96% of patients developed some toxicity, but this was generally grade 1 or 2 and was noted to be dependent on the initial dose (minimal in those who started at 90 µg weekly). The most frequent grade 3 or 4 toxicity, which occurred in 20% of patients, was represented by neutropenia. A total of 22% of the PV patients experienced related events necessitating discontinuation of therapy. On the other hand, of the 37 PV patients reported by Kiladjian et al. (2006a), 13 (35%) had to discontinue the treatment. Another preparation of pegylated interferon, alpha-2b, seems to be even less tolerated compared to the previous one. This interferon has been used in 36 patients with high-risk ET (Langer et al. 2005); treatment was stopped in ten patients (28%) due to grade 1–2 toxicity. In another study, 11 ET patients, either high-risk or refractory to hydroxyurea or anagrelide, received pegylated interferon-alpha-2b for a median duration of 9 months. One patient discontinued therapy at 4 months because of persistent grade 3 fatigue and a second at 5 months because of anxiety and depression (Alvarado et al. 2003). Finally, in the study of Samuelsson et al. (Samuelsson et al. 2006), that enrolled 21 patients each with PV and ET, the rate of discontinuation was as high as 30% and 55%, respectively. In brief, it can be expected that at least 20–25% of the patients who receive pegylated interferon as first-line therapy have to switch to second-line drugs due to poor tolerance or severe side effects.

11.4.2 Aspirin

The use of aspirin in PV had been discouraged in the past based on the results of the PVSG05 trial that randomized patients to treatment with radioactive phosphorus (^{32}P) or phlebotomy plus "high-dose" aspirin (300 mg orally three times per day) and dipyridamole (75 mg orally three times per day); indeed the trials were stopped after short follow-up due to an increase in hemorrhage (Tartaglia et al. 1986). The ECLAP study established the efficacy and demonstrated the safety of low-dose aspirin (100 mg daily) with no significant difference in the rates of major or minor bleeding compared to placebo (Landolfi et al. 2004). Intolerance to low-dose aspirin can develop in subjects who are allergic to the drug, manifest gastric disturbances, present frequent minor cutaneous or mucosal bleeding, or suffer from major bleeding, usually from the gastrointestinal tract. These side effects force to stop treatment at least in some of the subjects. A major bleeding is an indication to stop prescribing aspirin.

In summary, according to the ELN recommendations:

> Low-risk patients with polycythemia vera who [become] older than 60 years or develop major thrombotic or hemorrhagic complications require the introduction of cytoreductive therapy. In such patients, progressively increasing leukocyte and/or platelet count, enlarging spleen, uncontrolled disease-related symptoms, and poorly tolerated phlebotomy regimen may also justify the introduction

of cytoreductive therapy. In high-risk patients [with polycythemia vera], first-line therapy should be changed when intolerance has been demonstrated.

Low-risk untreated patients [with essential thrombocythemia] should start a cytoreductive treatment as soon as they move to the high-risk category as a result of increasing age, the occurrence of a major thrombotic or hemorrhagic event, or increasing platelet count greater than 1,500x10⁹/L. In high-risk patients [with essential thrombocythemia], treatment with hydroxyurea should be changed in case of intolerance. In patients with disease resistant to hydroxyurea, changing therapy may be an option.

[In both polycythemia vera and essential thrombocythemia] aspirin should be withdrawn in the event of major bleeding, most frequently gastrointestinal, or in the rare cases of allergy or intolerance.

11.5 Second-Line Drugs for the Treatment of PV or ET

Properties, indications, and toxicities of *hydroxyurea* and *interferon-alpha* have been described in the previous chapters dealing with first-line therapy and in the paragraphs above; their use as second-line agents in the categories of patients identified by ELN criteria does not require further discussion. Second-line drugs in those who develop resistance or refractoriness to hydroxyurea or interferon-alpha are anagrelide (for ET patients), busulphan, pipobroman, and radioactive phosphorus; possible alternatives to aspirin are also briefly discussed.

11.5.1 Anagrelide

Anagrelide is an imidazo-quinazolin derivative, initially developed as a platelet function inhibitor, that has selective inhibitory activity on the megakaryocytic cell lineage (Silverstein et al. 1988). The recommended starting dose is 0.5 mg four times a day, or 1 mg twice a day, with a gradual dose increase up to the dose required for maintaining the platelet count at target level (Birgegard 2006, 2009; Emadi and Spivak 2009).

Although the action mechanism at the molecular level still remains to be clarified, anagrelide reduces platelet production through inhibition of colony formation by committed megakaryocyte-colony-forming progenitors, reduction of megakaryocyte size and ploidy, and by overall affecting terminal megakaryocyte maturation (Mazur et al. 1992; Solberg et al. 1997; Tefferi et al. 1997; Tomer 2002). At high doses, anagrelide also prevents platelet aggregation, an effect that at least in part is mediated by inhibition of phosphodiesterase III (Balduini et al. 1992). The platelet inhibitory properties of anagrelide likely account for the increased rate of hemorrhages reported in the PT-1 trial (see below) where anagrelide was used in association with low-dose aspirin (HR 2.61, 95% CI 1.27–5.33; $P = 0.008$ vs. hydroxyurea) (Harrison et al. 2005). Therefore, the combined use of aspirin and anagrelide should be routinely avoided or at minimum be very cautious and weighted case-by-case.

Drug-induced inhibition of phosphodiesterase III is also largely consistent with the main side effects of anagrelide, represented by palpitations (10–20%), headache (13–35%), fluid retention, and possible occurrence or worsening of congestive cardiac failure. Usually, these occur in the first few months of treatment, are moderate in severity, often manageable with dose reduction, and usually subside with continued treatment (Birgegard 2009). However, in the above mentioned PT-1 trial, anagrelide was less tolerated than hydroxyurea with more frequent gastrointestinal, neurological, cardiovascular, and systemic complains (Harrison et al. 2005). Anagrelide is considered not mutagenic nor leukemogenic. The PT-1 trial did not reveal differences in leukemia occurrence between hydroxyurea and anagrelide, although the low number of cases prevents firm conclusions at this regard. Published detailed information about long-term safety for anagrelide is available for a small series of patients; in a study from Mayo Clinic, 35 young ET patients were treated for about 10 years without evidence of toxicity (Storen and Tefferi 2001). Anemia was the only new side effect that emerged after long-term therapy, with 24% of the patients experiencing a more than 3 g/dL decrease in hemoglobin level.

In one study in which anagrelide was tested in 577 patients with various myeloproliferative diseases (335 with ET, 114 chronic myelogenous leukemia, 68 PV, and 60 unclassifiable myeloproliferative disorders with thrombocytosis), anagrelide reduced the platelet count by 50% or to $<600 \times 10^9$/L for at least 28 days in 93% of evaluable patients, proving effectiveness in lowering platelet count (No-Author-listed 1992). The largest study concerning effectiveness of anagrelide in the management of high-risk patients with ET has been performed as a randomized comparison with hydroxyurea in 809 subjects in the PT-1 study (Harrison et al. 2005). Anagrelide proved significantly less effective than hydroxyurea in preventing arterial thrombosis ($P = 0.008$) or progression to myelofibrosis ($P = 0.01$) but conversely more effective against venous thrombosis ($P = 0.006$). A more detailed discussion about the PT-1 trial is presented.

In Europe, anagrelide is licensed only for patients with ET who are refractory or intolerant to first-line therapy with hydroxyurea, according to the previously outlined ELN criteria. On the contrary, anagrelide has been approved by the Food and Drug Administration as a first-line agent for the control of thrombocytosis associated with a myeloproliferative disorder.

11.5.2 Busulphan

Busulphan is a cell cycle nonspecific alkylating agent of the class of alkyl sulfonates. When used at low doses (usually, 2–4 mg daily), it can produce prolonged control of hematologic parameters in patients with PV or ET with relative safety and ease management. Toxicity may include interstitial pulmonary fibrosis, skin hyperpigmentation, and less frequently seizures, veno-occlusive disease of the liver, and wasting syndrome. The leukemogenic risk associated with low-dose busulphan is probably small, as shown in the study by Van de Pette et al. in ET patients (Van de Pette et al. 1986). However, the sequential use of busulphan and hydroxyurea resulted in a significant increase in the risk of second malignancies, including leukemias (Finazzi et al. 2000).

11.5.3 Pipobroman

Pipobroman is a piperazine derivative structurally linked to alkylating agents that acts as a competitive inhibitor of pyrimidines. The initial dose of pipobroman is usually at 1 mg/kg/die, and the maintenance dose is 0.3–0.6 mg/kg/die.

Passamonti et al. (2002) reported on 118 high-risk ET patients who were treated with this agent as first-line therapy at the starting dose of 0.8–1 mg/kg/day with a median follow-up of 10 years. Control of platelet count $<400 \times 10^9$/L was obtained in 91% of the patients, and the 10-year cumulative risk of thrombosis was 14%. Acute myeloid leukemia, myelofibrosis, and solid tumors occurred at a 10-year cumulative risk of 3%, 2%, and 7%, respectively. The duration of treatment with pipobroman did not correlate with the occurrence of second malignancies. In another study from the same group, 163 patients with PV were treated with pipobroman (at 1 mg/day) as first-line drug for a median follow-up of 120 months (Passamonti et al. 2000). Hematological remission was achieved in 94% of patients in a median time of 13 weeks (range, 6–48) of treatment. The cumulative risk of thrombotic events was 6%, 16%, and 20% at 3, 10, and 12 years, respectively. Acute leukemia occurred in 11 patients (6.7%), myelofibrosis in 7 (4.2%), and solid tumors in 11 (6.7%). The 10-year cumulative risk of leukemia, myelofibrosis, and solid tumors was 5%, 4%, and 8%, respectively. The only significant risk factor for leukemia and for solid tumors was age, while the duration of treatment did not influence these risks. Overall, these studies suggested that pipobroman is effective in the long-term control of ET and PV and, when used as first-line therapy, did not cause a significant increase of cases of leukemia or second neoplasia. In another retrospective study, 164 ET patients treated with pipobroman as first-line therapy for a median treatment time of 100 months (range, 25–243) were evaluated for occurrence of acute leukemia (De Sanctis et al. 2003) and for overall survival. Acute leukemia developed in nine patients (5.5%) after a median treatment time of 153 months (range, 79–227). The overall survival and the event-free survival at 120 months were 95% and 97%, whereas at 180 months, they were 84% and 76%, respectively.

In conclusion, these retrospective analyses showed a low incidence of leukemia in a large number of ET or PV patients treated with pipobroman as first-line chemotherapy.

The efficacy and safety of pipobroman in the long-term control of ET in 33 consecutive young patients at high risk of thrombosis followed for a median of 15.8 years was also evaluated in a single center study (Passamonti et al. 2004). Hematological control was obtained in all the patients, and there was no single case of thrombosis; however, one transformation to leukemia was recorded.

A randomized comparison of pipobroman and hydroxyurea used as first-line therapy was performed in 292 young (less than 65 years) PV patients by the French Polycythemia Study Group (FPSG) (Najean and Rain 1997a). Patients were randomized to receive treatment with hydroxyurea (25 mg/kg/day, followed by low-dose maintenance) or pipobroman (1.2 mg/kg/day, followed by low-dose maintenance). Patients were followed until death or up to 17 years, whichever first. Although hydroxyurea was slightly less effective in controlling hematological parameters, particularly platelet count, the risk of thromboembolic events as well as actuarial survival was similar in both arms. The risk of leukemia (10% at 13 years) and carcinoma (with the exclusion of skin cancers) was no different between the two arms. On the other hand, the risk of progression to myelofibrosis was higher in the hydroxyurea arm. An update of this trial after a median follow-up of 16.3 years in 285 patients has recently been reported (Kiladjian et al. 2011a). Patients treated with pipobroman had significantly higher rate of transformation to acute leukemia or myelodysplasia compared to hydroxyurea; at 10 and 20 years, the cumulative incidence of acute leukemia/myelodysplasia was 13% and 52%, respectively, in the pipobroman arm compared to 6.6% and 24% in the hydroxyurea arm ($P=0.004$). Conversely, pipobroman was more effective than hydroxyurea in preventing evolution to myelofibrosis: cumulative incidence of myelofibrosis was 5% and 21% at 10 and 20 years, respectively, compared to 15% and 32% for hydroxyurea arm ($P=0.02$).

Overall, these data indicate that pipobroman is an effective drug for hematological control and prevention of cardiovascular events in both ET and PV patients, but the significantly increased odds of transformation to leukemia strongly advocate its use as second-line therapy, with a preference for older patients (Kiladjian et al. 2006b).

11.5.4 Radioactive Phosphorus

The use of radioactive phosphorus (^{32}P) has been evaluated by the Polycythemia Vera Study Group in comparison with chlorambucil or phlebotomy-only arms in subjects with PV (Berk et al. 1986). Patients treated with ^{32}P had significantly less thrombotic events compared to the phlebotomy group, but survival was reduced from 13.9 to 11.8 years, at least in part because of more leukemias in the treatment arm.

The French Polycythemia Study Group explored the use of ^{32}P alone or in combination with hydroxyurea as maintenance therapy in PV patients older than 65 years (Najean and Rain 1997b). Four hundred sixty-one patients were randomized to receive (or not) low-dose hydroxyurea (5–10 mg/kg/day) after the first ^{32}P-induced remission. Hydroxyurea produced significant prolongation of the ^{32}P-induced remission and reduced the annual mean dose received to one-third. However, platelet count was not optimally controlled, and the rate of serious vascular complications was not decreased. On the other hand, there was a significant increase of transformation to leukemia beyond 8 years, as well a significant excess of carcinomas, while the risk of progression to myelofibrosis was not reduced at all. Life expectancy was shorter in the combined treatment arm (a median of 9.3 years vs. 10.9 years with ^{32}P alone), except in cases where the initial ^{32}P-induced remission lasted less than 2 years. Thus, notwithstanding the considerable reduction of the mean dose of ^{32}P received to produce a steady control of PV, the combined use with hydroxyurea as maintenance therapy significantly increased the leukemia and cancer risk and reduced the mean life expectancy by 15%.

11.5.5 Antiplatelet Drugs Other than Aspirin

No study has evaluated the safety and efficacy of drugs alternative to low-dose aspirin in case of intolerance in a controlled fashion.

Ticlopidine, a member of the thienopyridine family such as clopidogrel, was studied in 27 MPN patients with thrombocytosis who had contraindications to aspirin in a comparative fashion with 31 patients who received aspirin, with a median follow-up of 2 years (Ruggeri et al. 1993). Aspirin (at 300 mg/day) was associated with a high incidence of gastrointestinal hemorrhages (16%), while ticlopidine resulted better tolerated with no bleeding complications. Both drugs were similarly effective in relieving erythromelalgia and painful paresthesia.

On the other hand, it is appropriate in this setting to underline that the rate of gastrointestinal bleeding was significantly reduced among 320 patients with previous ulcer bleeding randomized to receive combination therapy of aspirin with a proton pump inhibitor compared to clopidogrel (Chan et al. 2005). Thus, the use of proton pump inhibitors should be tried in patients with poor gastric tolerance, including previous bleeding from a healed ulcer, to aspirin before shifting to alternative therapies, whose effectiveness and safety has not been proved yet while their cost is significantly higher.

In summary, according to the ELN recommendations:

Second-line therapy of polycythemia vera is IFN-alpha in patients intolerant or resistant to hydroxyurea therapy. Conversely, hydroxyurea is the second-line therapy for patients who are intolerant or refractory to first-line therapy with IFN-alpha. Pipobroman, busulphan, and 32P are second-line therapies reserved for patients with short life expectancy.

Anagrelide is the recommended second-line therapy for essential thrombocythemia. Interferon-alpha is an experimental therapy and should be reserved for selected patients, such as young females or patients who have contraindications to anagrelide therapy. Pipobroman, busulphan, and 32P are secondline therapies reserved for patients with short life expectancy.

The choice of second-line myelosuppressive drugs for PV should be carefully evaluated because some drugs administered after hydroxyurea may enhance the risk of acute leukemia. [Similarly], patients with ET who receive more than one cytotoxic agent do have a significantly higher risk of developing acute myeloid leukemia/myelodysplastic syndromes.

References

Alvarado Y, Cortes J, Verstovsek S, Thomas D, Faderl S, Estrov Z, Kantarjian H, Giles FJ (2003) Pilot study of pegylated interferon-alpha 2b in patients with essential thrombocythemia. Cancer Chemother Pharmacol 51:81–86

Bader U, Banyai M, Boni R, Burg G, Hafner J (2000) Leg ulcers in patients with myeloproliferative disorders: disease- or treatment-related? Dermatology 200:45–48

Balduini CL, Bertolino G, Noris P, Ascari E (1992) Effect of anagrelide on platelet count and function in patients with thrombocytosis and myeloproliferative disorders. Haematologica 77:40–43

Barbui T, Finazzi G (2005) When and how to treat essential thrombocythemia. N Engl J Med 353:85–86

Barbui T, Barosi G, Birgegard G, Cervantes F, Finazzi G, Griesshammer M, Harrison C, Hasselbalch HC, Hehlmann R, Hoffman R, Kiladjian J-J, Kröger N, Mesa R, McMullin MF, Pardanani A, Passamonti F, Vannucchi AM, Reiter A, Silver RT, Verstovsek S, Tefferi A (2011) Philadelphia-negative classical myeloproliferative neoplasms: critical concepts and management recommendations from European LeukemiaNet. J Clin Oncol 29:761–770

Barosi G, Besses C, Birgegard G, Briere J, Cervantes F, Finazzi G, Gisslinger H, Griesshammer M, Gugliotta L, Harrison C, Hasselbalch H, Lengfelder E, Reilly JT, Michiels JJ, Barbui T (2007) A unified definition of clinical resistance/intolerance to hydroxyurea in essential thrombocythemia: results of a consensus process by an international working group. Leukemia 21:277–280

Barosi G, Birgegard G, Finazzi G, Griesshammer M, Harrison C, Hasselbalch HC, Kiladjian JJ, Lengfelder E, McMullin MF, Passamonti F, Reilly JT, Vannucchi AM, Barbui T (2009) Response criteria for essential thrombocythemia and polycythemia Vera: result of a European LeukemiaNet consensus conference. Blood 113:4829–4833

Barosi G, Birgegard G, Finazzi G, Griesshammer M, Harrison C, Hasselbalch H, Kiladijan JJ, Lengfelder E, Mesa R, Mc Mullin MF, Passamonti F, Reilly JT, Vannucchi AM, Barbui T (2010) A unified definition of clinical resistance and intolerance to hydroxycarbamide in polycythaemia vera and primary myelofibrosis: results of a European LeukemiaNet (ELN) consensus process. Br J Haematol 148:961–963

Berk PD, Goldberg JD, Donovan PB, Fruchtman SM, Berlin NI, Wasserman LR (1986) Therapeutic recommendations in polycythemia vera based on

Polycythemia Vera Study Group protocols. Semin Hematol 23:132–143

Best PJ, Petitt RM (1998) Multiple skin cancers associated with hydroxyurea therapy. Mayo Clin Proc 73:961–963

Best PJ, Daoud MS, Pittelkow MR, Petitt RM (1998) Hydroxyurea-induced leg ulceration in 14 patients. Ann Intern Med 128:29–32

Birgegard G (2006) Anagrelide treatment in myeloproliferative disorders. Semin Thromb Hemost 32:260–266

Birgegard G (2009) Long-term management of thrombocytosis in essential thrombocythaemia. Ann Hematol 88:1–10

Chan FK, Ching JY, Hung LC, Wong VW, Leung VK, Kung NN, Hui AJ, Wu JC, Leung WK, Lee VW, Lee KK, Lee YT, Lau JY, To KF, Chan HL, Chung SC, Sung JJ (2005) Clopidogrel versus aspirin and esomeprazole to prevent recurrent ulcer bleeding. N Engl J Med 352:238–244

De Sanctis V, Mazzucconi MG, Spadea A, Alfo M, Mancini M, Bizzoni L, Peraino M, Mandelli F (2003) Long-term evaluation of 164 patients with essential thrombocythaemia treated with pipobroman: occurrence of leukaemic evolution. Br J Haematol 123:517–521

Emadi A, Spivak JL (2009) Anagrelide: 20 years later. Expert Rev Anticancer Ther 9:37–50

Finazzi G, Barbui T (2007) How I treat patients with polycythemia vera. Blood 109:5104–5111

Finazzi G, Ruggeri M, Rodeghiero F, Barbui T (2000) Second malignancies in patients with essential thrombocythaemia treated with busulphan and hydroxyurea: long-term follow-up of a randomized clinical trial. Br J Haematol 110:577–583

Harrison CN, Campbell PJ, Buck G, Wheatley K, East CL, Bareford D, Wilkins BS, van der Walt JD, Reilly JT, Grigg AP, Revell P, Woodcock BE, Green AR (2005) Hydroxyurea compared with anagrelide in high-risk essential thrombocythemia. N Engl J Med 353:33–45

Karincaoglu Y, Kaya E, Esrefoglu M, Aydogdu I (2003) Development of large genital ulcer due to hydroxyurea treatment in a patient with chronic myeloid leukemia and Behcet's disease. Leuk Lymphoma 44:1063–1065

Kiladjian JJ, Cassinat B, Turlure P, Cambier N, Roussel M, Bellucci S, Menot ML, Massonnet G, Dutel JL, Ghomari K, Rousselot P, Grange MJ, Chait Y, Vainchenker W, Parquet N, Abdelkader-Aljassem L, Bernard JF, Rain JD, Chevret S, Chomienne C, Fenaux P (2006a) High molecular response rate of polycythemia vera patients treated with pegylated interferon alpha-2a. Blood 108:2037–2040

Kiladjian JJ, Rain JD, Bernard JF, Briere J, Chomienne C, Fenaux P (2006b) Long-term incidence of hematological evolution in three French prospective studies of hydroxyurea and pipobroman in polycythemia Vera and essential thrombocythemia. Semin Thromb Hemost 32:417–421

Kiladjian JJ, Chomienne C, Fenaux P (2008) Interferon-alpha therapy in bcr-abl-negative myeloproliferative neoplasms. Leukemia 22:1990–1998

Kiladjian J-J, Mesa RA, Hoffman R (2011) The renaissance of interferon therapy for the treatment of myeloid malignancies. Blood 117:4706–4715

Kiladjian JJ, Chevret S, Dosquet C, Chomienne C, Rain JD (2011a) Treatment of polycythemia vera with hydroxyurea and pipobroman: final results of a randomized trial initiated in 1980. J Clin Oncol 29:3907–3913

Landolfi R, Marchioli R, Kutti J, Gisslinger H, Tognoni G, Patrono C, Barbui T (2004) Efficacy and safety of low-dose aspirin in polycythemia vera. N Engl J Med 350:114–124

Langer C, Lengfelder E, Thiele J, Kvasnicka HM, Pahl HL, Beneke H, Schauer S, Gisslinger H, Griesshammer M (2005) Pegylated interferon for the treatment of high risk essential thrombocythemia: results of a phase II study. Haematologica 90:1333–1338

Lannemyr O, Kutti J (1999) Hydroxyurea as a cause of drug fever in essential thrombocythaemia. Eur J Haematol 62:354–355

Loo PS, Khan M, Currie GP, Husain E, Kerr KM (2009) Hydroxycarbamide-inducedpneumonitis.Histopathology 55:234–236

Lossos IS, Matzner Y (1995) Hydroxyurea-induced fever: case report and review of the literature. Ann Pharmacother 29:132–133

Mazur EM, Rosmarin AG, Sohl PA, Newton JL, Narendran A (1992) Analysis of the mechanism of anagrelide-induced thrombocytopenia in humans. Blood 79:1931–1937

Najean Y, Rain JD (1997a) Treatment of polycythemia Vera: the use of hydroxyurea and pipobroman in 292 patients under the age of 65 years. Blood 90:3370–3377

Najean Y, Rain JD (1997b) Treatment of polycythemia Vera: use of 32P alone or in combination with maintenance therapy using hydroxyurea in 461 patients greater than 65 years of age. The French Polycythemia Study Group. Blood 89:2319–2327

No-Author-listed (1992) Anagrelide, a therapy for thrombocythemic states: experience in 577 patients. Anagrelide Study Group. Am J Med 92:69–76

Paleri V, Lindsey L (2000) Oral ulcers caused by hydroxyurea. J Laryngol Otol 114:976–977

Passamonti F, Brusamolino E, Lazzarino M, Barate C, Klersy C, Orlandi E, Canevari A, Castelli G, Merante S, Bernasconi C (2000) Efficacy of pipobroman in the treatment of polycythemia vera: long-term results in 163 patients. Haematologica 85:1011–1018

Passamonti F, Malabarba L, Orlandi E, Pascutto C, Brusamolino E, Astori C, Barate C, Canevari A, Corso A, Bernasconi P, Cazzola M, Lazzarino M (2002) Pipobroman is safe and effective treatment for patients with essential thrombocythaemia at high risk of thrombosis. Br J Haematol 116:855–861

Passamonti F, Rumi E, Malabarba L, Arcaini L, Orlandi E, Brusamolino E, Pascutto C, Cazzola M, Lazzarino M (2004) Long-term follow-up of young patients with essential thrombocythemia treated with pipobroman. Ann Hematol 83:495–497

Quintas-Cardama A, Kantarjian H, Manshouri T, Luthra R, Estrov Z, Pierce S, Richie MA, Borthakur G, Konopleva M, Cortes J, Verstovsek S (2009) Pegylated interferon alfa-2a yields high rates of hematologic and molecular response in patients with advanced essential thrombocythemia and polycythemia Vera. J Clin Oncol 27:5418–5424

Randi ML, Ruzzon E, Tezza F, Luzzatto G, Fabris F (2005) Toxicity and side effects of hydroxyurea used for primary thrombocythemia. Platelets 16:181–184

Ruggeri M, Castaman G, Rodeghiero F (1993) Is ticlopidine a safe alternative to aspirin for management of myeloproliferative disorders? Haematologica 78: 18–21

Ruzzon E, Randi ML, Tezza F, Luzzatto G, Scandellari R, Fabris F (2006) Leg ulcers in elderly on hydroxyurea: a single center experience in Ph- myeloproliferative disorders and review of literature. Aging Clin Exp Res 18:187–190

Salmon-Ehr V, Grosieux C, Potron G, Kalis B (1998) Multiple actinic keratosis and skin tumors secondary to hydroxyurea treatment. Dermatology 196:274

Samuelsson J, Hasselbalch H, Bruserud O, Temerinac S, Brandberg Y, Merup M, Linder O, Bjorkholm M, Pahl HL, Birgegard G (2006) A phase II trial of pegylated interferon alpha-2b therapy for polycythemia vera and essential thrombocythemia: feasibility, clinical and biologic effects, and impact on quality of life. Cancer 106:2397–2405

Sandhu HS, Barnes PJ, Hernandez P (2000) Hydroxyurea-induced hypersensitivity pneumonitis: a case report and literature review. Can Respir J 7: 491–495

Silver RT (2006) Long-term effects of the treatment of polycythemia vera with recombinant interferon-alpha. Cancer 107:451–458

Silverstein MN, Petitt RM, Solberg LA Jr, Fleming JS, Knight RC, Schacter LP (1988) Anagrelide: a new drug for treating thrombocytosis. N Engl J Med 318:1292–1294

Solberg LA Jr, Tefferi A, Oles KJ, Tarach JS, Petitt RM, Forstrom LA, Silverstein MN (1997) The effects of anagrelide on human megakaryocytopoiesis. Br J Haematol 99:174–180

Storen EC, Tefferi A (2001) Long-term use of anagrelide in young patients with essential thrombocythemia. Blood 97:863–866

Tartaglia AP, Goldberg JD, Berk PD, Wasserman LR (1986) Adverse effects of antiaggregating platelet therapy in the treatment of polycythemia vera. Semin Hematol 23:172–176

Tefferi A, Silverstein MN, Petitt RM, Mesa RA, Solberg LA Jr (1997) Anagrelide as a new platelet-lowering agent in essential thrombocythemia: mechanism of actin, efficacy, toxicity, current indications. Semin Thromb Hemost 23:379–383

Tomer A (2002) Effects of anagrelide on in vivo megakaryocyte proliferation and maturation in essential thrombocythemia. Blood 99:1602–1609

Van de Pette JE, Prochazka AV, Pearson TC, Singh AK, Dickson ER, Wetherley-Mein G (1986) Primary thrombocythaemia treated with busulphan. Br J Haematol 62:229–237

Vannucchi AM, Guglielmelli P (2010) Advances in understanding and management of polycythemia vera. Curr Opin Oncol 22:636–641

Vannucchi AM, Guglielmelli P, Tefferi A (2009) Advances in understanding and management of myeloproliferative neoplasms. CA Cancer J Clin 59:171–191

Blastic Transformation of BCR-ABL-Negative Myeloproliferative Neoplasms

12

Madappa N. Kundranda, Raoul Tibes, and Ruben A. Mesa

Contents

Abbreviations

aCML	Atypical chronic myeloid leukemia
AML	Acute myeloid leukemia
ASCT	Allogeneic stem cell transplant
ASXL1	Additional sex combs-like 1
ATP	Adenosine triphosphate
CMML	Chronic myelomonocytic leukemia
CR	Complete response
ESA	Erythroid stimulating agent
ET	Essential thrombocythemia
HDAC	Histone deacetylase
HPI	Hedgehog pathway inhibitors
HSCT	Hematopoietic stem cell transplant
ICSBP	Interferon consensus sequence binding protein
IDH	Isocitrate dehydrogenase
IKZF1	IKAROS family zinc finger 1
IPSS	International Prognostic Scoring System
IWG-MRT	International Working Group for Myelofibrosis Research and Treatment

M.N. Kundranda, R. Tibes, and R.A. Mesa (✉)
Division of Hematology and Oncology, Mayo Clinic,
Scottsdale, AZ, USA
e-mail: mesa.ruben@mayo.edu

MPL   Myeloproliferative leukemia
MPN   Myeloproliferative neoplasm
MPN-BP   Myeloproliferative neoplasm blast phase
mTOR   Mammalian target of rapamycin
NHEJ   Nonhomologous end joining
Ph   Philadelphia (chromosome)
PMV   Primary myelofibrosis
PV   Polycythemia vera
ROS   Reactive oxygen species
SNP-A   Single nucleotide polymorphism analysis
WHO   World Health Organization

12.1 Introduction

The myeloproliferative neoplasms (MPNs) are a distinct group of hematological disorders which exhibit terminal myeloid cell expansion in the peripheral blood. Based on the 2008 WHO Classification System, they are categorized into "classic" and "atypical" MPNs (Vardiman et al. 2009). The classic MPNs are further functionally classified based on the presence or absence of the t(9:22) chromosomal translocation in the Philadelphia (Ph) chromosome resulting in the BCR-ABL 1 fusion protein.

Although first described in 1951 by William Dameshek purely based on clinical and bone marrow similarities (Dameshek 1951), the BCR-ABL-negative MPNs (polycythemia vera [PV], essential thrombocythemia [ET], and primary myelofibrosis [PMF]) are currently in a period of rapid discovery regarding their pathogenetic mechanisms. The defining moment occurred for MPNs in 2005 with the discovery of JAK2 V617F mutation (Baxter et al. 2005; James et al. 2005; Kralovics et al. 2005; Levine et al. 2005). This gain-of-function mutation in the pseudokinase domain of the Janus kinase 2 gene (a key component of the cell growth and differentiation in the JAK-STAT pathway) results in the constitutive activation of the pathway. Since then, several additional genetic mutations with potential pathogenetic implications have been described; however, what leads to disease progression remains unclear.

The MPNs have a variable period of risk of vascular events and a long-term risk of transformation to an overt myelofibrotic phase, acute leukemia, or death (Fig. 12.1). Current available therapies have rarely been able to impact this natural history beyond palliating symptoms or decreasing the risk of vascular events. In this chapter, we will focus on the most advanced clinical scenario for MPN patients, the biology and consequence of blastic transformation.

12.2 Phenotype of Leukemic Transformation in the MPNs

Disease progression in MPNs is variable and based on risk factors; however, eventually most patients develop overt acute leukemia or most appropriately what is called a blast phase (Mesa et al. 2007b) (see Fig. 12.1). Clinically, as patients progress, they tend to experience a decrease in the efficacy of intramedullary hematopoiesis as manifested by worsening thrombocytopenia, worsening constitutional symptoms, and the potential development of functional neutropenia (Mesa et al. 2005). Patients most commonly will reach a blast phase after first having gone through a myelofibrotic phase whether PMF or post-ET/PV MF (Mesa et al. 2005). However, patients with PV or ET have been known to develop a blast phase without a clearly distinct prodrome of myelofibrosis developing (Finazzi et al. 2005).

12.3 Pathogenesis of Blastic Transformation in MPNs

The pathogenetic mechanisms of transformation to MPN-BP remain unclear. There are a growing number of MPN-associated mutations including JAK2, MPL, TET2, ASXL1, IDH1, IDH2, CBL, IKZF1, LNK, and EZH2 (Tefferi and Vainchenker 2011). The mechanisms by which these mutations can lead to widely varying disease phenotypes or what leads to disease progression (Fig. 12.1) remains unclear. Although most of these mutations originate at a progenitor cell

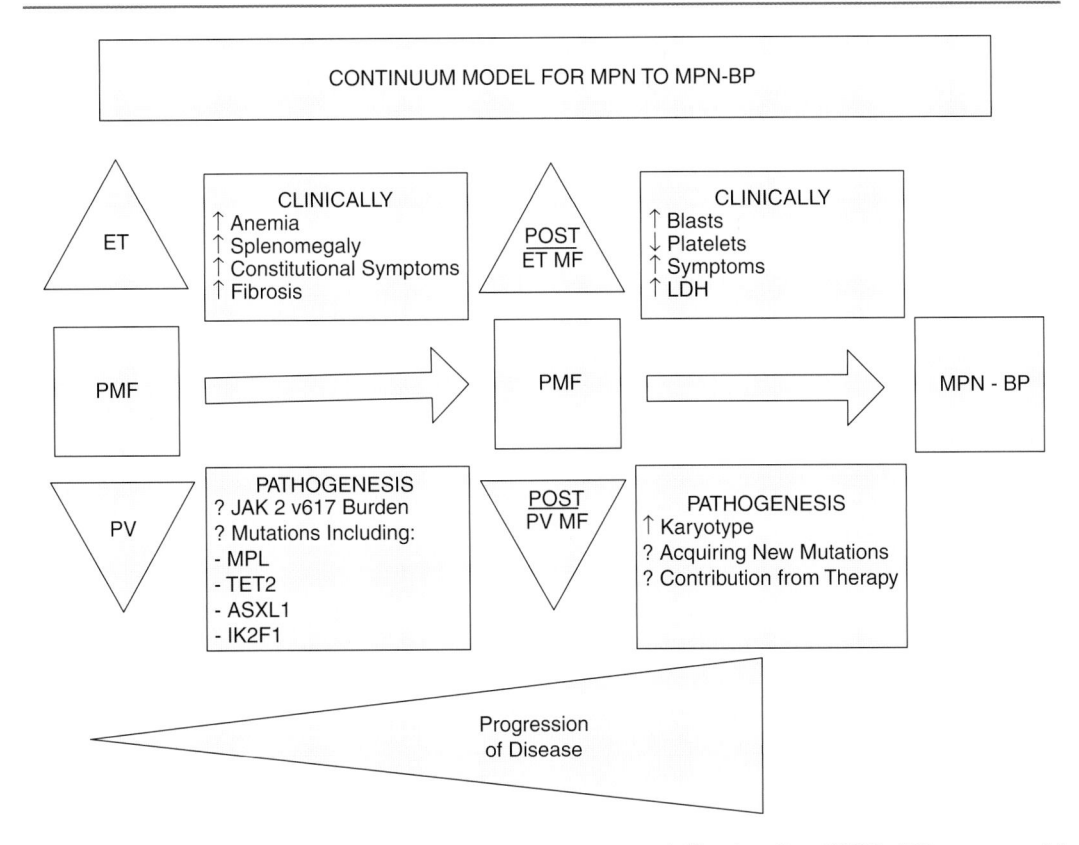

Fig. 12.1 Clinical and pathogenetic changes occurring during myeloproliferative disorder progression. *ET* essential thrombocythemia, *PV* polycythemia vera, *PMF* primary myelofibrosis, *Post-ET/PV MF* post-essential thrombocythemia/polycythemia vera myelofibrosis

level, they neither represent the primary clonogenic event nor are they mutually exclusive (Tefferi and Vainchenker 2011).

12.3.1 JAK2 Mutations

JAK2 located on chromosome 9p24 is one of the members of the Janus family of nonreceptor protein tyrosine kinases. JAK2 is ubiquitously expressed in mammalian cells and is an integral part of signal transduction and activation of the JAK-STAT pathway (which is involved in cell growth, proliferation, and survival) (Aaronson and Horvath 2002).

12.3.1.1 JAK2 V617F

JAK2 V617F is the most common mutation in BCR-ABL1-negative MPNs (Mesa et al. 2007b) and is seen in ~95% of patients with PV, in ~50%

of patients with ET, in ~65% of patients with PMF, and in ~50% of patients in blast phase MPN. This gain-of-function mutation (G to T) involving exon 14 leading to the substitution of valine with phenylalanine (V to F) at codon 617 results in the constitutive activation of the JAK-STAT pathway (Lu et al. 2005). Although preclinical data suggested the likely possibility of the JAK2 V617F mutation in disease progression (Tiedt et al. 2008), there is evidence that neither the presence of a JAK2 V617F mutation (Mesa et al. 2006b) nor an increased allele burden (Tefferi et al. 2008b) is more common in those who transform to MPN-BP. In addition, the majority (Theocharides et al. 2007), but not all (Swierczek et al. 2007), isolated acute leukemia clones obtained from previously JAK2-V167F mutant patients will have reverted to a JAK-wild type state. Clinical observations from series of MPN-BP patients further support that JAK2 V617F allele burden does not increase (or likely decreases) after transformation (Tam et al. 2008). In a recent observation of 778 patients with BCR-ABL1-negative MPNs of whom 7 transformed to BP, the JAK2 V617F mutation was noted in approximately 50% of those cases. However, although all JAK2 V617F-positive patients remained positive for this mutation after leukemic transformation, the mutation itself did not appear to alter the course of the disease, suggesting that JAK2 V617F is not essential for transformation in these cases (Lopes da Silva et al. 2011).

Other recent observations further demonstrate that perhaps different pathways for leukemic transformation occur in MPNs (a MF phenotypic step in JAK2 V617F-mutated patients, a direct MPN-BP from ET/PV in JAK2 wild type patients) (Beer et al. 2010). To further complicate this picture, there have been reports of multiple mutations occurring in the same patient, reiterating the fact that these mutations are neither mutually exclusive nor confined to a predictable pattern of occurrence (Schaub et al. 2010; Kralovics 2008).

12.3.1.2 JAK2 Exon 12 Mutations

The JAK2 exon 12 mutations are usually specific to the JAK2 V617F-negative PV patients. Initially identified in 2007 (Scott et al. 2007b) till date, >10 JAK2 exon 12 mutations have been described in the literature (Pietra et al. 2008). The mutational frequency in blast phase MPN is unknown, and the clinical course appears to be similar to that of JAK2 V617F mutated patients.

12.3.2 Myeloproliferative Leukemia Virus Oncogene (MPL) Mutations

MPL, found at chromosome 1p34, encodes the thrombopoietin receptor that works in concert with thrombopoietin for platelet production. Acquired MPL mutations (e.g., W515L and W515K) are associated with severe anemia and have been detected in patients with ET or MF, but not in patients with PV (Pancrazzi et al. 2008; Pikman et al. 2006). The incidence of MPL

mutations in blast phase MPN is unknown and so is its pathogenetic relevance.

12.3.3 TET2 Mutations

TET2 mutations found on chromosome 4q24 are thought to play a pivotal role in epigenetic regulation of transcription (Tahiliani et al. 2009). The incidence of TET2 mutations in blast phase MPN has been reported to be approximately 17% (Tefferi et al. 2009a). In a recent report using single nucleotide polymorphism analysis (SNP-A), all patients with TET2 mutations had additional chromosomal lesions. In addition, no TET2 mutations were noted in chronic phase MPN (Makishima et al. 2011). However, from a prognostic standpoint in patients with PV and PMF, the presence of a mutant TET2 did not affect leukemic transformation or survival (Tefferi et al. 2009a).

12.3.4 Additional Sex Combs-Like 1 (ASXL1) Mutations

ASXL1 mutations are found on chromosome 20q11.1 and belong to the enhancer of trithorax and polycomb gene family (Carbuccia et al. 2009). They are believed to affect regulation of transcription and RAR-mediated signaling (Carbuccia et al. 2009). The incidence of ASXL1 mutation in blast phase MPN is noted to be between 10% and 19% (Boultwood et al. 2010; Makishima et al. 2011; Abdel-Wahab et al. 2011). Currently, it is unclear whether ASXL1 mutations are an early or secondary event, and recent data are conflicting regarding its role with clinical outcome (Abdel-Wahab et al. 2011).

12.3.5 Isocitrate Dehydrogenase (IDH1 and IDH2) Mutations

IDH1 and IDH2 are located on chromosomes 2q33.3 and 15q26.1, respectively (Dang et al. 2009; Gross et al. 2010). These mutations confer an enzymatic gain of function that increases

2-hydroxyglutarate, eventually leading to malignant transformation (Dang et al. 2009; Gross et al. 2010). They were originally described in gliomas (Parsons et al. 2008), and the presence of the mutations was associated with superior survival (Weller et al. 2009). The mutational frequency of IDH in patients with blast phase MPN is approximately 21% (Pardanani et al. 2010). In a recent report using SNP-A, Makishima et al. (2011) detected canonical IDH mutations (R132 [IDH1] and R 172 [IDH2]) in blast phase CML, suggesting its role to predict a more malignant phenotype.

12.3.6 IKAROS Family Zinc Finger 1 (IKZF1) Mutations

IKZF1 mutations located on chromosome 7p12 encode for Ikaros transcription factors, which are key regulators of lymphoid differentiation. In a single study, IKZF1 mutational frequency in blast phase MPN has been reported as 19% (Jager et al. 2010). Given the low mutational frequency (<0.5%) that has been observed in chronic phase disease, it is certainly enticing to assume its relevant role in blast phase MPN; however, more studies will be required to establish this.

Based on our current knowledge of the pathogenesis of blast phase MPN, it is clear that we have made significant strides in identifying mutations in just the last couple of years. Unlike CML, pathogenetic mechanisms in BP-MPL are far more complex than originally estimated when the JAK2 V617F mutation was diagnosed and targeted. The transformation of CML from CP to BP is typically associated with additional karyotypic abnormalities which are independent of the BCR-ABL translocation (Vardiman et al. 2001). However, as we have previously demonstrated, patients with MPNs who eventually transform are more likely to have karyotypic abnormalities at diagnosis and develop new abnormalities prior to MPN-BP (Mesa et al. 2005, 2007b). The presence of chromosomal instability and acquisition of additional mutations are crucial for blastic transformation.

12.4 Defining Blastic Transformation from the MPNs

Historically, it has been noted that a better definition of BP-MPN (based on clinical and hematological characteristics) was required for determining therapeutic interventions (Karanas and Silver 1968). The majority of these patients (~75%) died within 6 months, and they were noted to have >30% myeloblasts and promyelocytes in the peripheral blood or bone marrow. Approximately four decades later and with the advent of newer molecular technology, we still continue to strive toward developing a clinically meaningful classification.

The reason why this is so difficult is because BP in patients with a prior MPN in part arises from lack of clear diagnostic guidance as to what constitutes acute leukemia in these patients. Patients with all chronic myeloid neoplasms exist in a spectrum of disease severity from the point of their diagnosis to acute leukemia. What constitutes this latter threshold in between is an arbitrary set point in a biological continuum. The World Health Organization's (WHO) updated classification in 2008 of myeloid neoplasms classified MPN-BP in an attempt to address some of these issues (Vardiman et al. 2009).

12.5 WHO Definition of Acute Leukemia

The World Health Organization's (WHO) updated classification in 2008 of myeloid neoplasms classified MPN-BP as acute myeloid leukemia with multilineage dysplasia (Vardiman et al. 2009). This subgroup was further divided into those who had a prior case of MDS or an MPN/MDS overlap disorder (Vardiman et al. 2009). This definition is most pertinent to those with an MPN/MDS overlap disorder (chronic myelomonocytic leukemia [CMML], atypical chronic myeloid leukemia [aCML], or MPN/MDS unclassifiable) yet does not really address those with prior PMF, post-ET/PV MF, or prior ET/PV.

The threshold for a diagnosis of achieving BP was either 20% blood or marrow blasts or the presence of an acute leukemia defining karyotypic lesions despite blast percentage (t[8;21][q22:q22], inv[16][p13q22], t[16;16] [p13;q22], or t[15;17][q22;q12]) (Vardiman et al. 2009). However, it does not address the issue that although karyotypic abnormalities are quite common among patients with MPN-BP (Mesa et al. 2005), it is less clear whether these defining mutations play any role in a transformed MPN (Mesa et al. 2005) as opposed to de novo AML.

12.6 Assessing the Importance of Peripheral Blast Percentage

Patients with MPNs, particularly PMF and post-ET/PV MF, are predisposed to circulating myeloblasts in the peripheral blood (Cervantes 2007; Cervantes et al. 2007). This latter phenomenon is true even when there is not a clear increase in bone marrow blast percentage. Reasons for this phenomenon relate to the abnormal trafficking of immature myeloid cells in these patients which may originate from abnormalities of the marrow stroma and is likely responsible for the increased circulating CD34+ cells in these patients (Barosi et al. 2001). Clinically, patients have been shown to have increased peripheral blood blasts for long periods of time without evidence of BP occurring (Cervantes et al. 1997). Based upon this phenomenon, the International Working Group for Myelofibrosis Research and Treatment (IWG-MRT) has included among their clinical trial criteria that a patient on a trial must have a sustained peripheral blood blast percentage of >20% for 4 weeks sustained before acute leukemia can be declared (Tefferi et al. 2006a). Until more is known regarding the biological underpinnings of a change from an MPN to MPN-BP, arbitrary clinical cutoffs will remain somewhat cumbersome. Indeed, some patients can have a clinical phenotype of MPN-BP with 15% blasts and succumb to their disease, while others with a higher blast "burden" may have a more indolent course.

12.7 Risk Factors for Blastic Transformation

The evaluation and assessment of risk factors in MPN patients is very important as they are at a higher risk over the course of their illness to transform into acute leukemia. The purpose of risk stratification is twofold. One, to identify patients at high risk of death from their disease in order to employ more aggressive therapy such as allogeneic stem cell transplantation earlier in the course of their disease (Kroger et al. 2005). Two, to avoid unnecessary introduction of therapy (in a particular subset of patients) earlier in the course of their disease which could exacerbate this underlying predisposition to acute leukemia (Finazzi et al. 2005; Wolanskyj et al. 2006). Analysis of risk factors for MPN-BP are features present (i.e., intrinsic to their MPN) at diagnosis or during the course of disease (including therapy).

Prognostication for patients with MPNs done at the time of diagnosis can look at risk of vascular events (mainly for ET and PV), death, and development of blast phase (which unfortunately usually leads to rapid death). Of these latter endpoints, we will focus on mortality and transformation. The International Working Group for Myelofibrosis Research and Treatment (IWG-MRT) recently published an International Prognostic Scoring System (IPSS-MF) to aid in assessing MF prognosis. Five features are independently associated with decreased survival age (>65), anemia (hemoglobin <10 g/dL), leukocytes >25×10^9, constitutional symptoms (night sweats, fever, significant weight loss), and the presence of circulating blasts in the peripheral blood. The IPSS-MF defines four risk groups (0, 1, 2, or more than 2 of the 5 adverse features) with projected survival medians for each group ranging from a median of 27 months for high-risk to 135 months for low-risk disease (Cervantes et al. 2009).

Although limited data exist on predicting eventual leukemic transformation, our group has shown that (1) low JAK2 V617F allele burden (Tefferi et al. 2008b), (2) peripheral blast percentage >3% (Huang et al. 2008), and (3) thrombocytopenia present at diagnosis (Huang et al. 2008) were associated with higher risk of MPN-BP in these patients.

Table 12.1 Risk factors at presentation of primary myelofibrosis, which suggest high risk of eventual transformation (MPN-BP)

Risk factor	Association with developing MPN-BP	References
Demographics		
Age at diagnosis	None	Huang et al. 2008
Sex	None	Huang et al. 2008
Peripheral blood		
Hemoglobin	Yes – univariate only	Huang et al. 2008; Tefferi et al. 2008a
Leukocyte count	Yes ($>15 \times 10^9$/L) – univariate	Tefferi et al. 2008a
Platelet count	$<100 \times 10^9$/L	Huang et al. 2008
Presence of blasts	Yes – univariate	Huang et al. 2008
Blast percentage	Yes (greatest when >3%)	Huang et al. 2008
Physical exam features		
Splenomegaly	None	Huang et al. 2008
Bone marrow		
Cellularity	None	Mesa et al. 2007a
Reticulin fibrosis	None	Mesa et al. 2007a
Blast percentage	Yes	Mesa et al. 2007a
Karyotypic abnormalities (complex >2 lesions)	Yes	Mesa et al. 2007a
Molecular lesions		
JAK2 V617F	Low allele burden	Tefferi et al. 2008b; Swierczek et al. 2007
MPL mutations	No data available	
Myelofibrosis prognostic scores		
Lille (Dupriez 1996)	None	Huang et al. 2008
Cervantes (Cervantes 2001)	Yes – univariate only	Huang et al. 2008
Mayo (Dingli 2006)	Yes – univariate only	Huang et al. 2008

Analysis of our institutional experience of eventual MPN-BP in PV and ET patients demonstrated that PV patients with baseline leukocytosis and ET patients with baseline anemia are most predisposed to development of either post-ET/PV MF or MPN-BP (Tefferi et al. 2008a). Additionally, our IWG-MRT analysis would suggest patients who eventually transform are more likely to have higher LDH levels and more karyotypic abnormalities (Mesa et al. 2007a). No uniform prognostic score for MPN-BP yet exists (Table 12.1).

12.8 Influence of Therapy upon Development of MPN-BP

No matter what type of cancer is treated, treatments such as radiation and chemotherapy have the potential to lead to the development of a second cancer in the long run. Therapy-related acute leukemia has long been a concern with chemotherapy of malignant neoplasms and is of greater concern in patients with underlying myeloid neoplasms (see Table 12.2). Also, because it can take many years for treatment-related cancers to develop, they are of greatest concern in those patients that have chronic neoplasms such as MPNs. Hence, the role of therapy to accelerate the development of MPN-BP has long been a concern in MPN patients.

Specific to MPNs, the use of myelosuppressive therapy with radioactive phosphorus (P-32) (Osgood 1964; Parmentier 2003) is most clearly associated with increased risk of MPN-BP along with alkylator therapy such as melphalan (Petti et al. 2002) and pipobroman (Kiladjian et al. 2006; Najean and Rain 1997). Much controversy exists regarding the agent hydroxyurea, a valid

Table 12.2 MPN therapies and their association with MPN-BP

Therapy	Association	References
Medical		
Hydroxyurea	Only as combination therapy	Finazzi et al. 2005
Erythropoiesis stimulating agents	Higher rate of blastic transformation in PMF patients treated with ESAs	Huang et al. 2008
Androgens	Higher rates of transformation in PMF, especially with danazol	Huang et al. 2008
Melphalan	Higher rates of transformation in trial of patients with PMF	Petti et al. 2002
Pipobroman	Higher leukemia rates in treated PV patients	Najean and Rain 1997; Kiladjian et al. 2006
Phosphorus-32	Clear and undisputed increased risk of transformation with use	Osgood 1964; Parmentier 2003
Thalidomide	No increase rate seen	Huang et al. 2008
Azacitidine	Only therapy paper in MPN-BP. ORR 52%, CR 24%, median duration of response 9 months	Thepot et al. 2010
Surgical		
Splenectomy	Conflicting reports, but no clear link established	Barosi et al. 1998; Mesa et al. 2006a

and efficacious myelosuppressive agent demonstrated to decrease risk of vascular events in patients with ET and PV. Despite much discussion, evidence now suggests that single-agent hydroxyurea is not a significant contributor to leukemic transformation. Indeed, hydroxyurea has not been shown to be leukemogenic in the unrelated disorder of sickle cell anemia (Steinberg et al. 2003). However, there may be a synergistic leukemogenic potential role of hydroxyurea in patients who then go on to receive other treatments (Finazzi et al. 2005). In the end, there is no way to definitively negate a slight role of hydrea on the risk of leukemic transformation, and therefore, patients should be counseled accordingly. There are other agents with no suggestion of leukemogenicity (aspirin, anagrelide, and interferon) (Huang et al. 2008). Our analysis suggested an independently increased risk of MPN-BP among patients exposed to erythroid stimulating agents (ESAs) and androgen (particularly danazol) (Huang et al. 2008). This risk was independent of anemia and was significant in multifactorial analysis. Whether there is a causal role remains unclear, and these single-institution observations do require further validation. Finally, patients who have been splenectomized for PMF have been reported in some series to have higher rates

of transformation (Barosi et al. 1998), but it remains unclear whether this may be merely an association in patients with a more aggressive disease course (Mesa et al. 2006a).

12.9 Clinical Course and Therapy of MPN-BP

Ph-negative MPNs usually follow an erratic but rather aggressive course once they start to progress. The absence of a uniform prognostic score to predict this progression makes it more difficult to manage these patients. Molecular events at the transformation from MPN to AML are not only complex but poorly defined. As outlined earlier in this chapter, several mutations occurring in MPNs can be found at transformation to AML at the same higher or lower frequency. However, 5–10% of MPNs progress to develop acute myeloid leukemia (AML) after 10 years of onset of disease (Finazzi et al. 2005), and this number maybe even higher with longer follow-up. Once a patient progresses to MPN-BP, significant morbidity and mortality usually follow (Mesa et al. 2005). Clinically, patients will have all of the challenging peripheral blood cytopenias typical in de novo acute leukemia. Additionally, they face

Table 12.3 Medical options for myeloproliferative neoplasm blast phase (MPN-BP) (Mesa et al. 2005)

Therapy	Composition	Median survival (months) (Mesa et al. 2005)
Supportive care	Transfusions +/− Hydroxyurea +/− Antibiotic support	2.1 (1.1–3.4)
Noninduction chemotherapy	Weekly vincristine Oral alkylators Low-dose cytarabine Oral etoposide	2.9 (0.8–5.3)
Induction chemotherapy	Cytarabine + anthracycline (7 days) High-dose cytarabine (>1,000 mg/m^2/dose) Mitoxantrone/VP-16/high-dose cytarabine	3.9 (1.6–8.9)
Antibody therapy	Gemtuzumab	2.5 (0.7–3.5)

[a]Median survivals according to Mayo Clinic series

the significant debilitation, cachexia, and poor performance status already present from their MPN. Additionally, they will frequently have significant splenomegaly contributing both symptomatically and to transfusion resistance (Table 12.3).

Patients with MPN-BP will frequently have multiple features which are considered characteristic of high-risk acute leukemia, specifically, advanced age, antecedent myeloid disorder, and complex and poor-risk karyotypic abnormalities (Mesa et al. 2005). Therefore, it is not surprising that therapy for these patients has been quite disappointing. We have previously demonstrated that aggressive therapy (with myelosuppressive induction intent) did not seem to offer any survival benefit over purely supportive care (transfusions +/− hydroxyurea) (Mesa et al. 2005). Patients who underwent induction therapy had a 40% chance of returning to a more chronic appearing phase of PMF, but without any clear impact on survival. Therefore, it was thought that induction therapy may well only provide a cosmetic cytoreduction in blasts without meaningful impact (Mesa et al. 2005).

In a recent study, 54 BCR-ABL1-negative MPNs who had progressed to either AML or MDS were treated with azacitidine (Thepot et al. 2010). The overall response rate was 52% (24% CR) with a median duration of response being 9 months. This is the only therapy paper that exists in the field to date; however, although the use of azacitidine is encouraging, the response duration is short, and hence other consolidation therapies need to be evaluated.

At the current time, hematopoietic stem cell transplant (HSCT) appears to the best chance for a cure in a majority of these patients. In a study by MD Anderson Cancer Center (Tam et al. 2008), resolution of blasts through induction chemotherapy was achieved in 46% of those in whom that therapy was delivered, with 8/40 patients undergoing stem cell transplant. Among these latter patients who were successfully transplanted, 73% were alive 31 months after transplant. The transplant results appear to be impacted by several features including comorbidities, conditioning regimens, and disease burden (Scott et al. 2007a). As is noted in MDS, cytoreductive therapy is associated with improved outcomes in certain patient populations (Saberwal et al. 2009; Scott and Deeg 2010). It is unclear if that is the case with MPN-BP. In any event, an overall management plan that incorporates the possibility of HSCT should be developed for patients with MPN-BP at the time of diagnosis.

The reasons for the lack of success of therapy in MPN-BP are many and include intrinsic drug resistance, lack of tolerability, death from exacerbation of comorbidities and, most importantly, the complete understanding of the molecular pathogenesis of the role of mutations to progression to blastic phase. Given the dismal consequence of transformation and the dire outcomes with conventional therapy, the interest in novel therapeutic options is great.

12.10 Investigational Therapies in MPN-BP

In the last 6 years, several new drugs are undergoing evaluation and are in various stages of development. Though most of these drugs are being evaluated in MPNs, they may have a role in MPN-BP. These include thalidomide analogs, JAK2 inhibitor adenosine triphosphate (ATP) mimetics, histone deacetylase (HDAC) inhibitors, and mammalian target of rapamycin (mTOR) inhibitors. We will discuss some of the most promising agents below.

12.10.1 Pomalidomide

Pomalidomide is a second-generation immunomodulatory drug (IMiD) that appears to have activity in myelofibrosis (Tefferi et al. 2009b) without the severe toxicity that is seen both in thalidomide (Tefferi and Elliot 2000) and lenalidomide (Tefferi et al. 2006b). Recently, we reported the results of a phase II trial of low-dose pomalidomide (0.5 mg/day); 9 of the 10 JAK2 V617F-positive patients with anemia became transfusion independent (Bejar et al. 2011). The drug was very well tolerated, and no neuropathy or grade 4 myelosuppression was observed.

12.10.2 JAK2 Inhibitors

There is preliminary evidence from JAK2 inhibitor trials suggesting that leukemic transformation may be decreased when compared to historical studies (Eghtedar et al. 2010). Although JAK2 allele burden may not play a direct role in transformation to MPN-BP, it does correlate with overall worsened disease features. This constant proliferative drive may generate cellular stress that leads to formation of reactive oxygen species (ROS) and other cellular insults with subsequent genomic damage and instability as a pathway during progression. It is therefore conceivable that JAK2 inhibitors may delay

progression. However, if JAK2 inhibitors indeed can prevent or reduce transformation to AML remains to be shown. Given the overall more benign course of PV and ET, compared, for example, to myelodysplastic syndrome patients, it will require large patient populations treated with these drugs to answer those questions. Stratifying patients at higher risk for progression to AML, especially patients with PMF, may allow the reduction in sample size of patients. Conceptually, patients demonstrating increased or rising JAK2 allele burden (as a harbinger of disease progression) may be candidates for JAK2 inhibitor combination trials.

Some of the new agents targeting putative underlying molecular mechanisms are, for example, hedgehog pathway inhibitors (HPI), the first of which have completed clinical trials (Lorusso et al. 2011; Von Hoff et al. 2009). These agents are being tested in hematological malignancies including CML as well as studies which are planned in MPNs. Survivin inhibitors have been tested in hematological malignancies and have shown some activity in lymphomas (Tolcher et al. 2008) as well as CML and AML in an early clinical trial performed by our group (Tibes et al. 2009b). With the increasing availability of targeted agents, many of these have been and are currently tested in various stages and phases of MPNs. For example, mTOR inhibitors have shown clinical activity in PMF and post-PV/ET MF patients with response rates for spleen size reduction of up to 46% and resolution of systemic symptoms by 52–74% (Vannucchi et al. 2010). Epigenetic modulation HDAC inhibitors seem promising and have been assessed in small studies, for example, with LBH589 (Mascarenhas et al. 2009). Overall, six patients experienced clinical improvement (Mascarenhas et al. 2009), and with another HDAC inhibitor ITF2357 (Rambaldi et al. 2008), six of eight patients had significant clinical responses. Responses were seen in ET, PV, and PMF patients. Spleen size reduction was seen in six of eight patients with splenomegaly at baseline, and pruritus was relieved in most patients. Both agents were generally well tolerated.

Other agents currently being tested include GSK3beta, TGFB, and HSP90 inhibitors. Novel agents are commonly tested in advanced stages and leukemic phase of MPNs first, and thereafter, clinical activity is assessed in chronic phase MPNs. Alternatively, agents may also be introduced earlier in the disease process which may yield better response rates.

12.11 Novel Investigational Concepts in MPN-BP

Much of the work of MPN to AML progression is derived from mouse models, and selected relevant data will be briefly summarized with a focus on therapeutic targeting of the underlying molecular mechanisms.

One proposed mechanism and gene involved include the interferon consensus sequence binding protein (ICSBP). ICSBP deficiency induces a MPN phenotype with progression to AML over time. Saberwal et al. demonstrated that in mouse models, the ICSBP has a leukemia suppressor effect by binding and regulating Fanconi F gene which is involved in DNA damage repair and maintaining genomic integrity (Saberwal et al. 2009). ICSBP deficiency leads to accumulation of chromosomal damage and aberrations over time. Interestingly, ICSBP expression is decreased in AML and CML in blast crisis (Saberwal et al. 2009). Interferon-alpha-2a yielded complete clinical as well as 33–58% molecular remissions in patients with PV and ET (Kiladjian et al. 2008; Quintas-Cardama et al. 2009). A connected candidate gene is the tyrosine phosphatase SHP2 (Konieczna et al. 2008). Constitutive activation of SHP2 in conjunction with ICSBP haploinsufficiency leads to an accelerated myeloproliferative picture with apoptosis resistance and rapid progression to AML in mouse models in a cytokine-dependent manner (Konieczna et al. 2008).

Additional genes linked to progression are PU.1, an essential myeloid transcription factor, leading to accelerated MPN to AML progression in mouse models (Bejar et al. 2011). The inhibitor of apoptosis protein survivin is overexpressed in patients with chronic myelomonocytic leukemia (CMML) and other MPNs (Invernizzi et al. 2006), suggesting a role in altering the balance of proliferative, differentiation, and apoptotic signals resulting in myeloproliferation.

Further areas of research possibly connecting several underlying mechanisms focus around generation of reactive oxygen species (ROS). ROS formation leads to increased DNA damage with resulting genomic instability as a driving factor in pathogenesis of progression from MPNs to more aggressive myeloid malignancies (Sallmyr et al. 2008). It is speculated that defects in some of the major cellular repair pathways such as nonhomologous end joining (NHEJ) activate compensatory repair pathways that are error prone, creating structural chromosomal abnormalities such as deletions or translocations (Sallmyr et al. 2008). This higher degree of genomic instability and karyotypic abnormalities are noted in patients with more aggressive disease, and blastic transformation has been observed in patient samples (Mesa et al. 2005, 2007b). In MPN-BP patients, there was a threefold increase in genomic alterations when compared with samples in chronic phase. The alterations included known recurrent deletions of chromosome 7 and 5, and trisomy 8 (+8, i.e., C-MYC) among others (Thoennissen et al. 2010). Altered chromosomal regions involved in disease progression harbor established myeloid target genes (ETV6, TP53, and RUNX1). As outlined earlier in more detail, for most of the well-characterized clinical mutations encountered in chronic phase MPNs, there is insufficient evidence to suggest a contribution to leukemic transformation. However, for some mutations/deletions like TET2, IDH1 and IDH2 (Green and Beer 2010; Tefferi et al. 2010), IKAROS family zinc finger 1 (IKZF1) (Jager et al. 2010), and possibly RUNX1 (Ding et al. 2009) mutations, higher frequency of mutations are found in the blast phase indicating their potential in the pathogenesis of progression to AML. How this increasing knowledge of involved genes and pathogenesis affects treatment decisions in MPN-BP is currently unknown. This is mainly because most of the identified genes and targets do not have candidate drugs that are available as of yet. However, it opens avenues for research and development of new clinical treatment strategies with currently available drugs or agents in development for targeting putative candidate genes. For example, TET2 mutations are involved in epigenetic regulation (Ko et al. 2010); 5-Azacytidine has shown promising results in patients with AML and MDS transformed from Ph-negative MPNs. As described previously, overall and complete response (CR) rates were 52% and 24%, respectively (Thepot et al. 2010); 5-azacytidine has been demonstrated to be less active in chronic phase MPNs (Mesa et al. 2009). There is limited but encouraging clinical experience with 5-Azacytidine in erythroid leukemias with CR rates of 58% (*n* = 10/17 patients) accompanied by frequent cytogenetic responses (Vigil et al. 2009). With our increased molecular understanding and clinical activity data, this can be integrated into treatment strategies and, for example, to assess patients with TET2 mutations for their response to 5-Azacytidine.

In direct extension of the above described data and work, applying high-throughput RNA interference, we identified the BCL-2 family members and specifically BCL-XL as potent sensitizers to 5-Azacytidine (Bogenberger et al. 2010; Tibes et al. 2009a). BCL-XL is a lineage-specific oncogene in an erythroid and megakaryocytic lineage (Silva et al. 1998), and its targeting alone or in combination has a strong scientific rationale. A potent BCL-XL inhibitor is ABT-263 with which we have proposed a clinical trial in combination with 5-Azacytidine or interferon-alpha-2a. Altogether, there seems to be a strong component of epigenetic regulation, and 5-Azacytidine has already demonstrated encouraging clinical activity in patients with AML and MDS transformed from MPNs.

With the increasing molecular understanding of MPNs, new knowledge of genomic events occurring at transformation into leukemic phase as well as with the increasing number of targeted agents, it seems hopeful that improvement in treatment and outcome for patients with MPNs at all stages will be made over the next years.

Conclusion

Though rare, the progression of patients to MPN-BP is an extremely serious development for patients both symptomatically and prognostically. Salvage of patients through induction chemotherapy followed by allogeneic stem cell transplant is possible, but likely an option only in a small number of MPN-BP patients.

Although we have a partial understanding of risk factors for eventual transformation, we have an incomplete understanding as to the pathogenetic mechanisms of disease progression. Given the rapid mortality and resistance to current therapies seen in patients with MPN-BP, the need for novel and targeted therapy for these patients is great. A better understanding of mechanisms of clonal progression is required to identify valid therapeutic targets. Hopefully, blockade of JAK2 earlier in the course of an MPN will delay or inhibit disease progression, yet whether this will occur depends upon long-term follow-up on current JAK2 inhibitor trials. Given the uncertain role that the JAK-STAT pathway maintains in the process of leukemic transformation, the need for further study into mechanisms of disease progression is crucial.

References

Aaronson DS, Horvath CM (2002) A road map for those who don't know JAK-STAT. Science 296:1653–1655

Abdel-Wahab O, Pardanani A, Patel J et al (2011) Concomitant analysis of EZH2 and ASXL1 mutations in myelofibrosis, chronic myelomonocytic leukemia and blast-phase myeloproliferative neoplasms. Leukemia 25(7):1200–1202

Barosi G, Ambrosetti A, Centra A et al (1998) Splenectomy and risk of blast transformation in myelofibrosis with myeloid metaplasia. Italian Cooperative Study Group on Myeloid with Myeloid Metaplasia. Blood 91:3630–3636

Barosi G, Viarengo G, Pecci A et al (2001) Diagnostic and clinical relevance of the number of circulating CD34(+) cells in myelofibrosis with myeloid metaplasia. Blood 98:3249–3255

Baxter EJ, Scott LM, Campbell PJ et al (2005) Acquired mutation of the tyrosine kinase JAK2 in human myeloproliferative disorders. Lancet 365:1054–1061

Beer PA, Delhommeau F, LeCouedic JP et al (2010) Two routes to leukemic transformation after a JAK2 mutation-positive myeloproliferative neoplasm. Blood 115:2891–2900

Bejar R, Levine R, Ebert BL (2011) Unraveling the molecular pathophysiology of myelodysplastic syndromes. J Clin Oncol 29:504–515

Bogenberger JM, Hagelstrom RT, Gonzales I et al (2010) Synthetic lethal RNAi screening identified inhibition of Bcl-2 family members as sensitizers to 5-Azacytidine in myeloid cells. Late Breaking Abstract LB-128, AACR annual meeting, Washington, DC

Boultwood J, Perry J, Zaman R et al (2010) High-density single nucleotide polymorphism array analysis and ASXL1 gene mutation screening in chronic myeloid leukemia during disease progression. Leukemia 24:1139–1145

Carbuccia N, Murati A, Trouplin V et al (2009) Mutations of ASXL1 gene in myeloproliferative neoplasms. Leukemia 23:2183–2186

Cervantes F (2007) Myelofibrosis: biology and treatment options. Eur J Haematol Suppl 79(68):13–17

Cervantes F, Pereira A, Esteve J et al (1997) Identification of 'short-lived' and 'long-lived' patients at presentation of idiopathic myelofibrosis. Br J Haematol 97:635–640

Cervantes F, Mesa R, Barosi G (2007) New and old treatment modalities in primary myelofibrosis. Cancer J 13:377–383

Cervantes F, Dupriez B, Pereira A et al (2009) New prognostic scoring system for primary myelofibrosis based on a study of the International Working Group for Myelofibrosis Research and Treatment. Blood 113:2895–2901

Cervantes F (2001) Prognostic factors and current practice in treatment of myelofibrosis with myeloid metaplasia: an update anno 2000. Pathologie-biologie 49(2):148–152

Dameshek W (1951) Some speculations on the myeloproliferative syndromes. Blood 6:372–375

Dang L, White DW, Gross S et al (2009) Cancer-associated IDH1 mutations produce 2-hydroxyglutarate. Nature 462:739–744

Dingli D, Schwager SM et al (2006) Prognosis in transplant-eligible patients with agnogenic myeloid metaplasia: a simple CBC-based scoring system. Cancer 106(3):623–630

Ding Y, Harada Y, Imagawa J et al (2009) AML1/RUNX1 point mutation possibly promotes leukemic transformation in myeloproliferative neoplasms. Blood 114:5201–5205

Dupriez B, Morel P et al (1996). Prognostic factors in agnogenic myeloid metaplasia: a report on 195 cases with a new scoring system. Blood 88(3):1013–1018

Eghtedar A, Verstovsek S, Cortes JE et al (2010) Phase II study of the JAK 2 inhibitor, INCB018424, in patients with refractory leukemias including post-myeloproliferative disorder (MPD) acute myeloid leukemia (sAML). Blood 116:abstract 509

Finazzi G, Caruso V, Marchioli R et al (2005) Acute leukemia in polycythemia vera: an analysis of 1638 patients enrolled in a prospective observational study. Blood 105:2664–2670

Green A, Beer P (2010) Somatic mutations of IDH1 and IDH2 in the leukemic transformation of myeloproliferative neoplasms. N Engl J Med 362:369–370

Gross S, Cairns RA, Minden MD et al (2010) Cancer-associated metabolite 2-hydroxyglutarate accumulates in acute myelogenous leukemia with isocitrate dehydrogenase 1 and 2 mutations. J Exp Med 207:339–344

Huang J, Li CY, Mesa RA et al (2008) Risk factors for leukemic transformation in patients with primary myelofibrosis. Cancer 112:2726–2732

Invernizzi R, Travaglino E, Benatti C et al (2006) Survivin expression, apoptosis and proliferation in chronic myelomonocytic leukemia. Eur J Haematol 76:494–501

Jager R, Gisslinger H, Passamonti F et al (2010) Deletions of the transcription factor Ikaros in myeloproliferative neoplasms. Leukemia 24:1290–1298

James C, Ugo V, Le Couedic JP et al (2005) A unique clonal JAK2 mutation leading to constitutive signalling causes polycythaemia vera. Nature 434:1144–1148

Karanas A, Silver RT (1968) Characteristics of the terminal phase of chronic granulocytic leukemia. Blood 32:445–459

Kiladjian JJ, Rain JD, Bernard JF, Briere J, Chomienne C, Fenaux P (2006) Long-term incidence of hematological evolution in three French prospective studies of hydroxyurea and pipobroman in polycythemia vera and essential thrombocythemia. Semin Thromb Hemost 32:417–421

Kiladjian JJ, Cassinat B, Chevret S et al (2008) Pegylated interferon-alfa-2a induces complete hematologic and molecular responses with low toxicity in polycythemia vera. Blood 112:3065–3072

Ko M, Huang Y, Jankowska AM et al (2010) Impaired hydroxylation of 5-methylcytosine in myeloid cancers with mutant TET2. Nature 468:839–843

Konieczna I, Horvath E, Wang H et al (2008) Constitutive activation of SHP2 in mice cooperates with ICSBP deficiency to accelerate progression to acute myeloid leukemia. J Clin Invest 118:853–867

Kralovics R (2008) Genetic complexity of myeloproliferative neoplasms. Leukemia 22:1841–1848

Kralovics R, Passamonti F, Buser AS et al (2005) A gain-of-function mutation of JAK2 in myeloproliferative disorders. N Engl J Med 352:1779–1790

Kroger N, Zabelina T, Schieder H et al (2005) Pilot study of reduced-intensity conditioning followed by allogeneic stem cell transplantation from related and unrelated donors in patients with myelofibrosis. Br J Haematol 128:690–697

Levine RL, Wadleigh M, Cools J et al (2005) Activating mutation in the tyrosine kinase JAK2 in polycythemia vera, essential thrombocythemia, and myeloid metaplasia with myelofibrosis. Cancer Cell 7:387–397

Lopes da Silva R, Ribeiro P, Lourenco A et al (2011) What is the role of JAK2 V617F mutation in leukemic transformation of myeloproliferative neoplasms? Lab Hematol 17:12–16

Lorusso PM, Rudin CM, Reddy JC (2011) Phase I trial of hedgehog pathway inhibitor GDC-0449 in patients with refractory, locally-advanced or metastatic solid tumors. Clin Cancer Res 17(8):2502–2511

Lu X, Levine R, Tong W et al (2005) Expression of a homodimeric type I cytokine receptor is required for JAK2 V617F-mediated transformation. Proc Natl Acad Sci USA 102:18962–18967

Makishima H, Jankowska AM et al (2011) CBL, CBLB, TET2, ASXL1, and IDH1/2 mutations and additional chromosomal aberrations constitute molecular events in chronic myelogenous leukemia. Blood 117(21):198–206

Mascarenhas J, Wang X, Rodriguez A et al (2009) A phase I study of LBH589, a novel histone deacetylase inhibitor in patients with primary myelofibrosis (PMF) and post-polycythemia/essential thrombocythemia myelofibrosis (Post-PV/ET MF). ASH annual meeting abstracts 114:308

Mesa RA, Li CY, Ketterling RP et al (2005) Leukemic transformation in myelofibrosis with myeloid metaplasia: a single-institution experience with 91 cases. Blood 105:973–977

Mesa RA, Nagorney DS, Schwager S et al (2006a) Palliative goals, patient selection, and perioperative platelet management: outcomes and lessons from 3 decades of splenectomy for myelofibrosis with myeloid metaplasia at the Mayo Clinic. Cancer 107:361–370

Mesa RA, Powell H, Lasho T et al (2006b) JAK2(V617F) and leukemic transformation in myelofibrosis with myeloid metaplasia. Leuk Res 30:1457–1460

Mesa RA, Cervantes F, Verstovsek S et al (2007a) Clinical evolution to primary myelofibrosis – blast phase: an international working group for myelofibrosis research and treatment (IWG-MRT) collaborative retrospective analysis. Blood 110:682

Mesa RA, Verstovsek S, Cervantes F et al (2007b) Primary myelofibrosis (PMF), post polycythemia vera myelofibrosis (post-PV MF), post essential thrombocythemia myelofibrosis (post-ET MF), blast phase PMF (PMF-BP): consensus on terminology by the international working group for myelofibrosis research and treatment (IWG-MRT). Leuk Res 31:737–740

Mesa RA, Verstovsek S, Rivera C et al (2009) 5-Azacitidine has limited therapeutic activity in myelofibrosis. Leukemia 23:180–182

Najean Y, Rain JD (1997) Treatment of polycythemia vera: the use of hydroxyurea and pipobroman in 292 patients under the age of 65 years. Blood 90: 3370–3377

Osgood EE (1964) Contrasting incidence of acute monocytic and granulocytic leukemias in P32-treated patients with polycythemia vera and chronic lymphocytic leukemia. J Lab Clin Med 64:560–573

Pancrazzi A, Guglielmelli P, Ponziani V et al (2008) A sensitive detection method for MPLW515L or MPLW515K mutation in chronic myeloproliferative disorders with locked nucleic acid-modified probes and real-time polymerase chain reaction. J Mol Diagn 10:435–441

Pardanani A, Lasho T, Finke C et al (2010) LNK mutation studies in blast-phase myeloproliferative neoplasms, and in chronic-phase disease with TET2, IDH, JAK2 or MPL mutations. Leukemia 24:1713–1718

Parmentier C (2003) Use and risks of phosphorus-32 in the treatment of polycythaemia vera. Eur J Nucl Med Mol Imaging 30:1413–1417

Parsons DW, Jones S, Zhang X et al (2008) An integrated genomic analysis of human glioblastoma multiforme. Science 321:1807–1812

Petti MC, Latagliata R, Spadea T et al (2002) Melphalan treatment in patients with myelofibrosis with myeloid metaplasia. Br J Haematol 116:576–581

Pietra D, Li S, Brisci A et al (2008) Somatic mutations of JAK2 exon 12 in patients with JAK2 (V617F)-negative myeloproliferative disorders. Blood 111: 1686–1689

Pikman Y, Lee BH, Mercher T et al (2006) MPLW515L is a novel somatic activating mutation in myelofibrosis with myeloid metaplasia. PLoS Med 3:e270

Quintas-Cardama A, Kantarjian H, Manshouri T et al (2009) Pegylated interferon alfa-2a yields high rates of hematologic and molecular response in patients with advanced essential thrombocythemia and polycythemia vera. J Clin Oncol 27:5418–5424

Rambaldi A, Dellacasa CM, Salmoiraghi S et al (2008) A phase 2A study of the histone-deacetylase inhibitor ITF2357 in patients with JAK2 V617F positive chronic myeloproliferative neoplasms. ASH annual meeting abstracts 112:100

Saberwal G, Horvath E, Hu L et al (2009) The interferon consensus sequence binding protein (ICSBP/IRF8) activates transcription of the FANCF gene during myeloid differentiation. J Biol Chem 284: 33242–33254

Sallmyr A, Fan J, Rassool FV (2008) Genomic instability in myeloid malignancies: increased reactive oxygen species (ROS), DNA double strand breaks (DSBs) and error-prone repair. Cancer Lett 270:1–9

Schaub FX, Looser R, Li S et al (2010) Clonal analysis of TET2 and JAK2 mutations suggests that TET2 can be a late event in the progression of myeloproliferative neoplasms. Blood 115:2003–2007

Scott BL, Deeg HJ (2010) Myelodysplastic syndromes. Annu Rev Med 61:345–358

Scott BL, Storer BE, Greene JE et al (2007a) Marrow fibrosis as a risk factor for posttransplantation outcome in patients with advanced myelodysplastic syndrome or acute myeloid leukemia with multilineage dysplasia. Biol Blood Marrow Transplant 13:345–354

Scott LM, Tong W, Levine RL et al (2007b) JAK2 exon 12 mutations in polycythemia vera and idiopathic erythrocytosis. N Engl J Med 356:459–468

Silva M, Richard C, Benito A et al (1998) Expression of Bcl-x in erythroid precursors from patients with polycythemia vera. N Engl J Med 338:564–571

Steinberg MH, Barton F, Castro O et al (2003) Effect of hydroxyurea on mortality and morbidity in adult sickle cell anemia: risks and benefits up to 9 years of treatment. JAMA 289:1645–1651

Swierczek SI, Yoon D, Prchal JT (2007) Blast transformation in a patient with primary myelofibrosis initiated from JAK2 V617F progenitor. Blood 110:a4665

Tahiliani M, Koh KP, Shen Y et al (2009) Conversion of 5-methylcytosine to 5-hydroxymethylcytosine in mammalian DNA by MLL partner TET1. Science 324:930–935

Tam CS, Nussenzveig RM, Popat U et al (2008) The natural history and treatment outcome of blast phase BCR-ABL-myeloproliferative neoplasms. Blood 112:1628–1637

Tefferi A, Elliot MA (2000) Serious myeloproliferative reactions associated with the use of thalidomide in myelofibrosis with myeloid metaplasia. Blood 96:4007

Tefferi A, Vainchenker W (2011) Myeloproliferative neoplasms: molecular pathophysiology, essential clinical understanding, and treatment strategies. J Clin Oncol 29(5):573–582

Tefferi A, Barosi G, Mesa RA et al (2006a) International Working Group (IWG) consensus criteria for treatment response in myelofibrosis with myeloid metaplasia, for the IWG for Myelofibrosis Research and Treatment (IWG-MRT). Blood 108:1497–1503

Tefferi A, Cortes J, Verstovsek S et al (2006b) Lenalidomide therapy in myelofibrosis with myeloid metaplasia. Blood 108:1158–1164

Tefferi A, Gangat N, Wolanskyj AP et al (2008a) 20+ yr without leukemic or fibrotic transformation in essential thrombocythemia or polycythemia vera: predictors at diagnosis. Eur J Haematol 80:386–390

Tefferi A, Lasho TL, Huang J et al (2008b) Low JAK2 V617F allele burden in primary myelofibrosis, compared to either a higher allele burden or unmutated status, is associated with inferior overall and leukemia-free survival. Leukemia 22:756–761

Tefferi A, Pardanani A, Lim KH et al (2009a) TET2 mutations and their clinical correlates in polycythemia vera, essential thrombocythemia and myelofibrosis. Leukemia 23:905–911

Tefferi A, Verstovsek S, Barosi G et al (2009b) Pomalidomide is active in the treatment of anemia associated with myelofibrosis. J Clin Oncol 27:4563–4569

Tefferi A, Lasho TL, Abdel-Wahab O et al (2010) IDH1 and IDH2 mutation studies in 1473 patients with chronic-, fibrotic- or blast-phase essential thrombocythemia, polycythemia vera or myelofibrosis. Leukemia 24: 1302–1309

Theocharides A, Boissinot M, Girodon F et al (2007) Leukemic blasts in transformed JAK2 V617F-positive myeloproliferative disorders are frequently negative for the JAK2 V617F mutation. Blood 110:375–379

Thepot S, Itzykson R, Seegers V et al (2010) Treatment of progression of Philadelphia-negative myeloproliferative neoplasms to myelodysplastic syndrome or acute myeloid leukemia by azacitidine: a report on 54 cases on the behalf of the Groupe Francophone des Myelodysplasies (GFM). Blood 116:3735–3742

Thoennissen NH, Krug UO, Lee DH et al (2010) Prevalence and prognostic impact of allelic imbalances associated with leukemic transformation of Philadelphia chromosome-negative myeloproliferative neoplasms. Blood 115:2882–2890

Tibes R, Bogenberger J, Choudhary A et al (2009a) RNAi-based identification of novel sensitizers to 5-azacytidine in myeloid leukemias. Haematologica 94(Suppl 2):219, abstract 0536

Tibes R, McDonagh KT, Lekakis L et al (2009b) Phase I study of the novel survivin and cdc2/CDK1 inhibitor terameprocol in patients with advanced leukemias. Blood (ASH annual meeting abstracts #1039)

Tiedt R, Hao-Shen H, Sobas MA et al (2008) Ratio of mutant JAK2 V617F to wild-type Jak2 determines the MPD phenotypes in transgenic mice. Blood 111:3931–3940

Tolcher AW, Mita A, Lewis LD et al (2008) Phase I and pharmacokinetic study of YM155, a small-molecule inhibitor of survivin. J Clin Oncol 26:5198–5203

Vannucchi AM, Guglielmelli P, Lupo L et al (2010) A phase 1/2 study of RAD001, a mTOR inhibitor, in patients with myelofibrosis: final results. ASH annual meeting abstracts 116:314

Vardiman JW, Thiele J et al (2009). The 2008 revision of the World Health Organization (WHO) classification of myeloid neoplasms and acute leukemia: rationale and important changes. Blood 114(5):937–951

Vardiman JW, Brunning RD, Harris NL (2001) WHO histological classification of chronic myeloproliferative diseases. In: Jaffe ES, Harris NL, Stein H, Vardiman JW (eds) World health organization classification of tumors: tumours of the haematopoietic and lymphoid tissues. International Agency for Research on Cancer (IARC) Press, Lyon, pp 17–44

Vigil C, Cortes J, Kantarjian HM et al (2009) Hypomethylating therapy for the treatment of acute erythroleukemia patients. ASH annual meeting abstracts 114:2069

Von Hoff DD, LoRusso PM, Rudin CM et al (2009) Inhibition of the hedgehog pathway in advanced basal-cell carcinoma. N Engl J Med 361:1164–1172

Weller M, Felsberg J, Hartmann C et al (2009) Molecular predictors of progression-free and overall survival in patients with newly diagnosed glioblastoma: a prospective translational study of the German Glioma Network. J Clin Oncol 27:5743–5750

Wolanskyj AP, Schwager SM, McClure RF et al (2006) Essential thrombocythemia beyond the first decade: life expectancy, long-term complication rates, and prognostic factors. Mayo Clin Proc 81:159–166

Current Clinical Needs

13

Giovanni Barosi

Contents

G. Barosi
Unit of Clinical Epidemiology and Center
for the Study of Myelofibrosis, IRCCS Policlinico
S. Matteo Foundation, Pavia, Italy
e-mail: barosig@smatteo.pv.it

13.1 Introduction

Myeloproliferative neoplasms-associated myelo-fibrosis (MPN-MF) (Mesa et al. 2011a) may arise de novo (primary myelofibrosis, PMF) or may follow clinically overt polycythemia vera (PV) or essential thrombocythemia (ET) (post PV- and post ET-MF). Patients with MPN-MF may be entirely asymptomatic; however, in their major-ity, MPN-MF patients present a disabling disease that interferes with their quality of life and social activities. Thus, there are many clinical needs which doctors facing patients with MPN-MF must cope with (Table 13.1).

13.2 Caring Patients with Asymptomatic Disease

A minority of patients with MPN-MF come to medical attention because of an abnormal blood cell count or an enlarged spleen detected during routine physical examination without other signs or symptoms of the disease. The proportion of these asymptomatic patients ranges from 15% to 25% in the larger series of cases diagnosed according pre-WHO criteria. This proportion is also higher if one would include the WHO-established "prefibrotic myelofibrosis" category in the realm of PMF (Swerdlow et al. 2008). Prefibrotic myelofibrosis is a histological variant characterized by absent or only mild increase in reticulin fibers in bone marrow with dual mega-karyocytic and granulocytic myeloproliferation

T. Barbui and A. Tefferi (eds.), *Myeloproliferative Neoplasms*, Hematologic Malignancies,
DOI 10.1007/978-3-642-24989-1_13, © Springer-Verlag Berlin Heidelberg 2012

Table 13.1 Common clinical needs in MPN-MF

Relief of fatigue and constitutional symptoms
Relief of pruritus
Relief of severe anemia
Relief of transfusion dependent anemia
Treatment of transfusional iron overload
Relief of symptomatic splenomegaly
Relentless of spleen enlargement in progressive splenomegaly
Reversion of accelerated phase or blast transformation of the disease
Treatment of extramedullary nonhepatosplenic hematopoiesis
Treatment of pulmonary hypertension
Treatment of portal hypertension
Treatment of splanchnic vein thrombosis
Treatment of thrombotic or hemorrhagic complication

associated with typical morphological characteristics of megakaryocytes. Its phenotype resembles that of ET; thus, in the majority of the patients, diagnosis is made by chance, and patients remain asymptomatic for a long time. Patients with MPN-MF who are diagnosed in an asymptomatic phase need to be informed on the nature of their disease and to be clinically monitored every 3 or 6 months.

13.3 Relieving Symptoms of Disease Activity

A great proportion of patients with MPN-MF suffer from general symptoms, such as fatigue, constitutional symptoms, or pruritus, that reflect the biological activity of the underlying disease. The presence of such symptoms affects quality of life and represents a major medical need.

13.3.1 Fatigue

The National Comprehensive Cancer Network (NCCN) defines fatigue as a persistent, subjective sense of tiredness related to cancer or cancer therapy that interferes with usual functioning (Ahlberg et al. 2003). In an international survey including geographically diverse groups of MPN patients, fatigue was reported in 84% of those with MPN-MF (Mesa et al. 2007). The severity

of fatigue increased with the severity of anemia and the presence of constitutional symptoms. However, fatigue was a problem even in patients with early stage PMF. In fact, the majority of patients who denied any features typically thought to be signs of problematic disease suffered from the significant symptom of fatigue that was not easily explained by anemia or medication toxicity. The presence of this latter finding suggests that there is an aspect to the underlying myeloproliferative process that may well directly cause fatigue even in the absence of a clear source.

Various key cytokines have been implicated in exacerbating fatigue in cancer patients, such as tumor necrosis factor alpha (TNF-α), interleukin-1, and interleukin-6 (Ahlberg et al. 2003). Indeed, recent reports demonstrate that fatigue in cancer patients correlates with alteration of function in proinflammatory cytokines (Collado-Hidalgo et al. 2006). In MPN-MF patients, the proof of cytokine-induced fatigue must be translated from that in cancer, since no ad hoc studies on cytokine expression and fatigue are available for MPNs.

Fatigue is an unmet clinical need in MPN-MF. The lack of efficacy of currently available therapeutic options for MPN-MF patients to abrogate fatigue is striking, and this must be considered in prescribing palliative therapy for these patients. It is important to acknowledge that when novel pharmacologic therapies are evaluated in these patients, improvements in fatigue should be rigorously assessed and considered in judging these agents. In addition, nonpharmacologic interventions, such as exercise, should be considered as alternative strategies for alleviating MPN-MF-associated fatigue. Exercise has the ability to potentially improve fatigue, but published data remain limited in scope (Winningham et al. 1989, 1994; Hayes et al. 2004; Galvao and Newton 2005).

13.3.2 Constitutional Symptoms

Night sweats, low-grade fevers, and weight loss or cachexia are constitutional symptoms individually present in 18–56% of patients with MPN-MF (Mesa et al. 2011b). They largely compromise quality of life and are clearly associated with the prognosis of the disease (Cervantes et al. 2009).

Constitutional symptoms reflect primarily the biological activity of the disease. In a study that used multiplex bead-based Luminex technology in 127 patients with PMF, constitutional symptoms were found correlated with IL-6 and IL-8 expression (Tefferi et al. 2011). IL-8 (CXCL8) is a potent chemokine that exerts a profound effect on the tumor microenvironment, including the survival and proliferation of tumor cells through autocrine signaling, promotion of angiogenesis, and leukocyte chemotaxis and activation (Waugh and Wilson 2008). IL-8 is normally produced by monocytes and/or macrophages and endothelial cells in response to proinflammatory stimuli. Its production in MPN-MF and other hematologic malignancies appears to be constitutive (Francia di Celle et al. 1996; Emadi et al. 2005), and its intramedullary release is believed to contribute to endothelial proliferation, angiogenesis, and impaired megakaryocyte and myeloid progenitor cell proliferation and differentiation (Emadi et al. 2005; Negaard et al. 2009). The lack of any correlation between plasma levels of IL-8 and *JAK2* V617F mutational status (Tefferi et al. 2011) is consistent with the heterogeneity of MPN-MF in regard to its molecular pathogenesis.

Constitutional symptoms must be considered a key treatment indication for MPN-MF. Experimental therapies have been addressed to the relief of constitutional symptoms by interfering with putative responsible cytokines. The first study was published in 2002 by an anti-TGF drug (Steensma et al. 2002b). In an open-label pilot study, etanercept, a dimeric soluble recombinant form of the extracellular domain of human p75 TNF receptor fused to the Fc fragment of human immunoglobulin G1, was given to patients with MPN-MF complicated by anemia and/or constitutional symptoms. Patients self-administered 25 mg etanercept subcutaneously twice weekly. Overall, a constitutional improvement of one type or another was seen in 12 of 20 patients, and the drug was well tolerated.

Now, it is increasingly evident that new drugs for MPN-MF, e.g., thalidomide, lenalidomide, pomalidomide, and JAK inhibitors, have the potential to modulate host immune response and cytokine expression. For example, in a recent phase I/II study, a JAK1/JAK2 inhibitor drug (INCB018424) has induced a rapid decrease in MPN-MF-associated inflammatory cytokine levels (IL-1RA, MIP-1β, TNF-α, VEGF, IL-6, and IL-8), which coincided with improvement in constitutional symptoms and splenomegaly (Verstovsek et al. 2010; Mesa et al. 2011). The inflammatory cytokine suppressing activity of JAK1/JAK2 inhibition has also been demonstrated in a murine model of MPN, using another JAK1/JAK2 inhibitor (CYT387) (Tyner et al. 2010). These observations strongly suggest the contribution of abnormal JAK-STAT (signal transducer and activator of transcription) signaling not only to clonal myeloproliferation but also to cytokine-driven debility, and constitutional symptoms in MPN-MF. They also illustrate the feasibility of therapeutically targeting key MPN-MF-associated cytokines or their downstream signaling pathways.

The widespread use of biological drugs for MPN-MF-associated constitutional symptoms may be limited by their potential risks and high cost. Thus, patients with MPN-MF and bothersome constitutional symptoms may benefit from a trial of these medications with the primary endpoint of improving their quality of life and in which a rigorous risk-benefit analysis could be performed.

13.3.3 Pruritus

Pruritus is defined as an unpleasant sensory experience that leads to scratching. Intractable pruritus (typically aquagenic) can be a disabling condition in approximately 50% of patients with MPN-MF (Mesa et al. 2007). The pathogenesis is unknown. Cross talk between neuron terminals and the spatially closely related dermal mast cells is increasingly recognized as an important pathway in the pathophysiology of pruritus (Greaves 2007). A variety of mast cell mediators, including histamine, tryptase, prostaglandins (PGs), and leukotrienes, are important mediators of itching in inflammatory skin diseases (Greaves 2007). Interleukin (IL)-31, a cytokine mainly produced by activated T cells, is another known critical player in pruritogenesis (Dillon et al. 2004). The presence of pruritus in patients with MPNs has been found to be statistically correlated with a greater number of mast cells, a greater number of mast cell colonies, decreased apoptosis of cultured mast cells, decreased of antipruritogenic PGD_2 release by cultured mast cells, and higher plasma levels of IL-31 (Ishii et al. 2009). These data demonstrate that a functional abnormality exists in MPN's mast cells, and mast cells are involved in the pathogenesis of pruritus. Besides the role of mast cells, studies in MPN patients have documented that basophils are constitutively activated and hypersensitive to IL-3, favoring a direct role of *JAK2* V617F mutation in the pathogenesis of pruritus (Pieri et al. 2009).

Like in PV, where pruritus can be an agonizing aspect of the disease, in MPN-MF, pruritus may deprive patients of sleep and interferes with their social and physical activities (Diehn and Tefferi 2001; Mesa et al. 2007). The itching occurs spontaneously or appears when taking a hot shower or after other sudden environmental changes.

A number of small studies have tried to address this clinical problem (Saini et al. 2010). Antihistamines, such as cyproheptadine, may be beneficial. If unsuccessful, interferon alpha or pegylated interferon was reported to be effective in most patients. Other treatment options include paroxetine, a selective serotonin uptake inhibitor, and photochemotherapy using psoralen and ultraviolet A light. Novel targeted therapies with inhibitors of JAK2 V617F (Verstovsek et al. 2010), mammalian target of rapamycin (mTOR) (Vannucchi et al. 2010), and histone deacetylase (HDAC) (Rambaldi et al. 2010) were found to be useful in controlling this symptom in phase I/II study.

13.4 Fighting the Most Clinically Relevant Manifestations of MPN-MF

13.4.1 Anemia

Anemia is a cardinal manifestation of MPN-MF patients. Severe anemia (hemoglobin less than 10 g/dL) affects 20% of patients at diagnosis or develops in 50% of patients after 3.5 years from

the diagnosis (data from the Italian Registry of Myelofibrosis). Anemia may be aregenerative or may be caused by ineffective red cell production and shortened red blood cell survival. Because the disorder is heterogeneous in its molecular and biological features, it is reasonable to assume that multiple factors contribute to the associated erythropoietic defect. Abnormal expression of proinflammatory cytokines and other growth factors and presence of autoimmune mechanisms have been implicated in MPN-MF-associated anemia (Barosi et al. 2010). Additional contributing factors include mutation profile (presence of *JAK2* V617F might be favorable (Vannucchi et al. 2008) and *MPL* (Guglielmelli et al. 2007) and *TET2* (Tefferi et al. 2009b) mutations unfavorable in this regard), bone marrow stromal changes, hypersplenism, and chronic low-grade hemolysis.

The presence and severity of anemia in MPN-MF signify a clonally advanced and biologically more aggressive disease. This is the primary reason why anemia is a powerful risk factor in the disease (Passamonti et al. 2010a, b; Elena et al. 2011). The need of resolving anemia in MPN-MF relies on the major impact anemia exerts on the quality of life of patients and on the risk of iron overload red cell transfusions produce. Androgens, danazol, and erythropoietin are the drugs traditionally used for this aim. Immunomodulating agents (thalidomide, lenalidomide, pomalidomide) and categories of anti-JAK2 drugs have opened a new era for the treatment of anemia in this disorder.

13.4.2 Splenomegaly

Symptomatic splenomegaly, i.e., spleen extending more than 10 cm from the left costal margin, affects 10% of patients at diagnosis or develop in 50% of patients after approximately 4 years from the diagnosis (data from the Italian Registry of Myelofibrosis). Increase of spleen volume in MPN-MF is mostly acknowledged as the result of splenic extramedullary hematopoiesis. Neoangiogenesis, however, gives a significant contribution to the spleen volume expansion as documented by the measurement of capillary vascular density in spleen sections (Barosi et al. 2004). With enlargement of the spleen, abdominal discomfort ensues, characterized by pressure of the spleen on the stomach that may lead to delayed gastric emptying and early satiety. In addition, the bulk of the spleen can result in areas of ischemia and painful episodes of splenic infarction, simulating an acute abdominal emergency. Pressure of the spleen on the colon or small bowel may be responsible of severe disabling diarrhea. Finally, splenomegaly can result in development or exacerbation of cytopenias from spleen sequestration.

The need of preventing large splenomegaly or of treating symptomatic splenomegaly in MPN-MF relies on the symptoms burden it produces. In addition, a major clinical need is to prevent splenectomy, a necessary intervention in patients who progress to massive and otherwise unmanageable splenomegaly due to failure of medical therapy (Mesa 2009). A further stringent reason for preventing symptomatic spleen enlargement is the detrimental consequences large spleen exert on the outcome of stem cell transplantation. Even though it is not yet clearly documented that splenectomy is a beneficial measure before stem cell transplantation, transplanting with large splenomegaly produces delay in engraftment (Tefferi 2010).

The choice of first-line medical therapy for treatment of splenomegaly and the therapy for refractory cases represents a key therapeutic issue in MPN-MF.

13.4.3 Blast Transformation

Leukemic transformation of MPN-MF is the final phase of blast accumulation that occurs in approximately 10–15% of patients and bears a dramatic symptomatic burden of disease and short life expectancy. In a recent series of 91 consecutive MPN-MF patients who experienced leukemic transformation, the disease was fatal in 98% of patients after a median of 2.6 months (Mesa et al. 2005). The results of any treatment for blast-phase MPN are extremely poor, and

experimental or palliative therapy should be considered.

13.5 Fighting Disease Complications

Many disease complications occur in MPN-MF. Some of them, like nonhepatosplenic extramedullary hematopoiesis, derive from the clonal myeloproliferation, or are a consequence of therapy, like transfusional iron overload. Other complications are the result of the thrombotic and hemorrhagic propensity of the disease. Others, finally, have unrevealed or multiple pathogenetic mechanisms, like pulmonary or portal hypertension. Disease complications such as hemorrhagic or thrombotic events need treatments that are not specific for MPN-MF. On the contrary, treatment of extramedullary nonhepatosplenic hematopoiesis or of pulmonary or portal hypertension are specific clinical needs.

13.5.1 Extramedullary Nonhepatosplenic Hematopoiesis

Extramedullary nonhepatosplenic hematopoiesis might cause symptoms in various organs, particularly in advanced phases of the disease and after splenectomy. The most common sites are pulmonary, gastrointestinal, central nervous, and genitourinary systems. Low-dose radiation therapy is currently the treatment of choice for MPN-MF-associated nonhepatosplenic extramedullary hematopoiesis (Tefferi 2000).

13.5.2 Transfusional Iron Overload

Transfusion dependency is the fate of many MPN-MF anemic patients who do not respond to treatment for anemia. In thalassemia, significant iron overload occurs after as few as 10–20 red blood cell (RBC) units, and patients develop cardiac, hepatic, and endocrine dysfunction. In MPN-MF, the role of iron overload in morbidity and mortality remains largely undefined. Based on strictly retrospective data analysis and using surrogate markers, some investigators have considered the possibility that iron overload contributes to the association between poor survival and red blood cell transfusion need (Leitch et al. 2010). In a series of studies from the Mayo Clinic, iron overload, measured by both transfusion burden and serum ferritin level, did not carry an independent prognostic value in PMF (Tefferi et al. 2009a). Thus, the need of treating iron overload is questionable and clinical trials need to decide what is the real value of iron chelation therapy on the outcome of the patients.

13.5.3 Pulmonary Hypertension

MPN-MF may be associated with pulmonary hypertension, i.e., development of a mean pulmonary artery pressure (P_{pa}) ≥ 25 mmHg at rest. The epidemiology and prevalence of this disorder in MPN-MF and in MPNs in general is unknown because of the small number of case reports in the literature (Garypidou et al. 2004). Most of the studies on epidemiology of pulmonary hypertension in MPN-MF, moreover, have a major limitation, as the diagnosis of pulmonary hypertension was not established as recommended by expert guidelines (Galiè et al. 2009). Therefore, the rate of patients with pulmonary hypertension may be overestimated, as elevated pulmonary pressure might not be confirmed by invasive measures, or could be due to other causes such as left-sided heart disease. Indeed, Reisner et al. (1992) demonstrated that heart disease is common in patients with MPNs. In addition, some patients may have hypermetabolic state resulting in high cardiac output and passive elevation of the P_{pa} without elevation in pulmonary vascular resistance. Thus, it has been envisaged that transthoracic Doppler echocardiography can serve only as a screening tool, and a right heart study with full hemodynamic evaluation is mandatory for the correct diagnosis of pulmonary hypertension.

The pathophysiological mechanisms for this complication are not fully understood, although several theories have been proposed. Extramedullary hematopoiesis diffusely involving the lung and pulmonary fibrosis due to the elaboration of fibrogenic cytokines from dysfunctional circulating clonal cells is the mostly evoked pathogenetic mechanism. According to this vision, megakaryocytes and platelet play a central etiological role. The theory derives from the observation of several case reports (Halank et al. 2004; Hill et al. 1996; Dot et al. 2007; Marvin and Spellberg 1993), describing patients with MPNs and pulmonary hypertension, with pathological examination of the lung demonstrating an obstruction of the small vessels by conglomerates of megakaryocytes. Hibbin et al. (1984) reported that MPN-MF is associated with increased numbers of circulating megakaryocytes and myeloid progenitor cells which are poorly deformable and are much larger than the diameter of alveolar capillaries. Therefore, these cells may occlude the pulmonary microvasculature and secrete vasoactive cytokines, which may contribute to the development of pulmonary hypertension. Recently, a positive correlation between thrombopoietin levels and systolic P_{pa} was shown (Haznedaroglu et al. 2002). Since patients with MPNs exhibit increased circulating thrombopoietin levels, thrombopoietin may be related to the pathogenesis of pulmonary hypertension in this patient population. This hypothesis has been corroborated from the evidence that platelet-derived growth factor released from activated platelets is a strong stimulus for smooth muscle hyperplasia (Neville and Sidawy 1998; Perros et al. 2008), and in an animal model of pulmonary hypertension, the control of the platelet count slows down the development of pulmonary hypertension (White et al. 1989).

Recent studies have suggested that enhanced angiogenesis might be a possible pathogenetic link between MPN-MF and pulmonary hypertension (Zetterberg et al. 2008; Cortelezzi et al. 2008). In 36 patients, peripheral blood levels of endothelial progenitor cells (EPCs), circulating endothelial cells, and CD34+ cells were quantified by flow cytometry (Cortelezzi et al. 2008). The results of the study showed enhanced angiogenesis in the peripheral blood and bone marrow of MPN-MF patients as they were characterized by increased bone marrow microvascular density, serum VEGF levels, and circulating EPCs. Taken together, these data suggest the presence of a distinctive angiogenic phenotype associated with MPN-MF and pulmonary hypertension.

Patients with MPN-MF-associated pulmonary hypertension present with progressive dyspnea, signs of biventricular heart failure, and rapidly increasing hepatosplenomegaly. There is a need for increased awareness among physicians that anemia is not always the sole contributor for increasing dyspnea in MPN-MF, and pulmonary hypertension might be a contributor. The recognition of this complication is necessary mainly because of the poor prognosis associated with it. Also, early intervention might reverse the hypertension in some cases. There are multiple radiographic pulmonary presentations in patients with MPN-MF to make this rare diagnosis (Wyatt and Fishman 1994). This underscores the need for a heightened awareness that Technectium-99 (99 m Tc) sulfur colloid scintigraphy can be strongly suggestive of the diagnosis, although false-negatives have been reported (Coates et al. 1994). Tissue diagnosis of extramedullary hematopoiesis in the lung can be achieved by pleuroscopy, fine needle aspiration of mass lesions, transbronchial biopsy, and open surgical or video-assisted thoracoscopic biopsy. Transbronchial biopsies are not advised in cases with severe pulmonary hypertension because of the high risk of alveolar hemorrhage. The decision as to which approach to use must be individualized, and the decision to perform invasive tissue biopsy must be tempered by the increased risk of perioperative complications. Histology in all reported cases reveals trilineage hematopoiesis with granulocytic, erythroid, and megakaryocytic precursors, with varying degrees of adjacent fibrosis.

Treatment with hydroxyurea is generally not successful in modifying pulmonary hypertension. The current management of pulmonary hypertension includes vasodilators including phosphodiesterase-type 5 inhibitors (which increase nitric oxide levels, e.g., sildenafil) and prostacyclin analogues with a combination of these agents demonstrating better results (Pozner et al. 2005; Boutet et al. 2008). These agents will also inhibit platelet aggregation and thus thrombus formation, another risk factor for pulmonary hypertension. Several case reports suggest that in patients with MPN-MF and pulmonary hypertension and evidence for extramedullary hematopoiesis, a treatment trial with whole-lung, low-dose, external beam radiotherapy may be a useful palliative tool (Steensma et al. 2002a; Weinschenker et al. 2002). Cases of extramedullary hematopoiesis treated with low-dose, whole-lung radiation showed prompt and gratifying improvements in oxygenation, symptoms, pulmonary hypertension, and roentograms. There are no data on the role of anticoagulation and antiaggregants in patients with pulmonary hypertension associated with MPN-MF.

13.5.4 Splanchnic Vein Thrombosis

Splanchnic vein thrombosis (SVT), i.e., occlusions of veins that constitute either the portal vein system or the hepatic vein (Budd–Chiari syndrome), is a complication of MPN-MF, like that of other MPNs. Its incidence in MPN-MF is unknown, and reports are contradictory. In the three most recent large studies on the prevalence and distribution of thrombotic events in PMF with the exclusion of the so-called "prefibrotic" form (Cervantes et al. 2006; Barbui et al. 2010b; Elliott et al. 2010), the overall incidence of SVT was 3.8%, 0.7%, and 3.4%, respectively. Moreover, in one study (Elliott et al. 2010), out of seven episodes of SVT, five occurred postsplenectomy, one occurred on tamoxifen, and one occurred spontaneously. This brought the author to conclude that most of the events were provoked. On the contrary, Rosti et al. (2010), in a cross-sectional analysis on 214 patients with classical MPNs including a selected population of PMF patients, found that SVT occurred in 10% of the PMF cases having a fibrotic bone marrow, while in 40% of cases with prefibrotic type of disease. This would signify that SVT is preferentially associated with an early PMF.

Since the clinical course of SVT can be complicated by intestinal ischemia or bleeding from the gastrointestinal tract, it is a potentially life-threatening complication. Timely diagnosis is a major challenge because of a possible asymptomatic presentation as well as the low specificity of its principal symptoms. In general, portal vein thrombosis has a subtle clinical presentation and may be diagnosed incidentally, while the Budd–Chiari syndrome has a more aggressive presentation. With the advances in imaging techniques, especially Doppler ultrasonography, computed-assisted tomography, and magnetic resonance imaging, an SVT diagnosis can be established earlier.

Major identified risk factors for SVT in MPNs are somewhat different from risk factors associated with venous thrombosis in other sites. The clonal myeloproliferation is the major risk factor per se. The reason why patients with a mild and inactive phenotype of PMF are at high risk of SVT is unknown. Rosti et al. (2010) found a significant association of increased circulating endothelial progenitor cells (ECFCs) frequency with history of SVT. The authors interpreted these results as signifying the biological hallmark of a separate disease category of patients among MPNs. This could be also supported by the fact that high ECFC mobilizers were mostly females and had preferentially young age. This result suggests several important future directions for research addressing the role of ECFCs on the splanchnic thrombotic event.

Factors that were also associated with the risk of SVT were splenectomy as a leading cause of portal vein thrombosis and inherited thrombophilia (De Stefano and Martinelli 2010). Of interest, SVT appears to have a stronger association with G20210A prothrombin mutation than with factor V Leiden mutation. The reason for this inverse association, when compared with what was observed in patients with deep vein thrombosis of the lower limbs, deserves additional investigation.

Anticoagulation is recommended for all patients during the acute phase of SVT, and for at least 3 subsequent months, in the absence of major contraindications, but there is no consensus on the optimal duration of treatment (De Franchis 2005). Recent studies suggest that secondary prevention with vitamin K antagonists may reduce the risk of recurrent venous thromboembolism, with a low incidence of hemorrhagic complications (Dentali et al. 2009). These results can be explained by the fact that anticoagulation prevents thrombosis progression, preserving patients from the complications of portal hypertension, as shown in a recent study in which bleeding events were confined to patients not receiving lifelong anticoagulant (Amitrano et al. 2007). On the basis of these results, lifelong anticoagulant therapy should be recommended in MPN-MF-associated SVT.

In the Budd–Chiari syndrome, intensive medical management including anticoagulation is mandatory, and more aggressive procedures should be considered in the most severe cases. Examples of such procedures include transjugular intrahepatic portosystemic shunt (TIPS), angioplasty (with or without stenting), surgical shunts, and even liver transplantation (Menon et al. 2004). Joint management with a liver team, follow-up of varices, and warning about pregnancy are recommended by European Leukemia Net experts (Barbui et al. 2010a). For those patients with thrombocytosis, hydroxyurea should be used to restore platelet counts to 400×10^9/L or less as soon as possible.

13.5.5 Portal Hypertension

Portal hypertension, i.e., an increase in the pressure within the portal vein and its tributaries of 12 mmHg or more (compared with a normal figure of 5–8 mmHg), has been reported as a complication in MON-MF (Shaldon and Sherlock 1962; Mesa et al. 2006). The diagnosis of portal hypertension is usually based on clinical criteria in conjunction with imaging studies; thus, the assessment of the gradient between wedged and free hepatic venous pressure, that would provide a reliable measure of portal pressure, is deemed not necessary for diagnostic purposes. Since portal hypertension secondary to MPN-MF is usually asymptomatic, diagnosis in these patients is often made when they become symptomatic, i.e., they present either with acute upper gastrointestinal bleeding from ruptured varices or in the form of melena, or with ascites. Thus, the prevalence of 7–18% of symptomatic portal hypertension reported in literature (Silverstein et al. 1973; Ligumski et al. 1978) underestimates the true prevalence of portal hypertension in MPN-MF.

The mechanisms leading to portal hypertension in MPN-MF are controversial. In the absence of portal and/or hepatic vein thromboses, two mechanisms have been proposed. The first theory states that portal hypertension develops in MPN-MF patients due to sinusoidal narrowing and intrahepatic obstruction caused by extramedullary hematopoiesis and infiltration of the liver by myeloid cells leading to increased intrahepatic resistance (Escartín Marin et al. 1977; Roux et al. 1987; Dubois et al. 1993). The other theory states that portal hypertension develops in such patients due to increased portal blood flow through the enlarged spleen (Silverstein et al. 1973; Escartín Marin et al. 1977; Wanless et al. 1990). As a matter of fact, few cases of portal hypertension in MPN-MF patients secondary to increased splenic and/or portal flow with minimal hematopoiesis have been reported (Rosenbaum et al. 1966; Blendis et al. 1970). On the other hand, Sikuler et al. (1985) experimentally demonstrated that in the absence of structural alteration of the liver, portal hypertension does not develop as a consequence of an increased portal flow.

Patients with portal hypertension characteristically exhibit a hyperdynamic circulation with increased cardiac output and decreased peripheral resistance (Petz 1989). Overactivity of some vasodilator factors has been proposed, and there is a growing body of evidence suggesting that endogenous nitric oxide accounts for much of this activity (Pizcueta et al. 1992a, b). Anemia, which is a very common feature in patients with MPN-MF, has been shown to further worsen the hyperdynamic circulation associated with portal hypertension (Cirera et al. 1997; Lee et al. 1999; Hua et al. 2006).

The need of therapy for asymptomatic portal hypertension secondary to MPN-MF has not been well established. Based on the theory of increased portal flow due to splenomegaly as a mechanism for the portal hypertension, splenectomy would be a reasonable choice. In fact, splenectomy proved to effectively reverse portal hypertension in selected patients (Sullivan et al. 1974; Lukie

and Card 1977). However, increased blood flow from an enlarged spleen is not the sole mechanism for development of portal hypertension in MPN-MF patients. The risk of splenectomy, together with the knowledge that splenectomy has not been shown to improve overall survival in these patients, must be strongly considered before proceeding for splenectomy to manage portal hypertension.

Managing the acute bleeding episodes due to esophageal or gastric varices consists of general resuscitative measures such as volume and blood replacement and specific measures to stop bleeding. Symptomatic portal hypertension requires prevention and treatment of gastrointestinal variceal bleeding with beta-adrenergic blockade and endoscopic therapies. Endoscopic variceal band ligation (EVL) (Nikolaidis et al. 2004; Ghidirim et al. 2006; Goh et al. 2007) as well as endoscopic variceal sclerotherapy (EVS) (Takasaki et al. 1996) have been utilized successfully for the management of gastrointestinal bleeding in MPN-MF patients. EVL has been reported to have very good efficacy, with fewer therapeutic sessions and complications when compared to EVS in variceal bleeding due to other etiologies (Hou et al. 1995). Nevertheless, there is a paucity of data regarding the use of EVL in patients with MPN-MF-associated portal hypertension, and further studies are required.

Symptomatic portal hypertension caused by intrahepatic or portal obstruction, refractory to conventional therapies for preventing variceal bleeding or ascites, is an indication for invasive procedures such as angioplasty, with or without stenting, or TIPS (Perelló et al. 2002; Alvarez-Larrán et al. 2005). TIPS is an effective and well-established procedure that involves creation of a side-to-side portacaval shunt in the liver, and it has very good efficacy for intractable ascites. However, such a procedure needs ideal candidates who display normal liver synthetic function with little interventional risk. Only a few reports have been published regarding the use of TIPS for portal hypertension secondary to MPN-MF, but these have proved to be effective (Wiest et al. 2004).

References

Ahlberg K, Ekman T, Gaston-Johansson F et al (2003) Assessment and management of cancer-related fatigue in adults. Lancet 362:640–650

Alvarez-Larrán A, Abraldes JG, Cervantes F et al (2005) Portal hypertension secondary to myelofibrosis: a study of three cases. Am J Gastroenterol 100:2355–2358

Amitrano L, Guardascione MA, Scaglione M et al (2007) Prognostic factors in noncirrhotic patients with splanchnic vein thromboses. Am J Gastroenterol 102:2464–2470

Barbui T, Barosi G, Birgegard G et al (2010a) Philadelphia-negative classical myeloproliferative neoplasms: critical concepts and management recommendations from European LeukemiaNet. J Clin Oncol 29:761–770

Barbui T, Carobbio A, Cervantes F et al (2010b) Thrombosis in primary myelofibrosis: incidence and risk factors. Blood 115:778–782

Barosi G, Rosti V, Massa M et al (2004) Spleen neoangiogenesis in patients with myelofibrosis with myeloid metaplasia. Br J Haematol 124:618–625

Barosi G, Magrini U, Gale RP (2010) Does auto-immunity contribute to anemia in myeloproliferative neoplasms (MPN)-associated myelofibrosis? Leuk Res 34:1119–1120

Blendis LM, Banks DC, Ramboer C et al (1970) Spleen blood flow and splanchnic haemodynamics in blood dyscrasia and other splenomegalies. Clin Sci 38:73–84

Boutet K, Montani D, Jaïs X et al (2008) Therapeutic advances in pulmonary arterial hypertension. Ther Adv Respir Dis 2:249–265

Cervantes F, Alvarez-Larrán A, Arellano-Rodrigo E et al (2006) Frequency and risk factors for thrombosis in idiopathic myelofibrosis: analysis in a series of 155 patients from a single institution. Leukemia 20:55–60

Cervantes F, Dupriez B, Pereira A et al (2009) New prognostic scoring system for primary myelofibrosis based on a study of the International Working Group for Myelofibrosis Research and Treatment. Blood 113:2895–2901

Cirera I, Elizalde JI, Piqué JM et al (1997) Anemia worsens hyperdynamic circulation of patients with cirrhosis and portal hypertension. Dig Dis Sci 42:1697–1702

Coates GG, Eisenberg B, Dail DH (1994) Tc-99 m sulfur colloid demonstration of diffuse pulmonary interstitial extramedullary hematopoiesis in a patient with myelofibrosis. A case report and review of the literature. Clin Nucl Med 19:1079–1084

Collado-Hidalgo A, Bower JE, Ganz PA et al (2006) Inflammatory biomarkers for persistent fatigue in breast cancer survivors. Clin Cancer Res 12:2759–2766

Cortelezzi A, Gritti G, Del Papa N et al (2008) Pulmonary arterial hypertension in primary myelofibrosis is common and associated with an altered angiogenic status. Leukemia 22:646–649

De Franchis R (2005) Evolving consensus in portal hypertension: report of the Baveno IV Consensus Workshop on methodology of diagnosis and therapy in portal hypertension. J Hepatol 43:167–176

De Stefano V, Martinelli I (2010) Splanchnic vein thrombosis: clinical presentation, risk factors and treatment. Intern Emerg Med 5:487–494

Dentali F, Ageno W, Witt D et al (2009) Natural history of mesenteric venous thrombosis in patients treated with vitamin K antagonists: a multi-centre, retrospective cohort study. Thromb Haemost 102:501–504

Diehn F, Tefferi A (2001) Pruritus in polycythaemia vera: prevalence, laboratory correlates and management. Br J Haematol 115:619–621

Dillon SR, Sprecher C, Hammond A et al (2004) Interleukin 31, a cytokine produced by activated T cells, induces dermatitis in mice. Nat Immunol 5:752–760

Dot JM, Sztrymf B, Yaïci A et al (2007) Pulmonary arterial hypertension due to tumor emboli. Rev Mal Respir 24:359–366

Dubois A, Dauzat M, Pignodel C et al (1993) Portal hypertension in lymphoproliferative and myeloproliferative disorders: hemodynamic and histological correlations. Hepatology 17:246–250

Elena C, Passamonti F, Rumi E et al (2011) Red blood cell transfusion-dependency implies a poor survival in primary myelofibrosis irrespective of International Prognostic Scoring System and Dynamic International Prognostic Scoring System. Haematologica 961:167–170

Elliott MA, Pardanani A, Lasho TL et al (2010) Thrombosis in myelofibrosis: prior thrombosis is the only predictive factor and most venous events are provoked. Haematologica 95:1788–1791

Emadi S, Clay D, Desterke C et al (2005) IL-8 and its CXCR1 and CXCR2 receptors participate in the control of megakaryocytic proliferation, differentiation, and ploidy in myeloid metaplasia with myelofibrosis. Blood 105:464–473

Escartín Marin P, Arenas Mirave JI, Boixeda D et al (1977) Hemodynamic study of the portal system in 6 cases of myeloid metaplasia. Rev Clin Esp 145:271–273

Francia di Celle P, Mariani S, Riera L et al (1996) Interleukin-8 induces the accumulation of B-cell chronic lymphocytic leukemia cells by prolonging survival in an autocrine fashion. Blood 87:4382–4389

Galiè N, Hoeper MM, Humbert M et al (2009) Guidelines for the diagnosis and treatment of pulmonary hypertension. Eur Heart J 30:2493–2537

Galvao DA, Newton RU (2005) Review of exercise intervention studies in cancer patients. J Clin Oncol 23:899–909

Garypidou V, Vakalopoulou S, Dimitriadis D et al (2004) Incidence of pulmonary hypertension in patients with chronic myeloproliferative disorders. Haematologica 89:245–247

Ghidirim G, Corchmaru I, Mishin I et al (2006) Endoscopic rubber band ligation for bleeding oesophageal varices in portal hypertension due to idiopathic myelofibrosis. J Gastrointestin Liver Dis 15:322

Goh BK, Chen JJ, Tan HK et al (2007) Acute variceal bleed in a patient with idiopathic myelofibrosis successfully treated with endoscopic variceal band ligation. Dig Dis Sci 52:173–175

Greaves MW (2007) Recent advances in pathophysiology and current management of itch. Ann Acad Med Singapore 36:788–792

Guglielmelli P, Pancrazzi A, Bergamaschi G et al (2007) Anaemia characterises patients with myelofibrosis harbouring Mpl mutation. Br J Haematol 137:244–247

Halank M, Marx C, Baretton G et al (2004) Severe pulmonary hypertension in chronic idiopathic myelofibrosis. Onkologie 27:472–474

Hayes S, Davies PS, Parker T et al (2004) Quality of life changes following peripheral blood stem cell transplantation and participation in a mixed-type, moderate-intensity, exercise program. Bone Marrow Transplant 33:553–558

Haznedaroglu IC, Atalar E, Ozturk MA et al (2002) Thrombopoietin inside the pulmonary vessels in patients with and without pulmonary hypertension. Platelets 13:395–399

Hibbin JA, Njoku OS, Matutes E et al (1984) Myeloid progenitor cells in the circulation of patients with myelofibrosis and other myeloproliferative disorders. Br J Haematol 57:495–503

Hill G, McClean D, Fraser R et al (1996) Pulmonary hypertension as a consequence of alveolar capillary plugging by malignant megakaryocytes in essential thrombocythaemia. Aust N Z J Med 26:852–853

Hou MC, Lin HC, Kuo BI et al (1995) Comparison of endoscopic variceal injection sclerotherapy and ligation for the treatment of esophageal variceal hemorrhage: a prospective randomized trial. Hepatology 21:1517–1522

Hua R, Cao H, Wu ZY (2006) Effects of hemoglobin concentration on hyperdynamic circulation associated with portal hypertension. Hepatobiliary Pancreat Dis Int 5:215–218

Ishii T, Wang J, Zhang W et al (2009) Pivotal role of mast cells in pruritogenesis in patients with myeloproliferative disorders. Blood 1133:5942–5950

Lee WC, Lin HC, Hou MC et al (1999) Effect of anaemia on haemodynamics in patients with cirrhosis. J Gastroenterol Hepatol 14:370–375

Leitch HA, Chase JM, Goodman TA et al (2010) Improved survival in red blood cell transfusion dependent patients with primary myelofibrosis (PMF) receiving iron chelation therapy. Hematol Oncol 28:40–48

Ligumski M, Polliack A, Benbassat J (1978) Nature and incidence of liver involvement in agnogenic myeloid metaplasia. Scand J Haematol 21:81–93

Lukie BE, Card RT (1977) Portal hypertension complicating myelofibrosis: reversal following splenectomy. Can Med Assoc J 117:771–772

Marvin KS, Spellberg RD (1993) Pulmonary hypertension secondary to thrombocytosis in a patient with myeloid metaplasia. Chest 103:642–644

Menon KV, Shah V, Kamath PS (2004) The Budd-Chiari syndrome. N Engl J Med 350:578–585

Mesa RA (2009) How I treat symptomatic splenomegaly in patients with myelofibrosis. Blood 113:5394–5400

Mesa RA, Li CY, Ketterling RP et al (2005) Leukemic transformation in myelofibrosis with myeloid metaplasia: a single-institution experience with 91 cases. Blood 105:973–977

Mesa RA, Barosi G, Cervantes F et al (2006) Myelofibrosis with myeloid metaplasia: disease overview and non-transplant treatment options. Best Pract Res Clin Haematol 19:495–517

Mesa RA, Niblack J, Wadleigh M et al (2007) The burden of fatigue and quality of life in myeloproliferative disorders (MPDs): an international Internet-based survey of 1179 MPD patients. Cancer 109:68–76

Mesa RA, Green A, Barosi G et al (2011a) MPN-associated myelofibrosis (MPN-MF). Leuk Res 35:12–13

Mesa RA, Kantarjian H, Tefferi A et al (2011b) Evaluating the serial use of the myelofibrosis symptom assessment form for measuring symptomatic improvement: performance in 87 myelofibrosis patients on a JAK1 and JAK2 inhibitor (INCB018424) clinical trial. Cancer. doi:10.1002/cncr.26129

Negaard HF, Iversen N, Bowitz-Lothe IM et al (2009) Increased bone marrow microvascular density in haematological malignancies is associated with differential regulation of angiogenic factors. Leukemia 23:162–169

Neville RF, Sidawy AN (1998) Myointimal hyperplasia: basic science and clinical considerations. Semin Vasc Surg 11:142–148

Nikolaidis N, Giouleme O, Sileli M et al (2004) Endoscopic variceal ligation for portal hypertension due to myelofibrosis with myeloid metaplasia. Eur J Haematol 72:379–380

Passamonti F, Cervantes F, Vannucchi AM et al (2010a) A dynamic prognostic model to predict survival in primary myelofibrosis: a study by the IWG-MRT (International Working Group for Myeloproliferative Neoplasms Research and Treatment). Blood 115(9):1703–1708

Passamonti F, Rumi E, Elena C et al (2010b) Incidence of leukaemia in patients with primary myelofibrosis and RBC-transfusion-dependence. Br J Haematol 150: 719–721

Perelló A, García-Pagán JC, Gilabert R et al (2002) TIPS is a useful long-term derivative therapy for patients with Budd-Chiari syndrome uncontrolled by medical therapy. Hepatology 35:132–139

Perros F, Montani D, Dorfmüller P et al (2008) Platelet-derived growth factor expression and function in idiopathic pulmonary arterial hypertension. Am J Respir Crit Care Med 178:81–88

Petz LD (1989) Hematologic aspects of liver disease. Curr Opin Gastroenterol 5:372–377

Pieri L, Bogani C, Guglielmelli P et al (2009) The JAK2V617 mutation induces constitutive activation and agonist hypersensitivity in basophils from patients with polycythemia vera. Haematologica 94:1537–1545

Pizcueta P, Piqué JM, Fernández M et al (1992a) Modulation of the hyperdynamic circulation of cirrhotic rats by nitric oxide inhibition. Gastroenterology 103:1909–1915

Pizcueta MP, Piqué JM, Bosch J et al (1992b) Effects of inhibiting nitric oxide biosynthesis on the systemic and splanchnic circulation of rats with portal hypertension. Br J Pharmacol 105:184–190

Pozner RG, Negrotto S, D'Atri LP et al (2005) Prostacyclin prevents nitric oxide-induced megakaryocyte apoptosis. Br J Pharmacol 145:283–292

Rambaldi A, Dellacasa CM, Finazzi G et al (2010) A pilot study of the Histone-Deacetylase inhibitor Givinostat in patients with JAK2V617F positive chronic myeloproliferative neoplasms. Br J Haematol 150:446–455

Reisner SA, Rinkevich D, Markiewicz W et al (1992) Cardiac involvement in patients with myeloproliferative disorders. Am J Med 93:498–504

Rosenbaum DL, Murphy GW, Swisher SN (1966) Hemodynamic studies of the portal circulation in myeloid metaplasia. Am J Med 41:360–368

Rosti V, Bonetti E, Bergamaschi G et al (2010) High frequency of endothelial colony forming cells marks a non-active myeloproliferative neoplasm with high risk of splanchnic vein thrombosis. PLoS One 5:e15277

Roux D, Merlio JP, Quinton A, Lamouliatte H, Balabaud C, Bioulac-Sage P et al (1987) Agnogenic myeloid metaplasia, portal hypertension, and sinusoidal abnormalities. Gastroenterology 92:1067–1072

Saini KS, Patnaik MM, Tefferi A (2010) Polycythemia vera-associated pruritus and its management. Eur J Clin Invest 40:828–834

Shaldon S, Sherlock S (1962) Portal hypertension in the myeloproliferative syndrome and the reticuloses. Am J Med 32:758–764

Sikuler E, Kravetz D, Groszmann RJ (1985) Evolution of portal hypertension and mechanisms involved in its maintenance in a rat model. Am J Physiol 248:G618–G625

Silverstein MN, Wollaeger EE, Baggenstoss AH (1973) Gastrointestinal and abdominal manifestations of agnogenic myeloid metaplasia. Arch Intern Med 131:532–537

Steensma DP, Hook CC, Stafford SL et al (2002a) Low-dose, single fraction, whole-lung radiotherapy for pulmonary hypertension associated with myelofibrosis with myeloid metaplasia. Br J Haematol 118: 813–816

Steensma DP, Mesa RA, Li CY et al (2002b) Etanercept, a soluble tumor necrosis factor receptor, palliates constitutional symptoms in patients with myelofibrosis with myeloid metaplasia: results of a pilot study. Blood 99:2252–2254

Sullivan A, Rheinlander H, Weintraub LR (1974) Esophageal varices in agnogenic myeloid metaplasia: disappearance after splenectomy. A case report. Gastroenterology 66:429–432

Swerdlow SH, Campo E, Harris NL et al (2008) WHO classification of tumours of haemopoietic and lymphoid tissues. IARC, Lyon

Takasaki M, Takahashi I, Takamatsu M et al (1996) Endoscopic injection sclerotherapy for esophageal variceal hemorrhage in a patient with idiopathic myelofibrosis. J Gastroenterol 31:260–262

Tefferi A (2000) Myelofibrosis with myeloid metaplasia. N Engl J Med 342:1255–1265

Tefferi A (2010) Allogeneic hematopoietic cell transplantation versus drugs in myelofibrosis: the risk-benefit balancing act. Bone Marrow Transplant 45:419–421

Tefferi A, Mesa RA, Pardanani A et al (2009a) Red blood cell transfusion need at diagnosis adversely affects survival in primary myelofibrosis-increased serum ferritin or transfusion load does not. Am J Hematol 84:265–267

Tefferi A, Pardanani A, Lim KH et al (2009b) TET2 mutations and their clinical correlates in polycythemia vera, essential thrombocythemia and myelofibrosis. Leukemia 235:905–911

Tefferi A, Vaidya R, Caramazza D et al (2011) Circulating interleukin (IL)-8, IL-2R, IL-12, and IL-15 levels are independently prognostic in primary myelofibrosis: a comprehensive cytokine profiling study. J Clin Oncol 29:1356–1363

Tyner JW, Bumm TG, Deininger J et al (2010) CYT387, a novel JAK2 inhibitor, induces hematologic responses and normalizes inflammatory cytokines in murine myeloproliferative neoplasms. Blood 115:5232–5240

Vannucchi AM, Antonioli E, Guglielmelli P et al (2008) Clinical correlates of JAK2V617F presence or allele burden in myeloproliferative neoplasms: a critical reappraisal. Leukemia 22(7):1299–1307

Vannucchi AM, Guglielmelli P, Lupo L et al. (2010) A phase 1/2 study of RAD001, a mTOR inhibitor, in patients with myelofibrosis: final results. Blood (ASH Annual Meeting Abstracts) 116:314

Verstovsek S, Kantarjian H, Mesa RA et al (2010) Safety and efficacy of INCB018424, a JAK1 and JAK2 inhibitor, in myelofibrosis. N Engl J Med 363:1117–1127

Wanless IR, Peterson P, Das A et al (1990) Hepatic vascular disease and portal hypertension in polycythemia vera and agnogenic myeloid metaplasia: a clinicopathological study of 145 patients examined at autopsy. Hepatology 12:1166–1174

Waugh DJ, Wilson C (2008) The interleukin-8 pathway in cancer. Clin Cancer Res 14:6735–6741

Weinschenker P, Kutner JM, Salvajoli JV et al (2002) Whole-pulmonary low-dose radiation therapy in agnogenic myeloid metaplasia with diffuse lung involvement. Am J Hematol 69:277–280

White SM, Wagner JG, Roth RA (1989) Effects of altered platelet number on pulmonary hypertension and platelet sequestration in monocrotaline pyrrole-treated rats. Toxicol Appl Pharmacol 99:302–313

Wiest R, Strauch U, Wagner H et al (2004) A patient with myelofibrosis complicated by refractory ascites and portal hypertension: to tips or not to tips? A case report with discussion of the mechanism of ascites formation. Scand J Gastroenterol 39:389–394

Winningham ML, MacVicar MG, Bondoc M et al (1989) Effect of aerobic exercise on body weight and composition in patients with breast cancer on adjuvant chemotherapy. Oncol Nurs Forum 16:683–689

Winningham ML, Nail LM, Burke MB et al (1994) Fatigue and the cancer experience: the state of the knowledge. Oncol Nurs Forum 21:23–36

Wyatt SH, Fishman EK (1994) Diffuse pulmonary extramedullary hematopoiesis in a patient with myelofibrosis: CT findings. J Comput Assist Tomogr 18:815–817

Zetterberg E, Popat U, Hasselbalch H et al (2008) Angiogenesis in pulmonary hypertension with myelofibrosis. Haematologica 93:945–946

Risk Stratification in PMF

14

Francesco Passamonti

Contents

Primary myelofibrosis (PMF) is a Philadelphia-negative myeloproliferative neoplasm (MPN) whose diagnostic criteria have been recently updated (Tefferi et al. 2007). Among MPNs, PMF has the most heterogeneous clinical presentation, which may encompass anemia, splenomegaly, leukocytosis or leukopenia, thrombocytosis or thrombocytopenia, and constitutional symptoms. Median survival in PMF is estimated at 6 years, but it can range from few months to many years (Cervantes et al. 2009; Passamonti et al. 2010a; Gangat et al. 2011; Tam et al. 2009).

Causes of death may be recapitulated into bone marrow failure (severe anemia, bleeding due to thrombocytopenia, and infections due to leukopenia) in 25–30% of patients, leukemic transformation, named blast phase (BP), in 10–20% of patients, cardiovascular complications in 15–20%, and portal hypertension in 10%. Increasing rates of secondary malignancy have been reported in patients with a longer follow-up. However, all large series reported a 20–30% rate of unknown cause of death (Cervantes et al. 2009; Gangat et al. 2011).

An ideal prognostic model should include some patients-based parameters (age, performance status, and symptoms), disease-based parameters (hemoglobin level, leukocyte, and platelet count), and genetic-based factors (cytogenetic abnormalities and mutations).

Advanced age (Cervantes et al. 1997, 2009; Gangat et al. 2011; Barosi et al. 1988; Reilly et al. 1997; Tefferi et al. 2001a; Passamonti et al. 2010b), anemia (Cervantes et al. 1997, 2009; Passamonti et al. 2010a; Gangat et al. 2011; Tam et al. 2009; Barosi et al. 1988; Reilly et al. 1997; Dupriez et al. 1996; Rupoli et al. 1994), red blood cell transfusion need (Gangat et al. 2011; Tefferi et al. 2009a, 2010a; Elena et al. 2011), leukopenia (Dupriez et al. 1996), leukocytosis (Passamonti

F. Passamonti
Division of Hematology, Department of Internal Medicine, University Hospital Ospedale di Circolo e Fondazione Macchi, Varese, Italy
e-mail: francesco.passamonti@ospedale.varese.it

T. Barbui and A. Tefferi (eds.), *Myeloproliferative Neoplasms*, Hematologic Malignancies, DOI 10.1007/978-3-642-24989-1_14, © Springer-Verlag Berlin Heidelberg 2012

et al. 2010a; Dupriez et al. 1996; Morel et al. 2010), thrombocytopenia (Tam et al. 2009; Morel et al. 2010; Patnaik et al. 2010), peripheral blast count (Cervantes et al. 1997, 2009; Barosi et al. 1988; Reilly et al. 1997; Passamonti et al. 2010a, b), systemic symptoms (Cervantes et al. 1997, 2009; Rupoli et al. 1994), hepatic myeloid metaplasia (Pereira et al. 1988), decreased marrow cellularity with higher degree of fibrosis (Chelloul et al. 1976), higher degree of microvessel density (Mesa et al. 2000), high number of circulating CD34-positive cells (Barosi et al. 2001; Arora et al. 2005; Alchalby et al. 2011), cytogenetic abnormalities (Cervantes et al. 2009; Gangat et al. 2011; Tam et al. 2009; Reilly et al. 1997; Tefferi et al. 2001a; Rumi et al. 2010; Hussein et al. 2010; Caramazza et al. 2011; Vaidya et al. 2011), the *JAK2* (V617F) mutation (Cervantes et al. 2009; Guglielmelli et al. 2009; Tefferi et al. 2008; Barosi et al. 2007), and high level of some cytokines (Tefferi et al. 2011) were shown to be associated with poor outcome in patients with PMF. In the last years, many models have been published in PMF, but the most widely used at diagnosis of PMF are the Lille score (Dupriez et al. 1996) and the more recent International Prognostic Scoring System (IPSS) (Cervantes et al. 2009). The progressive nature of PMF generated interest in defining new so-called dynamic models, such as the dynamic-IPSS (DIPSS) and the most recent DIPSS-plus.

14.1 Prognostic Models at Diagnosis of PMF

14.1.1 The Lille Score

This model was published in 1996, and it was designed on 195 patients with PMF. All patients fulfilled the Polycythemia Vera Study Group criteria for PMF (splenomegaly, red cell poikilocytosis, leukoerythroblastosis, absence of monocytosis, bone marrow fibrosis without any identifiable cause, and absence of Philadelphia chromosome) and those with post-PV MF, acute MF, and myelodysplastic syndromes with MF were excluded.

Median survival was 42 months. Adverse prognostic factors identified for survival were age over 60 years, hepatomegaly, weight loss, low hemoglobin level, low or very high leukocyte count, high percentage of circulating blasts, male sex, and low platelet count. The final scoring system was based on two of them: hemoglobin less than 10 g/dL and leukocyte count less than 4×10^9/L or higher than 30×10^9/L. Patients were grouped into three categories with low (0 factor), intermediate (1 factor), and high (2 factors) risk, associated with a median survival of 93, 26, and 13 months, respectively.

The study also revealed that an abnormal karyotype (~35% of patients) was associated with a short survival, especially in the low-risk group: median survival was 50 months (abnormal karyotype) vs. 112 months (normal karyotype). BP evolution was predicted by leukocytosis (leukocyte count over 30×10^9/L) and abnormal karyotype.

Strengths of this staging system were the simplicity and the possibility to identify high-risk patients to be treated with investigative treatments or hematopoietic stem-cell transplantation. The weakness is that patients with a very good prognosis are lacking.

14.1.2 The IPSS Model

A new scoring system, named IPSS, was defined through the collaboration of seven centers under the auspices of the International Working Group on MPN Research and Treatment (IWG-MRT) in 2009 (Cervantes et al. 2009). After a systematic individual case review, the database included 1,054 patients with PMF defined according to the World Health Organization (WHO) classification system, excluding post-PV and post–ET MF and prefibrotic MF. This is the largest prognostic study ever performed in PMF.

Median survival was 69 months, longer than that reported by the Lille score, probably due to the more consistency of data of a multicenter study, as the date of diagnosis did not affect survival in IPSS. Multivariate analysis of parameters obtained at disease diagnosis identified age greater

Table 14.1 Score values for International Prognostic Scoring System (IPSS) (Cervantes et al. 2009) and Dynamic International Prognostic Scoring System (DIPSS)

Parameter	Scores	
	IPSS	DIPSS
Age > 60 years	1	1
Hemoglobin <10 g/dL	1	2
Leukocyte count >25×10⁹/L	1	1
Blast cells ≥1%	1	1
Constitutional symptoms	1	1

IPSS: score 0 for low risk, score 1 for intermediate-1 risk, score 2 for intermediate-2 risk, score ≥3 for high risk; DIPSS: score 0 for low risk, score 1–2 for intermediate-1 risk, score 3–4 for intermediate-2 risk, score 5–6 for high risk

than 65 years, presence of constitutional symptoms, hemoglobin level less than 10 g/dL, leukocyte count greater than 25×10^9/L, and circulating blast cells 1% or greater as predictors of shortened survival. Based on the presence of 0 (low risk), 1 (intermediate-1 risk), 2 (intermediate-2 risk), or greater than or equal to 3 (high risk) of these variables, four risk groups with no overlapping in their survival curves were generated (Table 14.1). The four risk categories were well balanced: 22% in low risk, 29% in intermediate-1 risk, 28% in intermediate-2 risk, and 21% in high risk. Median survivals were 135 months for low-risk patients, 95 months for intermediate-1 patients, 48 months for intermediate-2 patients, and 27 months for high-risk patients (Fig. 14.1a).

Among these 1,054 patients, 409 patients had available cytogenetic analysis at diagnosis, and authors found that carrying an abnormal karyotype implies a shorter survival. However, the independent contribution of abnormal karyotype to prognosis was restricted to patients in the intermediate-1 and intermediate-2 risk groups. It is of interest that abnormal karyotype was associated to anemia.

Concerning the *JAK2* (V617F) mutation, no association was observed between the *JAK2* status and the prognostic score or the survival. As JAK inhibitors have an effect on spleen size

(Pardanani et al. 2011), it is intriguing that patients without splenomegaly at diagnosis survived longer than the remainder, but the difference did not reach statistical significance, whereas the variable splenomegaly did not improve the PMF prognostic score.

The study also offers an update on causes of death in PMF. Among patients in whom the final cause of death was known, leukemic transformation was the most frequent cause (86 patients), followed by PMF progression without acute transformation (50), thrombosis and cardiovascular complications (37), infection (29) or bleeding (14) out of the setting of acute transformation, portal hypertension (12), secondary malignancies (12), and other causes (36).

Strengths of IPSS were the multicenter origin, the simplicity, the proven higher discriminating power than prior models, the possibility to identify low-risk patients to be monitored with conventional treatments, and higher risk patients to be treated with experimental treatments or hematopoietic stem-cell transplantation. The IPSS weakness is the non-integration with specific cytogenetic abnormalities.

Nowadays, the IPSS is the prognostic scoring system to be used in the clinical practice at diagnosis, as stated by the European Leukemia Net recommendation very recently (Barbui et al. 2011). The option of hematopoietic stem-cell transplantation is taken into consideration for patients with higher risk scores. In addition, it is also used to stratify patients to be enrolled in clinical trials with JAK inhibitors: until now, only patients with intermediate-2 or high-risk categories have been included in these investigative treatments.

14.1.3 The MD Anderson Score

This is a composite prognostic model including clinical parameters and specific cytogenetic abnormalities (Tam et al. 2009). Cytogenetic abnormalities and their relationship with survival are, however, discussed later in this chapter. The score was built on 256 patients with PMF. The

Fig. 14.1 Survival estimate according to four prognostic models. (**a**) International Prognostic Scoring System (IPSS) (Cervantes et al. 2009), (**b**) MD Anderson scoring system (Tam et al. 2009), (**c**) Dynamic International Prognostic Scoring System (DIPSS) (Passamonti et al. 2010b), (**d**) Dynamic International Prognostic Scoring System-plus (DIPSS-plus) (Gangat et al. 2011)

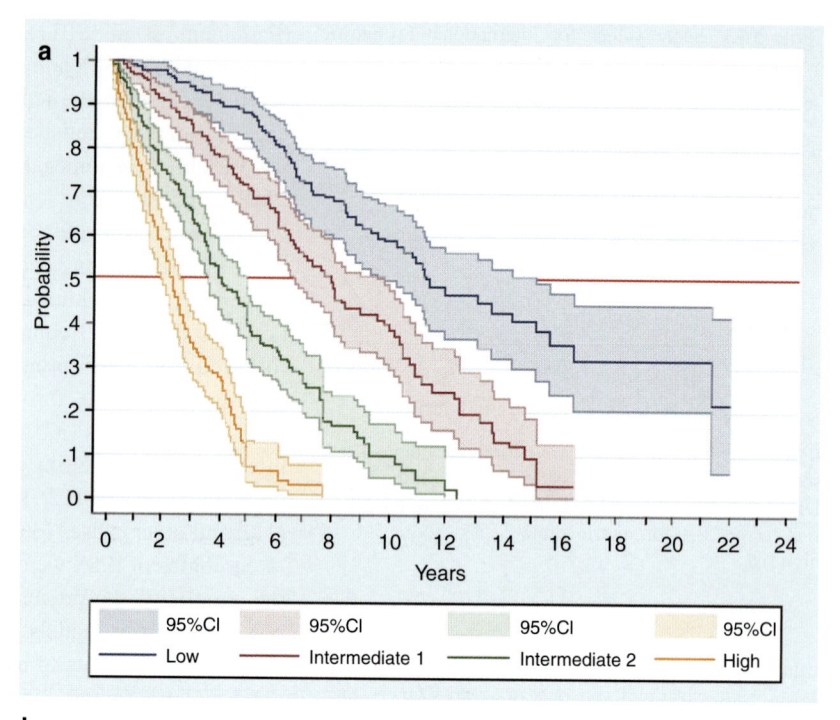

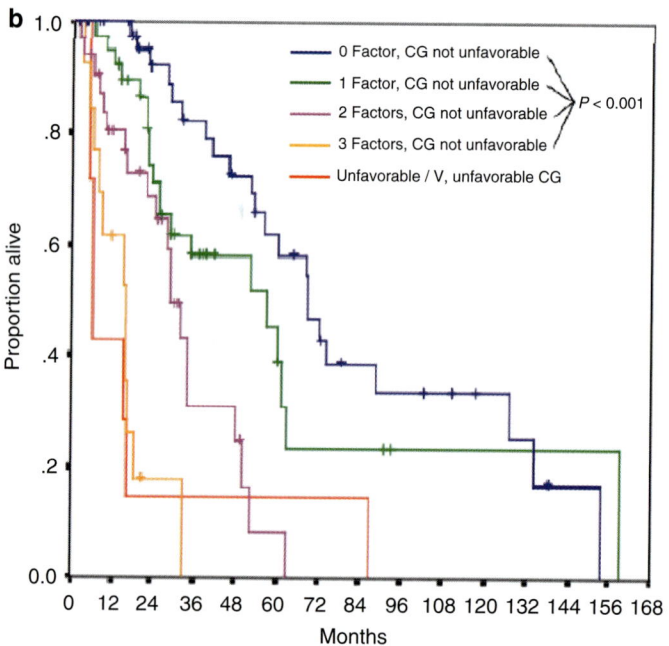

Fig. 14.1 (continued)

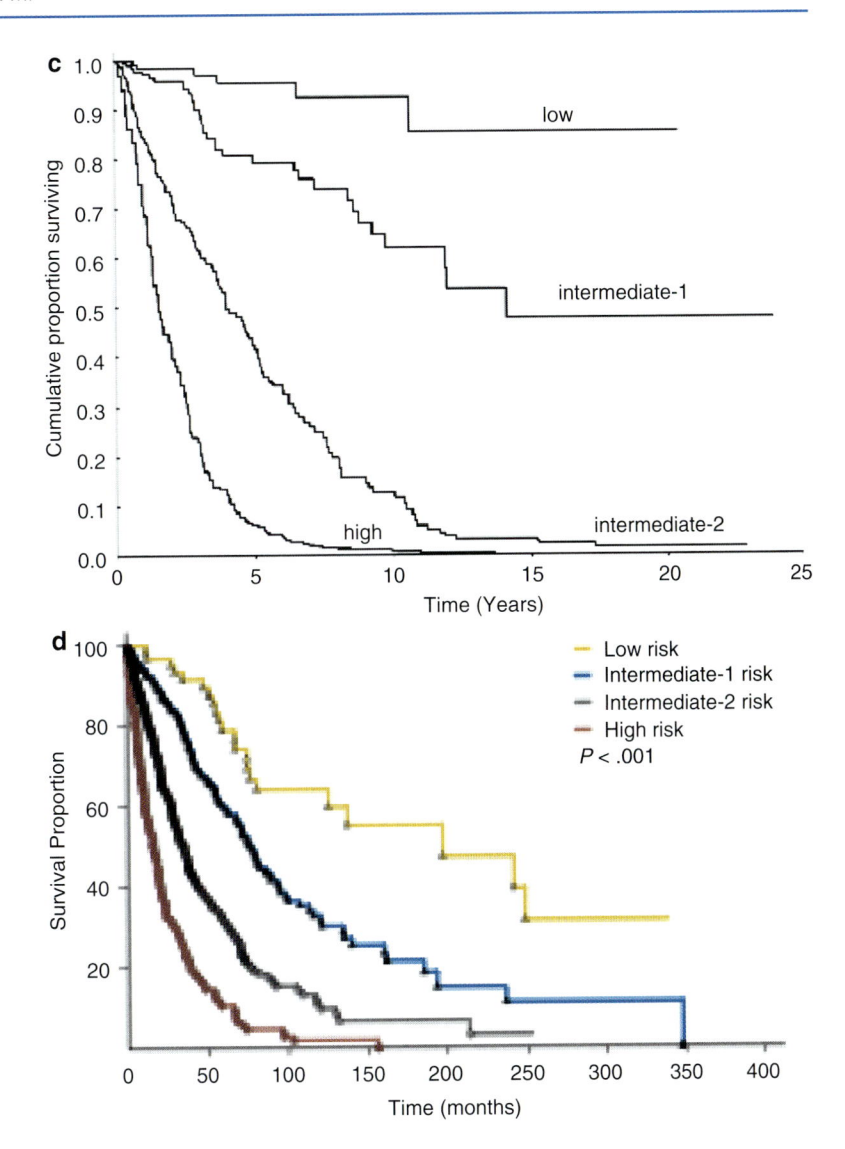

model contained unfavorable karyotype (rearrangement of chromosome 5 or 7, 17 or more than three abnormalities), hemoglobin level less than 10 g/dL, platelet count less than 100×10^9/L, performance status higher than 1, and effectively risk-stratified patients at initial evaluation (Fig. 14.1b). The study provided also some evidence that developing over time unfavorable karyotype or chromosome-17 abnormalities worsen survival in PMF. This suggests to endorse prospective studies on this topic.

Strength of this study is the composite nature of risk factors, while its weaknesses are the low number of patients with unfavorable-very unfavorable karyotype ($n = 25$) and the overall survival ranging from 7 months for very unfavorable to only 69 months for low-risk patients.

14.2   Other Prognostic Factors in PMF

14.2.1   *JAK2* (V617F) Mutation

The *JAK2* (V617F) mutation (Janus kinase 2), occurring within exon 14 of *JAK2* and located on 9p24, is the most frequent mutation in MPN, ranging from roughly 96% in PV to 65% in ET and PMF. This mutation affects the autoinhibitory domain (JH2, pseudokinase) of *JAK2* leading to constitutive activation of *JAK2* and JAK/STAT signaling. IN PMF, the prognostic role of the *JAK2* (V617F) mutation has been widely assessed, while the prognostic role of other mutations such as *TET2* or *MPL* are less investigated and seem not affecting survival (Tefferi et al. 2009b). As previously mentioned, in 345 patients of the IPSS project, no association was observed between the *JAK2* status and the prognostic score or the survival (Cervantes et al. 2009). A study including 152 patients with PMF showed that the presence of the *JAK2* (V617F) mutation was associated with inferior survival despite the finding that mutated patients were less likely to require red blood cell (RBC) transfusions during follow-up (Campbell et al. 2006). Some of the differences in survival may be explained by the fact that among the six patients with documented leukemic transformation, five were V617F-positive. In another series of 304 patients with PMF, 174 were genotyped, and this study showed that the V617F mutational status was associated with an increased risk of death from any cause, leukemic transformation, development of marked splenomegaly, and requirement for splenectomy or chemotherapy (Barosi et al. 2007). However, when adjusting for conventional risk factors, only progression to splenomegaly and acute myeloid leukemia (AML) transformation were independently predicted by the *JAK2* (V617F) mutation. Three more recent studies including 199, 186, and 174 patients each showed no significant correlation between the presence of the V617F mutation and survival or leukemic transformation (Caramazza et al. 2011; Guglielmelli et al. 2009; Tefferi et al. 2008).

Within *JAK2* (V617F)-positive patients, a potential prognostic role might be assigned to allele burden and its variation over PMF course. The first question concerns the conversion from a heterozygous to a homozygous status and its relationship with events. This remains an unsolved issue as two studies reported different results, one documenting a progression rate of 10 per 100 patient years (Barosi et al. 2007), the second basically reporting a stability (Mesa et al. 2006) with opposite results in terms of outcome. The second question concerns more properly the allele burden. Data from the literature indicate that having a lower allele burden implies a worse survival. In one study (Guglielmelli et al. 2009), patients in the lower quartile had shorter time to anemia and leukopenia and did not progress to large splenomegaly, meaning a more myelodepletive phenotype. Survival was significantly reduced in the lower quartile compared with upper quartiles and *JAK2* wild-type patients, mostly because of infections. In the second paper (Tefferi et al. 2008), Kaplan–Meier plots revealed significantly shortened overall and leukemia-free survival for the lower quartile allele burden group, mostly deputed to AML transformation.

After reports noted in 2009, describing an association between a *JAK2* haplotype (46/1) and *JAK2* (V617F)-positive MPN, 130 patients with PMF, assessed for the 46/1 haplotype, have been studied for survival (Tefferi et al. 2010b). Nullizygosity for the JAK2 46/1 haplotype, was associated with shortened survival, which was not accounted for IPSS. This result, which however needs further confirmation, raises the possibility that non-46/1 haplotypes are affiliated with a biologically more aggressive phenotype.

Very intriguing results have been reported on the prognostic relevance of the *JAK2* (V617F) mutation in the allogeneic stem-cell transplantation (ASCT) setting (Alchalby et al. 2010). In 139 out of 162 patients with known *JAK2* (V617F) mutation status who received ASCT after reduced-intensity conditioning, overall survival was significantly reduced in patients harboring *JAK2* wild type compared with *JAK2* mutated patients. No significant influence on outcome was reported for allele burden. Patients who cleared *JAK2* mutation level in peripheral blood 6 months after ASCT had a significant lower risk of relapse, shedding light for the first time to the clinical benefit of reducing V617F allele burden.

In conclusion, data on the *JAK2* (V617F) mutation in PMF show that having the mutation does not imply a different outcome respect to the contrary at least in patients under conventional treatments. In the transplant setting, the *JAK2* (V617F) mutations seems to have a protective effect, although this should be confirmed. Any conclusion on allele burden or its variation over time seems premature as data are in part conflicting and the method for quantification is not yet standardized.

14.2.2 Cytogenetic Abnormalities and Classes

Among MPN, PMF shows the highest aberration rate with approximately 30% of patients carrying an abnormal karyotype at diagnosis (Hussein et al. 2009a). Cytogenetic analysis has a role to identify an abnormal profile that provides evidence of clonality. However, most cytogenetic abnormalities observed may correspond to secondary sub-clones. Although most PMF patients' bone marrow aspirate is "dry tap," karyotype analysis can be performed on peripheral blood (Tefferi et al. 2001b).

The most frequent isolated abnormalities in PMF involve chromosome 1, 8, 9, 13, and 20 (Rumi et al. 2010; Caramazza et al. 2011). Recent studies have shown that the presence of abnormal karyotype in PMF patients has an IPSS-independent prognostic value (Cervantes et al. 2009; Rumi et al. 2010; Hussein et al. 2010) and predicts leukemia transformation (Tefferi et al. 2001a). The following is a list of chromosomes mostly involved in PMF cytogenetic abnormalities.

14.2.2.1 Chromosome 1

Chromosome 1 abnormalities are common in MPN; they are up to 28% in PMF (Caramazza et al. 2010). Specific abnormalities include duplications (e.g., 1q12→1q32 in PV, 1q21–32→1q32–44 in post-PV MF or PMF) and deletions (e.g., 1p13–36→pter in PV or PMF, 1q21 in PMF). Balanced t(1;6) involving 1q21 or 1q23 and 6p21.3 breakpoints are infrequent but must be relatively specific to PMF or post-PV/ET MF (Dingli et al. 2005). Unbalanced translocations are often accompanied by chromosomal loses that may occur independently as deletions (e.g., 1p13–36→pter in PV or PMF, 1q21 in PMF). Trisomy of chromosome 1q suggests that triplication of these genes likely contributes to the evolution in post-PV MF and may be a

secondary event, since it frequently coexists with other abnormalities present at disease presentation, such as del(20q) (Andrieux et al. 2003). Moreover, a study reported a case of PMF with t(1;2)(p34;p21) (Tefferi et al. 2001b), and it is interesting to note that the 1q breakpoint is the same that harbors the gene for thrombopoietin receptor (*MPL*). Approximately 11% of patients with PMF and a lesser percentage with ET carry es somatic activating *MPL* mutations (Pikman et al. 2006).

14.2.2.2 Chromosome 8

Trisomy 8 is associated with myeloid malignancies, mostly with PMF and PV (Reilly et al. 1997; Tefferi et al. 2001a; Hussein et al. 2009b). The genetic consequences of chromosome 8 duplication remain unclear. However, a recent in vitro study suggested a role for microRNAs (miRNAs). In cases of trisomy 8, miR-124a and miR-30d located on 8p21 and 8q23, respectively, are over-expressed suggesting that a gene dosage effect may be contributing to this finding. In PMF patients, the presence of trisomy 8 correlates with a bad prognosis.

14.2.2.3 Chromosome 9

Chromosome 9 abnormalities as sole or associated with other cytogenetic changes are frequent in MPN, mostly in PV and PMF. In the largest cytogenetic study on 433 PMF patients, trisomy 9 was detected in 2% ($n=9$) of cases, while unbalanced translocation involving chromosome 9 and 1 was found in two patients, and only one showed del(9)(q22q32) (Caramazza et al. 2010). Al-Assar et al., in a study incorporating comparative genomic hybridization (CGH), reported gains of 9p in 50% of PMF cases, involving 9p13 and 9p23 (Al-Assar et al. 2005). An amplification of such genes seems implicated in solid tumors and in a PV patient who transformed to acute myeloid leukemia (Helias et al. 2008). However, the role of chromosome 9 abnormalities in PMF is still unclear.

14.2.2.4 Chromosome 13

Del(13q) is a common abnormality in MPN, especially in PMF (Reilly et al. 1997; Caramazza et al. 2011; Hussein et al. 2009b). Del(13q) involves 13q12 and 13q14-q22 breakpoints, and the retinoblastoma susceptibility (*Rb-1*) gene is located in the critically deletion region. The inactivation of this gene could have a role in pathogenesis. FISH studies to detect *Rb-1* deletions have documented hemizygous gene deletion only in those cases with del(13q) on standard metaphases analysis (Sinclair et al. 2001). Moreover, additions and translocations involving chromosome 13 has been described in PMF (Caramazza et al. 2011; Sinclair et al. 2001).

14.2.2.5 Chromosome 20

Del(20q) is present as sole abnormality in approximately 7–10% of PMF patients (Hussein et al. 2010; Caramazza et al. 2011). In PMF, there is a highly significant association between sole del(20q) and both leukopenia and thrombocytopenia (Caramazza et al. 2011). This association suggests a 20q-haploinsufficient gene effect, which might also explain the previous association between myelodysplastic syndromes (MDS) and thrombocytopenia. Several studies have demonstrated that del(20q) did not affect adversely survival in PMF (Tefferi et al. 2001a; Hussein et al. 2010; Caramazza et al. 2011).

14.2.2.6 Prognostic Impact of Cytogenetic Abnormalities in PMF

Concerning prognostic relevance of cytogenetic changes in PMF, recent studies have been consistent in their report on prognostic impact of cytogenetic abnormalities (Tam et al. 2009; Rumi et al. 2010; Hussein et al. 2010; Caramazza et al. 2011; Hidaka et al. 2009). The latest study of 433 PMF patients, evaluated at diagnosis or within 1 year, refined a two-tired cytogenetic-risk stratification: unfavorable and favorable karyotype (Caramazza et al. 2011). Three previous studies, each comprising 202, 200, and 131 patients, reported similar results identifying the favorable prognostic value of sole 20q or sole 13q (Tam et al. 2009; Hussein et al. 2010; Hidaka et al. 2009). Then, two of these studies identified sole +9 as another favorable cytogenetic marker. In the two-tired cytogenetic risk (Caramazza et al.

2011), the high number of patients featured a sufficient number of cases with sole abnormalities of chromosome 1 including translocations and duplications ($n=12$) and $-7/7q$ ($n=5$) to examine their individual impact on survival and label the former as being prognostically favorable and the latter unfavorable. In summary, this study (Caramazza et al. 2011) identified a high-risk profile for cytogenetics when patients carry sole abnormalities of i(17q), -5/5q, 12p, 11q23 rearrangement, inv(3), sole +8 or sole $-7/7q$, complex karyotype, and a low-risk profile when patients carry normal dyploid, or sole abnormalities not included in high-risk profile. The respective 5-year survival rates were 8% and 51%, respectively. Multivariable analysis confirmed the IPSS-independent prognostic value of cytogenetic-risk categorization. Cytogenetic score combined with platelet count above $100 \times 10^9/L$ predicted leukemia-free survival; the 5-year leukemic transformation rates for unfavorable vs. favorable karyotype were 46% and 7%. This study was the basis for development of DIPSS-plus discussed above.

Recently in a large study of 793 PMF patients (Vaidya et al. 2011), monosomal karyotype (MK), which is defined as two or more autosomal monosomies or a single autosomal monosomy associated with at least one structural abnormality, identified a subset of patients with unfavorable karyotype ($n=17$, 42% of the 41 patients with complex karyotype) associated with extremely poor overall and leukemia-free survival. The MK is not incorporated in the DIPSS-plus.

14.2.3 RBC Transfusion Dependency

The term RBC transfusion dependence is widely used by clinicians to describe a condition of severe anemia typically arising when erythropoiesis is reduced such that a person continuously requires RBC transfusions. Recently, the criteria for RBC transfusion dependency in PMF has been published (Gale et al. 2011). Experts considered a volume of 2U RBC/month over 3 months to be the most appropriate observational interval and RBC transfusions frequency to define a person as RBC transfusion dependent. Several factors may influence the individual patient transfusion program and contribute to intersubject variation in transfusion needs. These include age, sex, baseline hemoglobin level, rate of hemoglobin decrease, performance status, extra-hematological comorbidity. In general, the cutoff level of hemoglobin to define the need of RBC transfusion is 8.5 g/dL.

Anemia is the most relevant clinical issue in the majority of patients with PMF, present in ~35% of patients at diagnosis and acquired in ~65% of patients during follow-up. Ineffective hematopoiesis, hypersplenism, and bone marrow fibrosis might explain anemia in PMF. More recent observations gave a mutational-based explanation of anemia in PMF, in fact, while the presence of *JAK2* (V617F) seems to be protective, *MPL* (Guglielmelli et al. 2007) and *TET2* (Tefferi et al. 2009b) mutations are associated with more severe anemia. Anemia as hemoglobin level less than 10 g/dL is one of the most widely accepted risk factors for survival in PMF, and once anemia becomes symptomatic, RBC transfusions are the mainstays of therapy.

The prognostic impact of RBC transfusion need was examined in 254 consecutive patients, of whom 24% required transfusions at diagnosis and 9% became RBC transfusion dependent during the first year post-diagnosis (Tefferi et al. 2010a). RBC transfusion need clearly separated two groups with different survivals: 35 months (transfused from diagnosis), 25 months (transfused after 1 years), and 117 months (not transfused). RBC transfusion need had an IPSS-independent prognostic power downgrading or upgrading prognosis within specific IPSS categories. This result was confirmed by a study on 288 consecutive patients with PMF (Elena et al. 2011): RBC transfusion dependency at diagnosis affected survival independently of IPSS. The study also assessed RBC transfusion need acquired anytime of the follow-up revealing that transfusion status may predict survival dynamically and independently from DIPSS categories.

Finally, transfusion-dependent patients invariably develop secondary iron overload, but, in PMF, differently from MDS (Malcovati et al. 2005), serum ferritin or transfusional load does not affect survival (Chee et al. 2008). However, no prospective data are available to elucidate whether iron loading may concur to the negative prognostic impact of transfusion dependency in MDS nor in PMF.

14.2.4 Proinflammatory Cytokines

Abnormal cytokine profile in PMF is considered to represent an inflammatory response and to contribute to clinical phenotype, bone marrow fibrosis, angiogenesis, extramedullary hematopoiesis, and constitutional symptoms. The interest on cytokines has recently arisen as a JAK inhibitor, named ruxolitinib, reduced a different pattern of proinflammatory cytokines (Verstovsek et al. 2010). Among 30 cytokines tested in a cohort of 90 treatment-naive patients with PMF, high levels of IL-8, IL-2R, IL-12, and IL-15 correlated with inferior survival independently from DIPSS-plus (Tefferi et al. 2011). Investigators found that the presence of threefold increased levels of one or both IL-8 and IL-2R may predict worse survival.

14.3 Dynamic Prognostic Models for Survival in PMF

In a non-time-dependent analysis (models at diagnosis), patients are assigned to a risk group on the basis of the assessment of risk factors at diagnosis and are followed in the same category irrespective of the acquisition of other risk factors during disease course. According to a dynamic model, patients contribute to the estimate of survival in a score category only as long as they do not acquire further risk factors, then they shift to a higher score category.

Dynamic prognostic models are based on the knowledge that the acquisition of additional risk factors during the disease course may substantially modify patients' outcome. In addition, using prognostic models developed at diagnosis to stratify patients during the follow-up is not a correct approach for prognostication.

14.3.1 The DIPSS Model

Among 1,054 patients evaluated to develop the IPSS, 525 patients were considered regularly followed and suitable for a time-dependent analysis. The IWG-MRT investigators firstly explored whether the acquisition anytime during follow-up of one or more within prognostic factors of the IPSS predicts survival and, then, generated a new prognostic score based on a time-dependent risk evaluation, named DIPSS (Passamonti et al. 2010a).

All IPSS risk factors (age greater than 65 years, presence of constitutional symptoms, hemoglobin level less than 10 g/dL, leukocyte count greater than 25×10^9/L, and circulating blast cells 1% or greater) maintained their impact on survival when dynamically acquired, but gaining anemia over time affects survival with a hazard ratio roughly double than that of other parameters. So, the scoring system of DIPSS is different from IPSS (Table 14.1). The resulting DIPSS risk categories are low (score = 0), intermediate-1 (score 1 or 2), intermediate-2 (score 3 or 4), and high (score 5 or 6). Median survival was not reached in low-risk patients; it was 14.2 years in intermediate-1, 4 years in intermediate-2, and 1.5 years in high risk (Fig. 14.1c).

From a practical point of view, anytime a decision has to be made on the basis of an updated prognostic status, the parameters of the DIPSS models will be checked, and corresponding values will be assigned (Table 14.1). The sum of the values will allow allocating the patient into a risk category (low, intermediate-1, intermediate-2, high), and cumulative survival can be estimated (Fig. 14.1c). It is obvious that the corresponding cumulative probability of survival at each time point of the follow-up should be read considering the time elapsed since diagnosis. This estimate remains applicable thereafter until patient changes risk category.

Strengths of DIPSS were the multicenter origin, the simplicity of the parameters, and the opportunity to define prognosis anytime during the follow-up, which, practically, means at each visit. Nowadays dynamic prognostication of patients is particularly critical as many investigative trials with JAK inhibitors are ongoing, and hematopoietic stem-cell transplantation still remains the only eradicating procedure (Barbui et al. 2011). The weakness is the non-integration with specific cytogenetic abnormalities, which remains a mirage as well as collecting sequential data on this parameter, regularly and consecutively, is lacking.

14.3.2 The DIPPS-Plus Model

This model was designed on a basis of 793 patients with PMF of which 428 were referred within and 365 after their first year of diagnosis: at these time points several parameters were checked for their impact on survival (Gangat et al. 2011). This composite model included as worse prognostic factors the unfavorable cytogenetics (complex, sole or two including +8, -7/7q, i(17q), inv (3), -5/5q, 12p, 11q23 rearrangements), RBC transfusion need, platelet count lower than 100×10^9/L, and DIPSS categories. According to the model, 1 point each was assigned to DIPSS intermediate-1 risk, unfavorable karyotype, platelets lower than 100×10^9/L, and red cell transfusion need, while DIPSS intermediate-2 and high risk were assigned 2 and 3 points, respectively (Table 14.2). On the basis of this scoring system, four categories were generated: low risk (0 adverse points; median survival, 185 months), intermediate-1 risk (1 adverse point; median survival, 78 months), intermediate-2 risk (2–3 adverse points; median survival, 35 months), and high risk (4–6 adverse points; median survival, 16 months), as shown in Fig. 14.1d.

It is interesting to note that DIPSS-plus investigators found a proportion of patients in each DIPSS risk category with red cell transfusion

Table 14.2 Score values Dynamic International Prognostic Scoring System-plus (DIPSS-plus)

Parameter	Score value
DIPSS intermediate-1	1
DIPSS intermediate-2	2
DIPSS high risk	3
Unfavorable cytogenetic	1
Red blood cell need	1
Platelet <100×10^9/L	1

DIPSS-plus: score 0 for low risk, score 1 for intermediate-1 risk, score 2–3 for intermediate-2 risk, score 4–6 for high risk need, unfavorable karyotype, and thrombocytopenia of 0%, 7%, and 7% for low risk; 13%, 12%, and 18% for intermediate-1 risk; 56%, 17%, and 32% for intermediate-2 risk; and 69%, 23%, and 47% for high risk, respectively. This shed light to the possibility to better stratify patients with intermediate-risk categories.

Strengths of DIPPS-plus are the introduction of cytogenetic categories in the model and the high number of patients accrued, while weakness is the difficulty of applying this system anytime. DIPSS-plus should be used at specific therapeutic checkpoints such as diagnosis or for better deciphering the time of hematopoietic stem-cell transplantation.

Conclusions

For the time being, IPSS at diagnosis and DIPSS anytime of disease course very well and easily define survival of PMF patients. DIPSS-plus adds critical prognostic information and suggests paying attention to cytogenetic categories, platelet count, and RBC transfusion need.

References

Al-Assar O, Ul-Hassan A, Brown R, Wilson GA, Hammond DW, Reilly JT (2005) Gains on 9p are common genomic aberrations in idiopathic myelofibrosis: a comparative genomic hybridization study. Br J Haematol 129:66–71

Alchalby H, Badbaran A, Zabelina T et al (2010) Impact of JAK2V617F-mutation status, allele burden and clearance after allogeneic stem cell transplantation for myelofibrosis. Blood 116(18):3572–3581

Alchalby H, Lioznov M, Fritzsche-Friedland U et al (2011) Circulating CD34(+) cells as prognostic and follow-up marker in patients with myelofibrosis undergoing allo-SCT. Bone Marrow Transplant. doi:10.1038/bmt.2011.17

Andrieux J, Demory JL, Caulier MT et al (2003) Karyotypic abnormalities in myelofibrosis following polycythemia vera. Cancer Genet Cytogenet 140:118–123

Arora B, Sirhan S, Hoyer JD, Mesa RA, Tefferi A (2005) Peripheral blood CD34 count in myelofibrosis with myeloid metaplasia: a prospective evaluation of prognostic value in 94 patients. Br J Haematol 128:42–48

Barbui T, Barosi G, Birgegard G et al (2011) Philadelphia-negative classical myeloproliferative neoplasms: critical concepts and management recommendations from European LeukemiaNet. J Clin Oncol 29:761–770

Barosi G, Berzuini C, Liberato LN, Costa A, Polino G, Ascari E (1988) A prognostic classification of myelofibrosis with myeloid metaplasia. Br J Haematol 70:397–401

Barosi G, Viarengo G, Pecci A et al (2001) Diagnostic and clinical relevance of the number of circulating CD34(+) cells in myelofibrosis with myeloid metaplasia. Blood 98:3249–3255

Barosi G, Bergamaschi G, Marchetti M et al (2007) JAK2 V617F mutational status predicts progression to large splenomegaly and leukemic transformation in primary myelofibrosis. Blood 110:4030–4036

Campbell PJ, Griesshammer M, Dohner K et al (2006) V617F mutation in JAK2 is associated with poorer survival in idiopathic myelofibrosis. Blood 107:2098–2100

Caramazza D, Hussein K, Siragusa S et al (2010) Chromosome 1 abnormalities in myeloid malignancies: a literature survey and karyotype-phenotype associations. Eur J Haematol 84:191–200

Caramazza D, Begna KH, Gangat N et al (2011) Refined cytogenetic-risk categorization for overall and leukemia-free survival in primary myelofibrosis: a single center study of 433 patients. Leukemia 25:82–88

Cervantes F, Pereira A, Esteve J et al (1997) Identification of 'short-lived' and 'long-lived' patients at presentation of idiopathic myelofibrosis. Br J Haematol 97:635–640

Cervantes F, Dupriez B, Pereira A et al (2009) New prognostic scoring system for primary myelofibrosis based on a study of the International Working Group for Myelofibrosis Research and Treatment. Blood 113:2895–2901

Chee CE, Steensma DP, Wu W, Hanson CA, Tefferi A (2008) Neither serum ferritin nor the number of red blood cell transfusions affect overall survival in refractory anemia with ringed sideroblasts. Am J Hematol 83:611–613

Chelloul N, Briere J, Laval-Jeantet M, Najean Y, Vorhauer W, Jacquillat C (1976) Prognosis of myeloid metaplasia with myelofibrosis. Biomedicine 24:272–280

Dingli D, Grand FH, Mahaffey V et al (2005) Der(6)t(1;6) (q21–23;p21.3): a specific cytogenetic abnormality in myelofibrosis with myeloid metaplasia. Br J Haematol 130:229–232

Dupriez B, Morel P, Demory JL et al (1996) Prognostic factors in agnogenic myeloid metaplasia: a report on 195 cases with a new scoring system. Blood 88:1013–1018

Elena C, Passamonti F, Rumi E et al (2011) Red blood cell transfusion-dependency implies a poor survival in primary myelofibrosis irrespective of IPSS and DIPSS. Haematologica 96:167–170

Gale RP, Barosi G, Barbui T et al (2011) What are RBC-transfusion-dependence and -independence? Leuk Res 35:8–11

Gangat N, Caramazza D, Vaidya R et al (2011) DIPSS plus: a refined Dynamic International Prognostic Scoring System for primary myelofibrosis that incorporates prognostic information from karyotype, platelet count, and transfusion status. J Clin Oncol 29:392–397

Guglielmelli P, Pancrazzi A, Bergamaschi G et al (2007) Anaemia characterises patients with myelofibrosis harbouring Mpl mutation. Br J Haematol 137:244–247

Guglielmelli P, Barosi G, Specchia G et al (2009) Identification of patients with poorer survival in primary myelofibrosis based on the burden of JAK2V617F mutated allele. Blood 114:1477–1483

Helias C, Struski S, Gervais C et al (2008) Polycythemia vera transforming to acute myeloid leukemia and complex abnormalities including 9p homogeneously staining region with amplification of MLLT3, JMJD2C, JAK2, and SMARCA2. Cancer Genet Cytogenet 180: 51–55

Hidaka T, Shide K, Shimoda H et al (2009) The impact of cytogenetic abnormalities on the prognosis of primary myelofibrosis: a prospective survey of 202 cases in Japan. Eur J Haematol 83:328–333

Hussein K, Huang J, Lasho T et al (2009a) Karyotype complements the International Prognostic Scoring System for primary myelofibrosis. Eur J Haematol 82:255–259

Hussein K, Van Dyke DL, Tefferi A (2009b) Conventional cytogenetics in myelofibrosis: literature review and discussion. Eur J Haematol 82:329–338

Hussein K, Pardanani AD, Van Dyke DL, Hanson CA, Tefferi A (2010) International Prognostic Scoring System-independent cytogenetic risk categorization in primary myelofibrosis. Blood 115:496–499

Malcovati L, Porta MG, Pascutto C et al (2005) Prognostic factors and life expectancy in myelodysplastic syndromes classified according to WHO criteria: a basis for clinical decision making. J Clin Oncol 23:7594–7603

Mesa RA, Hanson CA, Rajkumar SV, Schroeder G, Tefferi A (2000) Evaluation and clinical correlations of bone marrow angiogenesis in myelofibrosis with myeloid metaplasia. Blood 96:3374–3380

Mesa RA, Powell H, Lasho T, DeWald GW, McClure R, Tefferi A (2006) A longitudinal study of the JAK2(V617F) mutation in myelofibrosis with myeloid metaplasia: analysis at two time points. Haematologica 91:415–416

Morel P, Duhamel A, Hivert B, Stalniekiewicz L, Demory JL, Dupriez B (2010) Identification during the follow-up of time-dependent prognostic factors for the competing risks of death and blast phase in primary myelofibrosis: a study of 172 patients. Blood 115:4350–4355

Pardanani A, Vannucchi AM, Passamonti F, Cervantes F, Barbui T, Tefferi A (2011) JAK inhibitor therapy for myelofibrosis: critical assessment of value and limitations. Leukemia 25:218–225

Passamonti F, Cervantes F, Vannucchi AM et al (2010a) A dynamic prognostic model to predict survival in primary myelofibrosis: a study by the IWG-MRT (International Working Group for Myeloproliferative Neoplasms Research and Treatment). Blood 115:1703–1708

Passamonti F, Cervantes F, Vannucchi AM et al (2010b) Dynamic International Prognostic Scoring System (DIPSS) predicts progression to acute myeloid leukemia in primary myelofibrosis. Blood 116:2857–2858

Patnaik MM, Caramazza D, Gangat N, Hanson CA, Pardanani A, Tefferi A (2010) Age and platelet count are IPSS-independent prognostic factors in young patients with primary myelofibrosis and complement IPSS in predicting very long or very short survival. Eur J Haematol 84:105–108

Pereira A, Bruguera M, Cervantes F, Rozman C (1988) Liver involvement at diagnosis of primary myelofibrosis: a clinicopathological study of twenty-two cases. Eur J Haematol 40:355–361

Pikman Y, Lee BH, Mercher T et al (2006) MPLW515L is a novel somatic activating mutation in myelofibrosis with myeloid metaplasia. PLoS Med 3:e270

Reilly JT, Snowden JA, Spearing RL et al (1997) Cytogenetic abnormalities and their prognostic significance in idiopathic myelofibrosis: a study of 106 cases. Br J Haematol 98:96–102

Rumi E, Passamonti F, Bernasconi P et al (2010) Validation of cytogenetic-based risk stratification in primary myelofibrosis. Blood 115:2719–2720

Rupoli S, Da Lio L, Sisti S et al (1994) Primary myelofibrosis: a detailed statistical analysis of the clinicopathological variables influencing survival. Ann Hematol 68:205–212

Sinclair EJ, Forrest EC, Reilly JT, Watmore AE, Potter AM (2001) Fluorescence in situ hybridization analysis of 25 cases of idiopathic myelofibrosis and two cases of secondary myelofibrosis: monoallelic loss of RB1, D13S319 and D13S25 loci associated with cytogenetic deletion and translocation involving 13q14. Br J Haematol 113:365–368

Tam CS, Abruzzo LV, Lin KI et al (2009) The role of cytogenetic abnormalities as a prognostic marker in primary myelofibrosis: applicability at the time of diagnosis and later during disease course. Blood 113:4171–4178

Tefferi A, Mesa RA, Schroeder G, Hanson CA, Li CY, Dewald GW (2001a) Cytogenetic findings and their clinical relevance in myelofibrosis with myeloid metaplasia. Br J Haematol 113:763–771

Tefferi A, Meyer RG, Wyatt WA, Dewald GW (2001b) Comparison of peripheral blood interphase cytogenetics with bone marrow karyotype analysis in myelofibrosis with myeloid metaplasia. Br J Haematol 115:316–319

Tefferi A, Thiele J, Orazi A et al (2007) Proposals and rationale for revision of the World Health Organization diagnostic criteria for polycythemia vera, essential thrombocythemia, and primary myelofibrosis: recommendations from an ad hoc international expert panel. Blood 110:1092–1097

Tefferi A, Lasho TL, Huang J et al (2008) Low JAK2V617F allele burden in primary myelofibrosis, compared to either a higher allele burden or unmutated status, is associated with inferior overall and leukemia-free survival. Leukemia 22:756–761

Tefferi A, Mesa RA, Pardanani A et al (2009a) Red blood cell transfusion need at diagnosis adversely affects survival in primary myelofibrosis-increased serum ferritin or transfusion load does not. Am J Hematol 84:265–267

Tefferi A, Pardanani A, Lim KH et al (2009b) TET2 mutations and their clinical correlates in polycythemia vera, essential thrombocythemia and myelofibrosis. Leukemia 23(5):905–911

Tefferi A, Siragusa S, Hussein K et al (2010a) Transfusion-dependency at presentation and its acquisition in the first year of diagnosis are both equally detrimental for survival in primary myelofibrosis–prognostic relevance is independent of IPSS or karyotype. Am J Hematol 85:14–17

Tefferi A, Lasho TL, Patnaik MM et al (2010b) JAK2 germline genetic variation affects disease susceptibility in primary myelofibrosis regardless of V617F mutational status: nullizygosity for the JAK2 46/1 haplotype is associated with inferior survival. Leukemia 24: 105–109

Tefferi A, Vaidya R, Caramazza D, Finke C, Lasho T, Pardanani A (2011) Circulating interleukin (IL)-8, IL-2R, IL-12, and IL-15 levels are independently prognostic in primary myelofibrosis: a comprehensive cytokine profiling study. J Clin Oncol 29: 1356–1363

Vaidya R, Caramazza D, Begna KH et al (2011) Monosomal karyotype in primary myelofibrosis is detrimental to both overall and leukemia-free survival. Blood 117(21):5612–5615

Verstovsek S, Kantarjian H, Mesa RA et al (2010) Safety and efficacy of INCB018424, a JAK1 and JAK2 inhibitor, in myelofibrosis. N Engl J Med 363:1117–1127

Nontransplant Treatment Options for Myelofibrosis: How to Treat Anemia, Splenomegaly, Constitutional Symptoms, and Extramedullary Disease

15

Ayalew Tefferi

Contents

15.1 Introduction

15.1.1 Disease Classification

Myelofibrosis (MF) is a myeloid malignancy characterized by clonal myeloproliferation usually associated with bone marrow fibrosis. The World Health Organization (WHO) classification system recognizes five categories of myeloid malignancies: acute myeloid leukemia (AML), myelodysplastic syndromes (MDS), myeloproliferative neoplasms (MPN), MDS/MPN overlap, and PDGFR/*FGFR1*-rearranged myeloid/lymphoid neoplasms with eosinophilia (Vardiman et al. 2009). The WHO MPN category includes eight subcategories: polycythemia vera (PV), essential thrombocythemia (ET), primary myelofibrosis (PMF), chronic myelogenous leukemia (CML), chronic neutrophilic leukemia (CNL), chronic eosinophilic leukemia-not otherwise specified (CEL-NOS), mast cell disease (MCD), and MPN-unclassifiable. The first four are usually referred to as "classic" MPN (Dameshek 1951). Among these, PV, ET, and PMF are classified as "*BCR-ABL1*-negative MPN." Some patients with PV or ET can over time develop a clinical phenotype that is indistinguishable from PMF and referred to as post-PV and post-ET MF (Barosi et al. 2008). The term MF is used to encompass all three variants: PMF, post-PV MF, and post-ET MF.

15.1.2 Pathogenesis Overview

All MPN, including MF, originate from acquired mutations involving the hematopoietic stem cell (Lambert et al. 2009; Beer et al. 2009). The disease-causing mutation in MF is not known; however, the majority of the patients harbor *JAK2*V617F and a minority *MPL, LNK, CBL, TET2, ASXL1, IDH, IKZF1, EZH2,* or *DNMT3A* mutations (Tefferi 2010; Ernst et al. 2010). None of these mutations are disease initiating or disease specific, and their precise pathogenetic

A. Tefferi
Division of Hematology, Department of Medicine,
Mayo Clinic, Rochester, MN, USA
e-mail: tefferi.ayalew@mayo.edu

contribution is not known (Schaub et al. 2010). *JAK2*, *MPL*, and *LNK* mutations result in constitutive JAK-STAT activation and induce MPN-like disease in mice (James et al. 2005; Pikman et al. 2006; Oh et al. 2010; Bersenev et al. 2010). This is the basis for JAK inhibitor therapy in *BCR-ABL1*-negative MPN (Pardanani et al. 2011; Verstovsek et al. 2010). *TET2*, *ASXL1*, and *EZH2* mutations are suspected of playing a role in epigenetic dysregulation of transcription (Tahiliani et al. 2009; Lee et al. 2010; Ko et al. 2010). This is the basis for clinical trials involving hypomethylating agents and histone deacetylase inhibitors in MF and other MPN. In addition, clonal myeloproliferation in MF is accompanied by abnormal cytokine expression, which might explain the benefit of JAK inhibitors as well as support the use of anticytokine and immune modulatory drugs in MF (Vaidya et al. 2010).

15.1.3 Contemporary Diagnosis

Current diagnosis of PMF is based on WHO criteria and includes clinical, morphologic, cytogenetic, and molecular assessment (Tefferi et al. 2007a). The diagnosis of post-PV or post-ET MF is according to International Working Group for MPN Research and Treatment (IWG-MRT) criteria (Barosi et al. 2008). Typical clinical and laboratory features of MF include anemia, splenomegaly, constitutional symptoms, cachexia, extramedullary hematopoiesis (EMH), peripheral blood leukoerythroblastosis, dacryocytosis, leukocytosis, thrombocytosis, increased lactate dehydrogenase (LDH), bone marrow fibrosis, and osteosclerosis. The possibility of prefibrotic PMF, as opposed to ET, should be considered in the presence of persistently increased serum LDH, anemia, leukoerythroblastosis, and marked splenomegaly (Barbui et al. 2010). It is underscored that the distinction between ET and prefibrotic PMF is clinical relevant since both overall and leukemia-free survival are significantly inferior in the latter (Barbui et al. 2010). The differential diagnosis of PMF should also include bone marrow fibrosis associated with nonneoplastic or other neoplastic conditions including metastatic

cancer, lymphoid neoplasm, or another myeloid malignancy, especially CML, MDS, chronic myelomonocytic leukemia (CMML), or AML.

15.1.4 Current Risk Stratification

Current prognostication in primary MF is based on the *Dynamic International Prognostic Scoring System-plus* (*DIPSS-plus*) model, which uses eight independent predictors of inferior survival: age >65 years, hemoglobin <10 g/dL, leukocyte count >25×10^9/L, circulating blasts ≥1%, presence of constitutional symptoms, red cell transfusion need, platelet count <100×10^9/L, and unfavorable karyotype (Gangat et al. 2011). These parameters are used to classify patients into low (no risk factors), intermediate-1 (one risk factor), intermediate-2 (two or three risk factors), and high-risk (four or more risk factors) disease groups; the corresponding median survivals are estimated at 15.4, 6.5, 2.9, and 1.3 years (Gangat et al. 2011). Such information is used to plan a risk-adapted treatment strategy for the individual patient, which might include "observation alone," conventional or investigational (e.g., JAK inhibitors, pomalidomide) drug therapy, allogeneic stem cell transplant using reduced or conventional intensity conditioning, splenectomy, or radiotherapy.

15.2 Risk-Adapted Therapy for Myelofibrosis

Current drug therapy in PMF is not curative and has not been shown to prolong survival. Allogenic stem cell transplant (ASCT) is potentially curative but also associated with relatively high risk of death and morbidity. Therefore, one must first determine if a particular patient needs any form of therapy and carefully select the treatment strategy with the best chance of inducing disease control without compromising life expectancy (Table 15.1 and Fig. 15.1). According to the DIPSS-plus prognostic model (Gangat et al. 2011), the respective median survival of low- or intermediate-1-risk patients exceeds 15 and 6 years and even longer

Table 15.1 Palliative drug therapy in myelofibrosis

Problem	First line	Second line	Experimental
Anemia	ESA[a]	Danazol	Pomalidomide
	Lenalidomide[b]	Thalidomide ± prednisone	CYT387
	Androgen ± prednisone	Lenalidomide	
		Splenectomy	
Splenomegaly	Hydroxyurea	Splenectomy	JAK inhibitors
		Radiotherapy	
		Cladribine	
Constitutional symptoms	Hydroxyurea	Splenectomy	JAK inhibitors
		Etanercept	
Extramedullary disease (nonhepatosplenic)	Hydroxyurea	Radiotherapy	
	Radiotherapy		
Symptomatic portal hypertension (ascites, variceal bleed)	Hydroxyurea	Radiotherapy	JAK inhibitors
	Cladribine	TIPS	
		Splenectomy	

Keywords: *ESA* erythropoiesis-stimulating agents, *CYT387* a JAK1/JAK2 inhibitor, *TIPS* transjugular intrahepatic portosystemic shunt, *JAK* Janus kinase
[a]In the absence of marked splenomegaly and presence of a serum erythropoietin level <100 U/L
[b]Only in the presence of del(5q)

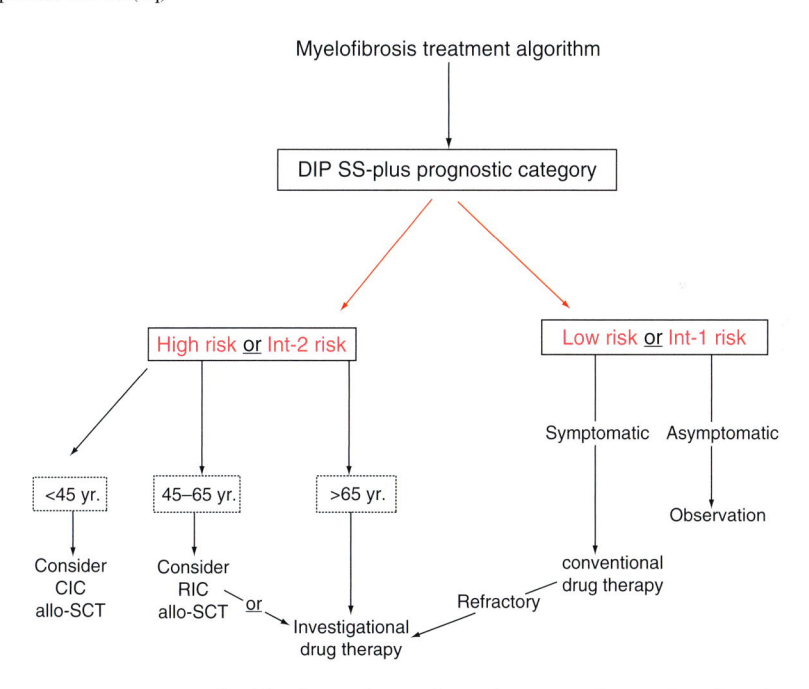

Fig. 15.1 A contemporary treatment algorithm for myelofibrosis. Keywords: *DIPSS*-plus, Dynamic International Prognostic Scoring System (DIPSS)-plus prognostic model for primary myelofibrosis (Gangat et al. 2011); *Int*, intermediate; *yrs*, years; *CIC*, conventional intensity conditioning; *RIC*, reduced intensity conditioning; *allo-SCT*, allogeneic stem cell transplantation. Conventional drug therapy includes erythropoiesis-stimulating agents, androgens, danazol, corticosteroids, thalidomide, lenalidomide, hydroxyurea, and cladribine. Please see text regarding which agent is used when

for patients below age 65 years. Therefore, the risk of allo-SCT-associated mortality and morbidity is not justified in such patients. Similarly, there is no evidence to support the value of conventional drug therapy in asymptomatic patients with low- or intermediate-1-risk disease. Therefore, a "watch and wait" treatment strategy is reasonable and usually preferred in asymptomatic low- or intermediate-risk patients with MF. MF patients with high- or intermediate-2-risk disease are usually symptomatic and can be managed by conventional drug therapy, splenectomy, radiotherapy, allo-SCT, or experimental drug therapy (Fig. 15.1). The goal of therapy in using allo-SCT is cure or prolongation of life. The goal of therapy in nontransplant candidates is disease palliation.

15.3   Treatment of Anemia

The management of symptomatic anemia depends on presence or absence of associated splenomegaly. In the absence of marked splenomegaly, the use of erythropoiesis-stimulating agents (ESA) is reasonable and is likely to benefit those who are not transfusion dependent and in whom serum Epo level is below 100 U/L (Huang and Tefferi 2009; Cervantes et al. 2004). The use of ESA is discouraged in the presence of marked splenomegaly because it might exacerbate splenomegaly. Other drugs for anemia include both conventional and experimental agents: corticosteroids (e.g., prednisone 0.5 mg/kg/day) (Tefferi et al. 2009), androgens (e.g., fluoxymesterone 10 mg TID) (Besa et al. 1982), danazol (600 mg/day) (Cervantes et al. 2005), thalidomide (50 mg/day)±prednisone (0.25 mg/day) (Mesa et al. 2003; Thomas et al. 2006), lenalidomide (10 mg/day)±prednisone (Tefferi et al. 2006; Quintas-Cardama et al. 2009; Mesa et al. 2010), pomalidomide (0.5 mg/day) (Tefferi et al. 2009; Begna et al. 2011), and CYT387 (150–300 mg/day) (Pardanani et al. 2010). Lenalidomide is the preferred agent in the presence of del(5q) and has the ability to induce a response in both anemia and splenomegaly in the majority of patients (Tefferi et al. 2007b). In the absence of del(5q), it is reasonable to start with androgens and prednisone as first-line therapy, and a response rate of approximately 20% is expected. Second-line therapy includes either thalidomide with prednisone or danazol with similar response rates that range from 15% to 30%. In most instances, responses last for about 1 year.

Pomalidomide and CYT387 are currently available only in a clinical trial setting. Pomalidomide is a thalidomide derivative. In a phase-2 study, approximately 25% of patients with anemia responded to pomalidomide alone (2 mg/day) or pomalidomide (0.5 or 2 mg/day) combined with prednisone (Tefferi et al. 2009). In a subsequent phase-2 study of single-agent pomalidomide (0.5 mg/day) (Begna et al. 2011), anemia response was documented only in the presence of *JAK2*V617F (24% vs. 0%) and predicted by the presence of pomalidomide-induced basophilia (38% vs. 6%) or absence of marked splenomegaly (38% vs. 11%). Platelet response was seen in 58% of patients with baseline platelet count of $50–100 \times 10^9$/L, but the drug had limited activity in reducing spleen size (Begna et al. 2011). JAK inhibitor therapy in MF is usually associated with anemia as a side effect. Rather unexpectedly, in a phase-1/phase-2 study using the JAK1/JAK2 inhibitor, CYT387 (150–300 mg/day), a close to 50% response rate in anemia accompanied equally remarkable response rates in splenomegaly and constitutional symptoms (Pardanani et al. 2010).

All of the above drugs are associated with important side effects. The side effects of corticosteroid use are well known and include diabetes and osteopenia. Androgen use can be associated with abnormal liver function tests, and the drug is best avoided in the presence of increased serum prostate-specific antigen level or history of prostate cancer. Both androgens and danazol can cause virilizing effects. Thalidomide, lenalidomide, or pomalidomide should be avoided in women of childbearing age. Thalidomide use is often complicated by peripheral neuropathy, and lenalidomide use, by myelosuppression (Thomas et al. 2006; Mesa et al. 2010). Higher doses of pomalidomide (>2 mg/day) are also myelosuppressive. Patients receiving thalidomide, lenalidomide, or pomalidomide should be on aspirin therapy and closely monitored for thrombosis, which is another side effect for this class of drugs. Side effects of CYT387 include thrombocytopenia and mild peripheral neuropathy.

15.3.1 Treatment of Splenomegaly

MF-associated splenomegaly is often associated with mechanical discomfort, early satiety, profound constitutional symptoms, and severe episodic pain crisis from splenic infarct. The first-line treatment of choice is hydroxyurea at a starting dose of 500 mg PO BID (Siragusa et al. 2009; Martinez-Trillos et al. 2010). In the presence of marked splenomegaly, a response rate of approximately 35% has been reported (Siragusa et al. 2009). Response rates to hydroxyurea were significantly lower (10%) in *JAK2*V617F-negative patients, compared to those with detectable *JAK2*V617F: 67% and 33% response rates in patients with mutant allele burdens of < or >50%, respectively (Siragusa et al. 2009). Spleen responses to hydroxyurea last for an average of 1 year, and treatment side effects include myelosuppression, xeroderma, and mucocutaneous ulcers. Other drugs for splenomegaly are usually reserved for hydroxyurea-refractory cases. These include intravenous cladribine (5 mg/m^2 by 2-h infusion daily × 5 days, to be repeated monthly) (Faoro et al. 2005), thalidomide (Thomas et al. 2006; Marchetti et al. 2004), lenalidomide (Tefferi et al. 2006), and most recently JAK inhibitors. Response rates for these latter agents range from 20% to 50%. Interferon-α is of limited value in the treatment of MF-associated splenomegaly (Tefferi et al. 2001).

Several JAK2 inhibitor ATP mimetics are currently in clinical trials (*clinicaltrials.gov*). I will discuss three such drugs as an example of what they can do for MF-associated splenomegaly. INCB018424 is a JAK1/JAK2 inhibitor. In a phase-1/phase-2 study of 153 patients with MF (Verstovsek et al. 2010), 44% experienced ≥50% decrease in palpable spleen size, and a similar proportion of patients experienced the same benefit, in two subsequent randomized studies. Adverse events included thrombocytopenia, anemia, and a "cytokine rebound reaction" upon drug discontinuation. TG101348 is a JAK2 selective inhibitor. In a phase-1/phase-2 study of 59 patients with MF (Pardanani et al. 2011), about 47% of patients achieved a ≥50% decrease in palpable spleen size. Adverse events included nausea, vomiting, diarrhea, asymptomatic increases in serum lipase, transaminases or creatinine, thrombocytopenia, and anemia. CYT387 is JAK1/JAK2 inhibitor. In a phase-1/phase-2 study of 60 patients from the Mayo Clinic, CYT387 induced an approximately 45% response rate in splenomegaly (Pardanani et al. 2010). Adverse events included thrombocytopenia and mild peripheral neuropathy.

Most patients with MF and symptomatic splenomegaly become drug resistant. Splenectomy is offered to such patients (Tefferi et al. 2000). The largest experience in splenectomy for the treatment of MF comes from the Mayo Clinic and involves a total of 314 patients who underwent open splenectomy between 1976 and 2004 (Mesa et al. 2006). Indications for splenectomy included mechanical symptoms (49%), frequent red cell transfusion requirements (25%), symptomatic portal hypertension (15%), and thrombocytopenia (11%). More than 75% of patients benefited from their splenectomy lasting for a median of 1 year (range 0–8 years); specific benefits included becoming transfusion independent, which was observed in the majority of informative patients, and resolution of moderate to severe thrombocytopenia. Perioperative complications occurred in 28% of the patients and included infections, thrombosis, and bleeding. Overall perioperative mortality rate was 9%. In addition, approximately 10% of patients experienced accelerated hepatomegaly and 29% thrombocytosis after splenectomy. After a median follow-up of 28 months from splenectomy, median overall survival was 19 months, and leukemic transformation was documented in 14% of patients. Some of the complications associated with splenectomy in patients with MF might be prevented by the presurgery use of hydroxyurea in patients with platelet count of $>200 \times 10^9$/L and postsurgery use of systemic anticoagulation. Approximately 20% of patients might experience progressive hepatomegaly after splenectomy.

Radiotherapy is useful in both hepatosplenic and nonhepatosplenic EMH. In one literature review of splenic radiation in patients with MPN (Weinmann et al. 2001), radiation doses ranged between 3 and 5 Gy in 0.1–0.5 Gy fractions and resulted in pain relief and reduction in spleen size in most treated patients. However, remissions were often transient lasting from 3 to 6 months. In a Mayo Clinic study of 23 MF patient undergoing splenic irradiation, a median dose of 2.8 Gy (range 0.3–14) was given in a median of 7.5 fractions (range 2–17); approximately a third of the patients received multiple treatment courses (Elliott et al. 1998). Approximately 94% of the patients achieved an objective response in spleen size, and the median duration of response was 6 months. Median survival after splenic irradiation was 22 months. Approximately 44% of treated patients experienced treatment-related cytopenia, which was protracted in 26% and fatal in 13% (Elliott et al. 1998). More recent studies suggest that the use of low-dose intermittent radiation therapy (e.g., 1 Gy in a single or fractionated doses given every 1–3 months) might allow long-term control of symptomatic splenomegaly or postsplenectomy hepatomegaly (Riesterer et al. 2008).

Current indications for Transjugular Intrahepatic Portosystemic Shunt (TIPS) include recurrent variceal bleeding and refractory ascites, both of which could accompany advanced MF. The therapeutic value of TIPS has not been systematically studied in MF, but relevant information is available from several case reports (Doki et al. 2007; Angermayr et al. 2002; Belohlavek et al. 2001; Tanaka et al. 2000; Alvarez-Larran et al. 2005; Wiest et al. 2004). These case reports confirm feasibility and efficacy (i.e., reduction in hepatic venous pressure gradient and regression of ascites and varices). Complications of TIPS such as encephalopathy might be less of a problem in such patients since their hepatic synthetic activity is usually preserved. At the same time, the cause of ascites in

MF is not always increased portal hypertension and might involve peritoneal EMH implants that would not be expected to respond to TIPS (Wiest et al. 2004). Budd-Chiari syndrome (i.e., hepatic venous outflow obstruction) in the setting of PV or other MPN is also amenable to treatment with TIPS, especially during its acute stage, and might avert the need for orthotopic liver transplantation (Watanabe et al. 2000; Zahn et al. 2010).

15.3.2 Treatment of Constitutional Symptoms

Treatment of constitutional symptoms in MF had, in the past, been difficult. An earlier study with a tumor necrosis factor (TNF) antagonist, etanercept, a soluble TNF receptor, reported a 60% response in constitutional symptoms associated with a 20% response in cytopenias or spleen size (Steensma et al. 2002a). A similar anticytokine activity appears to underlie the value of JAK inhibitors in alleviating constitutional symptoms. For example, INCB018424, a JAK1/JAK2 inhibitor discussed above, induced improvement in constitutional symptoms (fatigue, pruritus, abdominal discomfort, early satiety, night sweats) and promoted weight gain in the majority of treated patients (Verstovsek et al. 2010). Whereas the drug's effect on *JAK2*V617F allele burden or bone marrow pathology was negligible, a marked treatment-associated reduction in proinflammatory cytokines (e.g., IL-1RA, IL-6, TNF-a, MIP-1b) was documented and was temporally associated with the drug-induced improvement in constitutional symptoms. Many other JAK inhibitors were also effective in alleviating MF-associated constitutional symptoms, and they include TG101348, a more selective JAK2 inhibitor, and CYT387, another JAK1/JAK2 inhibitor (Pardanani et al. 2010, 2011). Interestingly, plasma cytokine levels were not significantly affected by treatment with TG101348. It is possible that the latter drug's effect is partly secondary to its better tumor-debulking activity and, in that regard, similar to what is sometimes seen with splenectomy or effective cytoreductive therapy.

15.3.3 Treatment of Nonhepatosplenic Extramedullary Hematopoiesis

Nonhepatosplenic EMH associated with MF is best managed with low-dose radiotherapy (100–500 cGy in 5–10 fractions) (Koch et al. 2003; Steensma et al. 2002b; Neben-Wittich et al. 2010a). Nonhepatosplenic EMH might involve the vertebral column (spinal cord compression), lymph nodes (lymphadenopathy), pleura (pleural effusion) peritoneum (ascites), skin (cutaneous nodules), or lung (pulmonary hypertension). In a Mayo Clinic study, 27 patients with antemortem diagnosis of nonhepatosplenic EMH were identified and included 18 patients with MF (Koch et al. 2003). The thoracic vertebrae were the most frequently affected region, and specific therapy was not indicated in almost a third of the patients. More than 70% of patients responded to involved-field radiotherapy given at a median dose of 1 Gy (range 1–10 given in one to five fractions) for paraspinal disease, 1.25 Gy (range 1–1.5 given at a median of five fractions) for pleural or pulmonary disease, and 2 Gy (range 1.5–4.5 given at a median of seven fractions) for abdominal or pelvic disease (Koch et al. 2003). Diffuse bone pain, especially affecting the upper and lower extremities, is sometimes seen in patients with MF and is usually refractory to treatment with NSAIDs or narcotics. The use of involved-field radiation therapy in such instances has also been reported to be effective and safe (Neben-Wittich et al. 2010a, b).

MF-associated pulmonary hypertension is suspected in the presence of clinical symptoms and signs including dyspnea/hypoxia on exertion and peripheral edema, increased systolic pulmonary artery pressure on echocardiography, and an abnormal pulmonary uptake during a technetium 99m sulfur colloid scintigraphy. It is important to rule out alternative causes such as thromboembolic, infectious, or inflammatory lung processes (high-resolution CT scanning helps in this regard). In the absence of an alternative explanation for pulmonary hypertension, in a patient with MF, treatment with single-fraction (100 cGy) whole-lung irradiation is reasonable even if the technetium scan was negative (Steensma et al. 2002b).

15.4 Concluding Remarks

Currently available conventional or investigational drugs in MF have not been shown to either cure the disease or prolong survival. The latter possibility can only be tested in a controlled study, and any attempt to use historical controls in that regard is inappropriate and unscientific. There is currently much hype regarding JAK inhibitor therapy in MF, but one should recognize the fact that none of the currently available JAK inhibitors induce complete or partial remissions, and because of the complex molecular pathogenesis of MF, it is unlikely that we will see an imatinib-CML-like therapeutic success any time soon. Regardless, there is still something we can do to improve the well-being of our patients with MF, but the trick is to know what to do for whom and when. I hope that this chapter is useful in that regard.

References

Alvarez-Larran A, Abraldes JG, Cervantes F et al (2005) Portal hypertension secondary to myelofibrosis: a study of three cases. Am J Gastroenterol 100: 2355–2358

Angermayr B, Cejna M, Schoder M et al (2002) Transjugular intrahepatic portosystemic shunt for treatment of portal hypertension due to extramedullary hematopoiesis in idiopathic myelofibrosis. Blood 99:4246–4247

Barbui T, Thiele J, Passamonti F, et al (2010) Survival and risk of leukemic transformation in essential thrombocythemia are significantly influenced by accurate morphologic diagnosis: an international study on 1,104 patients. ASH Annual Meeting Abstracts 116:457

Barosi G, Mesa RA, Thiele J et al (2008) Proposed criteria for the diagnosis of post-polycythemia vera and post-essential thrombocythemia myelofibrosis: a consensus statement from the International Working Group for myelofibrosis research and treatment. Leukemia 22:437–438

Beer PA, Jones AV, Bench AJ et al (2009) Clonal diversity in the myeloproliferative neoplasms: independent origins of genetically distinct clones. Br J Haematol 144:904–908

Begna KH, Mesa RA, Pardanani A et al (2011) A phase-2 trial of low-dose pomalidomide in myelofibrosis with anemia. Leukemia 25:301–304

Belohlavek J, Schwarz J, Jirasek A, Krajina A, Polak F, Hruby M (2001) Idiopathic myelofibrosis complicated by portal hypertension treated with a transjugular intrahepatic portosystemic shunt (TIPS). Wien Klin Wochenschr 113:208–211

Bersenev A, Wu C, Balcerek J et al (2010) Lnk constrains myeloproliferative diseases in mice. J Clin Invest 120: 2058–2069

Besa EC, Nowell PC, Geller NL, Gardner FH (1982) Analysis of the androgen response of 23 patients with agnogenic myeloid metaplasia: the value of chromosomal studies in predicting response and survival. Cancer 49:308–313

Caramazza D, Begna KH, Gangat N et al (2011) Refined cytogenetic risk categorization for overall and leukemia-free survival in primary myelofibrosis: a single center study of 433 patients. Leukemia 25(1):82–88

Cervantes F, Alvarez-Larran A, Hernandez-Boluda JC, Sureda A, Torrebadell M, Montserrat E (2004) Erythropoietin treatment of the anaemia of myelofibrosis with myeloid metaplasia: results in 20 patients and review of the literature. Br J Haematol 127: 399–403

Cervantes F, Alvarez-Larran A, Domingo A, Arellano-Rodrigo E, Montserrat E (2005) Efficacy and tolerability of danazol as a treatment for the anaemia of myelofibrosis with myeloid metaplasia: long-term results in 30 patients. Br J Haematol 129:771–775

Cervantes F, Dupriez B, Pereira A et al (2009) New prognostic scoring system for primary myelofibrosis based on a study of the International Working Group for myelofibrosis research and treatment. Blood 113: 2895–2901

Dameshek W (1951) Some speculations on the myeloproliferative syndromes. Blood 6:372–375

DeAngelo DJ, Spencer A, Fischer T, et al (2009) Activity of oral Panobinostat (LBH589) in patients with myelofibrosis. ASH Annual Meeting Abstracts 114:2898

Doki N, Irisawa H, Takada S, Sakura T, Miyawaki S (2007) Transjugular intrahepatic portosystemic shunt for the treatment of portal hypertension due to idiopathic myelofibrosis. Intern Med 46:187–190

Elliott MA, Chen MG, Silverstein MN, Tefferi A (1998) Splenic irradiation for symptomatic splenomegaly associated with myelofibrosis with myeloid metaplasia. Br J Haematol 103:505–511

Ernst T, Chase AJ, Score J et al (2010) Inactivating mutations of the histone methyltransferase gene EZH2 in myeloid disorders. Nat Genet 42:722–726

Faoro LN, Tefferi A, Mesa RA (2005) Long-term analysis of the palliative benefit of 2-chlorodeoxyadenosine for myelofibrosis with myeloid metaplasia. Eur J Haematol 74:117–120

Gangat N, Caramazza D, Vaidya R et al (2011) DIPSS-plus: a refined dynamic international prognostic scoring system (DIPSS) for primary myelofibrosis that incorporates prognostic information from karyotype, platelet count and transfusion status. J Clin Oncol 29(4):392–397

Huang J, Tefferi A (2009) Erythropoiesis stimulating agents have limited therapeutic activity in transfusion-dependent patients with primary myelofibrosis regardless of serum erythropoietin level. Eur J Haematol 83:154–155

James C, Ugo V, Le Couedic JP et al (2005) A unique clonal JAK2 mutation leading to constitutive signalling causes polycythaemia vera. Nature 434:1144–1148

Ko M, Huang Y, Jankowska AM et al (2010) Impaired hydroxylation of 5-methylcytosine in myeloid cancers with mutant TET2. Nature 468:839–843

Koch CA, Li CY, Mesa RA, Tefferi A (2003) Nonhepatosplenic extramedullary hematopoiesis: associated diseases, pathology, clinical course, and treatment. Mayo Clin Proc 78:1223–1233

Lambert JR, Everington T, Linch DC, Gale RE (2009) In essential thrombocythemia, multiple JAK2-V617F clones are present in most mutant-positive patients: a new disease paradigm. Blood 114:3018–3023

Lee SW, Cho YS, Na JM et al (2010) ASXL1 represses retinoic acid receptor-mediated transcription through associating with HP1 and LSD1. J Biol Chem 285: 18–29

Li G, Miskimen KL, Wang Z et al (2010) Effective targeting of STAT5-mediated survival in myeloproliferative neoplasms using ABT-737 combined with rapamycin. Leukemia 24:1397–1405

Marchetti M, Barosi G, Balestri F et al (2004) Low-dose thalidomide ameliorates cytopenias and splenomegaly in myelofibrosis with myeloid metaplasia: a phase II trial. J Clin Oncol 22:424–431

Martinez-Trillos A, Gaya A, Maffioli M et al (2010) Efficacy and tolerability of hydroxyurea in the treatment of the hyperproliferative manifestations of myelofibrosis: results in 40 patients. Ann Hematol 89:1233–1237

Marubayashi S, Koppikar P, Taldone T et al (2010) HSP90 is a therapeutic target in JAK2-dependent myeloproliferative neoplasms in mice and humans. J Clin Invest 120:3578–3593

Mesa RA, Steensma DP, Pardanani A et al (2003) A phase 2 trial of combination low-dose thalidomide and prednisone for the treatment of myelofibrosis with myeloid metaplasia. Blood 101:2534–2541

Mesa RA, Nagorney DS, Schwager S, Allred J, Tefferi A (2006) Palliative goals, patient selection, and perioperative platelet management: outcomes and lessons from 3 decades of splenectomy for myelofibrosis with myeloid metaplasia at the Mayo Clinic. Cancer 107:361–370

Mesa RA, Yao X, Cripe LD et al (2010) Lenalidomide and prednisone for myelofibrosis: Eastern Cooperative Oncology Group (ECOG) phase 2 trial E4903. Blood 116:4436–4438

Neben-Wittich MA, Brown PD, Tefferi A (2010a) Successful treatment of severe extremity pain in myelofibrosis with low-dose single-fraction radiation therapy. Am J Hematol 85:808–810

Neben-Wittich M, Brown P, Tefferi A (2010b) Successful treatment of severe extremity pain in myelofibrosis with Low-dose single-fraction radiation therapy. Am J Clin Oncol-Cancer Clin Trials 33:203–204

Oh ST, Simonds EF, Jones C et al (2010) Novel mutations in the inhibitory adaptor protein LNK drive JAK-STAT signaling in patients with myeloproliferative neoplasms. Blood 116:988–992

Oku S, Takenaka K, Kuriyama T et al (2010) JAK2 V617F uses distinct signalling pathways to induce cell proliferation and neutrophil activation. Br J Haematol 150:334–344

Pardanani A, George G, Lasho T, et al (2010) A phase I/II study of CYT387, an oral JAK-1/2 inhibitor, in myelofibrosis: significant response rates in anemia, splenomegaly, and constitutional symptoms. ASH Annual Meeting Abstracts 116:460

Pardanani A, Gotlib JR, Jamieson C et al (2011) Safety and efficacy of TG101348, a selective JAK2 inhibitor, in myelofibrosis. J Clin Oncol 29(7):789–796

Pikman Y, Lee BH, Mercher T et al (2006) MPLW515L is a novel somatic activating mutation in myelofibrosis with myeloid metaplasia. PLoS Med 3:e270

Quintas-Cardama A, Tong W, Kantarjian H et al (2008) A phase II study of 5-azacitidine for patients with primary and post-essential thrombocythemia/polycythemia vera myelofibrosis. Leukemia 22:965–970

Quintas-Cardama A, Kantarjian HM, Manshouri T et al (2009) Lenalidomide plus prednisone results in durable clinical, histopathologic, and molecular responses in patients with myelofibrosis. J Clin Oncol 27:4760–4766

Rambaldi A, Dellacasa CM, Finazzi G et al (2010) A pilot study of the histone-deacetylase inhibitor givinostat in patients with JAK2V617F positive chronic myeloproliferative neoplasms. Br J Haematol 150:446–455

Riesterer O, Gmur J, Lutolf U (2008) Repeated and pre-emptive palliative radiotherapy of symptomatic hepatomegaly in a patient with advanced myelofibrosis. Onkologie 31:325–327

Schaub FX, Looser R, Li S et al (2010) Clonal analysis of TET2 and JAK2 mutations suggests that TET2 can be a late event in the progression of myeloproliferative neoplasms. Blood 115:2003–2007

Siragusa S, Vaidya R, Tefferi A (2009) Hydroxyurea effect on marked splenomegaly associated with primary myelofibrosis: response rates and correlation with JAK2V617F allele burden. ASH Annual Meeting Abstracts 114:4971

Steensma DP, Mesa RA, Li CY, Gray L, Tefferi A (2002a) Etanercept, a soluble tumor necrosis factor receptor, palliates constitutional symptoms in patients with myelofibrosis with myeloid metaplasia: results of a pilot study. Blood 99:2252–2254

Steensma DP, Hook CC, Stafford SL, Tefferi A (2002b) Low-dose, single-fraction, whole-lung radiotherapy for pulmonary hypertension associated with myelofibrosis with myeloid metaplasia. Br J Haematol 118:813–816

Tahiliani M, Koh KP, Shen Y et al (2009) Conversion of 5-methylcytosine to 5-hydroxymethylcytosine in mammalian DNA by MLL partner TET1. Science 324:930–935

Tanaka N, Yamakado K, Kihira H, Hashimoto A, Murayama T, Takeda K (2000) Re: transjugular intra-hepatic portosystemic shunt for intractable esophageal-gastric variceal hemorrhage in a patient with idiopathic myelofibrosis. Cardiovasc Intervent Radiol 23:491–492

Tefferi A (2010) Novel mutations and their functional and clinical relevance in myeloproliferative neoplasms: JAK2, MPL, TET2, ASXL1, CBL, IDH and IKZF1. Leukemia 24:1128–1138

Tefferi A, Mesa RA, Nagorney DM, Schroeder G, Silverstein MN (2000) Splenectomy in myelofibrosis with myeloid metaplasia: a single-institution experience with 223 patients. Blood 95:2226–2233

Tefferi A, Elliot MA, Yoon SY et al (2001) Clinical and bone marrow effects of interferon alfa therapy in myelofibrosis with myeloid metaplasia. Blood 97:1896

Tefferi A, Cortes J, Verstovsek S et al (2006) Lenalidomide therapy in myelofibrosis with myeloid metaplasia. Blood 108:1158–1164

Tefferi A, Thiele J, Orazi A et al (2007a) Proposals and rationale for revision of the World Health Organization diagnostic criteria for polycythemia vera, essential thrombocythemia, and primary myelofibrosis: recommendations from an ad hoc international expert panel. Blood 110:1092–1097

Tefferi A, Lasho TL, Mesa RA, Pardanani A, Ketterling RP, Hanson CA (2007b) Lenalidomide therapy in del(5)(q31)-associated myelofibrosis: cytogenetic and JAK2V617F molecular remissions. Leukemia 21:1827–1828

Tefferi A, Verstovsek S, Barosi G et al (2009) Pomalidomide is active in the treatment of anemia associated with myelofibrosis. J Clin Oncol 27:4563–4569

Thomas DA, Giles FJ, Albitar M et al (2006) Thalidomide therapy for myelofibrosis with myeloid metaplasia. Cancer 106:1974–1984

Vaidya R, Caramazza D, Finke C, Lasho T, Pardanani A, Tefferi A (2010) Circulating IL-2R, IL-8, IL-15 and CXCL10 levels are independently prognostic in primary myelofibrosis: a comprehensive cytokine profiling study. ASH Annual Meeting Abstracts 116:3068

Vannucchi AM, Guglielmelli P, Gattoni E, et al (2009) RAD001, an inhibitor of mTOR, shows clinical activity in a phase I/II study in patients with primary myelofibrosis (PMF) and post polycythemia vera/essential thrombocythemia myelofibrosis (PPV/PET MF). ASH Annual Meeting Abstracts 114:307

Vardiman JW, Thiele J, Arber DA et al (2009) The 2008 revision of the World Health Organization (WHO) classification of myeloid neoplasms and acute leukemia: rationale and important changes. Blood 114:937–951

Verstovsek S, Kantarjian H, Mesa RA et al (2010) Safety and efficacy of INCB018424, a JAK1 and JAK2 inhibitor, in myelofibrosis. N Engl J Med 363:1117–1127

Wang Y, Fiskus W, Chong DG et al (2009) Cotreatment with panobinostat and JAK2 inhibitor TG101209 attenuates JAK2V617F levels and signaling and exerts synergistic cytotoxic effects against human myeloproliferative neoplastic cells. Blood 114:5024–5033

Watanabe H, Shinzawa H, Saito T et al (2000) Successful emergency treatment with a transjugular intrahepatic portosystemic shunt for life-threatening Budd-Chiari syndrome with portal thrombotic obstruction. Hepatogastroenterology 47:839–841

Weinmann M, Becker G, Einsele H, Bamberg M (2001) Clinical indications and biological mechanisms of splenic irradiation in chronic leukaemias and myeloproliferative disorders. Radiother Oncol 58:235–246

Wiest R, Strauch U, Wagner H et al (2004) A patient with myelofibrosis complicated by refractory ascites and portal hypertension: to tips or not to tips? A case report with discussion of the mechanism of ascites formation. Scand J Gastroenterol 39:389–394

Zahn A, Gotthardt D, Weiss KH et al (2010) Budd-Chiari syndrome: long term success via hepatic decompression using transjugular intrahepatic porto-systemic shunt. BMC Gastroenterol 10:25

Allogeneic Hematopoietic Stem Cell Transplantation for Myelofibrosis

16

Nicolaus Kröger

Contents

N. Kröger
Department of Stem Cell Transplantation,
University Hospital Hamburg-Eppendorf,
Hamburg, Germany
e-mail: nkroeger@uke.uni-hamburg.de

16.1 Introduction

Primary myelofibrosis (PMF) is a stem cell-derived clonal myeloproliferative disorder in which the primary disease process is a clonal proliferation of multiple cell elements especially the megakaryocytes. This proliferation is accompanied by an increased secretion of different cytokines with a secondary intramedullary fibrosis, osteosclerosis, angiogenesis, and extramedullary hematopoiesis (Tefferi 2005). Clinically, this disease is characterized with different degrees of cytopenias, hepatosplenomegaly, and constitutional symptoms (Smith et al. 1990). Myelofibrosis (MF) may occur at advanced stages of polycythemia vera (PV) and essential thrombocythemia (ET) and thus referred to as post-PV and post-ET MF (Mesa et al. 2007). This disease is challenging for both patients and physicians. The first challenge is the estimation of the potential natural history and life expectancy in every individual patient since the survival of PMF patients may vary widely from several months to many years (Cervantes et al. 2008). Second, due to the fact that PMF affects primarily the elderly group of patients, it is important as well to estimate the accompanying comorbidities which could influence the therapeutic decisions. Importantly, the pharmacomedical treatment options for this disease such as growth factors, androgens, interferon-α and conventional cytotoxic medications, and more recently so-called JAK2 inhibitors lead only to symptomatic palliation without altering the natural history of the disease (Kröger and Mesa 2008). Currently, the only available curative therapy for myelofibrosis is allogeneic hematopoietic stem cell transplantation (AHSCT) which is still associated with a substantial treatment-related morbidity and mortality (Kerbauy et al. 2007). Reduced-intensity conditioning offers an option to reduce treatment-related mortality (TRM) and leads to a broader HSCT applicability also to older patients. However, whether this approach could lead to increased posttreatment relapse risk is still unknown. When, how, and to which patients this therapeutic modality should be offered are critical issues which need to be explored.

16.2 Allogeneic Hematopoietic Stem Cell Transplantation After Myeloablative Conditioning

Application of AHSCT in PMF setting was relatively delayed due to the concern that advanced bone marrow fibrosis may prevent or complicate the engraftment of hematopoietic stem cells (Rajantie et al. 1986; Soll et al. 1995). In the late 1980s and the early 1990s, it could be shown through few small reports that even in the case of advanced and high-risk disease, sustained engraftment and regression of bone marrow were achievable (Dokal et al. 1989; Creemers et al. 1992). A larger study in 1999 by Guardiola et al. included 55 patients with myelofibrosis who received graft from HLA-identical sibling. The median age was 42 years, and the 1-year nonrelapse mortality was 27%, resulting in a 5-year estimated survival of 47% (Guardiola et al. 1999). Deeg et al. reported of 56 patients from the Fred Hutchinson Cancer Center who received stem cell graft from related or unrelated donor after either TBI ($n=12$) or busulfan-based conditioning regimen ($n=44$). The median age of the patients was 43 years, and the 3-year overall survival was 58% (Deeg et al. 2003). The results were updated by Kerbauy, including now 95 patients with a median age of 49 years and resulting in a 5-year nonrelapse mortality rate of 34% and a 7-year estimated

overall survival of 61 years (Kerbauy et al. 2007). Patriarca et al. reported for the GITMO about 48 patients with a median age of 49 years who received various standard myeloablative conditioning regimens. They reported of a nonrelapse mortality of 35% at 1 year and a 3-year overall survival of 42% (Patriarca et al. 2008). Ballen reported the results of CIBMTR including 229 patients who received various myeloablative conditioning regimens from HLA-identical sibling ($n=72$). The nonrelapse mortality at day 100 was 42% for the MUD and 22% for the HLA-identical sibling, resulting in a 5-year OS of 31% and 39% respectively (Ballen et al. 2005).

Stewart reported for the British Society for Blood and Marrow Transplantation on 27 patients who received stem cell graft from related or unrelated donors after busulfan/cyclophosphamide ($n=4$) or TBI-based ($n=23$) myeloablative conditioning regimens. The nonrelapse mortality at 3 years was 41%, and the 3-year overall survival was 44% (Stewart et al. 2010).

More recently, Robin et al. (2010) reported on behalf of the French Society of 147 patients with myelofibrosis who received an allograft between 1997 and 2008. Thirty-one percent received a myeloablative conditioning regimen. There was no significant difference between myeloablative and reduced-intensity conditioning, but the results for myeloablative were not given separately. Overall, the 4-year nonrelapse mortality was 39%, resulting in an overall survival at 4 years of 39%.

The major risk factors in the myeloablative studies were advanced age, advanced disease status according to Lille score, and mismatched unrelated donors.

Table 16.1 summarizes the results of the selected studies performed with standard myeloablative conditioning. TRM rates in these studies were 20–48% at 1 year posttransplant. The results were more favorable in young patients with less advanced disease and when targeted busulfan-based conditioning was used. In the elderly group in which MF is most frequently diagnosed, AHSCT was associated with a significant treatment-related risk.

Table 16.1 Allogeneic stem cell transplantation for myelofibrosis after standard myeloablative conditioning regimen

Author	No. of patients	Conditioning regimen		Median age	Nonrelapse mortality	Overall survival
Myeloablative conditioning						
Ballen et al. CIBMTR (2010)	n = 134 sibling	Various		45 years	22% at day 100	39% at 5 years
	n = 23 other related			40 years	27% at day 100	31% at 5 years
	n = 72 MUD			42 years	42% at day 100	31% at 5 years
Guardiola et al. (1999)	n = 55 sibling	Various TBI-based	n = 35 n = 20	42 years	27% at 1 year	47% at 5 years
Deeg et al. (2003)	n = 56 sibling + MUD	Busulfan-based TBI-based	n = 44 n = 12	43 years	31% after 3 years	58% at 3 years
Kerbauy et al. (2007)	n = 95 sibling + MUD	Busulfan-based TBI-based	n = 80 n = 15	49 years	34% at 5 years	61% at 7 years
Patriarca et al. (2008)	n = 48 sibling + MUD	Various		49 years	35% at 1 year	42% at 3 years
Stewart et al. (2010)	n = 27 sibling + MUD	Bu/Cy TBI-based	n = 4 n = 23	38 years	41% at 3 years	44% at 3 years
Lissandre et al. (2011)	n = 15 sibling + MUD	Various		49 years	20% at 3 years	47% at 3 years (RFS)

16.3   Allogeneic Hematopoietic Stem Cell Transplantation After Reduced-Intensity Conditioning

The rationale to use reduced-intensity conditioning in hematological malignancies relies on the assumption that eradication of malignant cells does not only depend on the intensity of conditioning but also on the posttransplant continuous action of alloreactive immunocompetent cells of donor origin. The evidence of existence of such a graft-versus-myelofibrosis effect came from two reports in which patients with relapse after AHSCT achieved regression of bone marrow fibrosis after infusion of donor lymphocytes (DLIs) (Byrne et al. 2000; Cervantes et al. 2000). AHSCT for myelofibrosis after dose-reduced conditioning was first reported in 2002 in two studies with three and four patients respectively (Hessling et al. 2002; Devine et al. 2002). The encouraging results of preliminary reports led to

the conduction of further larger studies. The results of ten European transplant centers on 20 patients were reported as an abstract (Hertenstein et al. 2002) from which four were previously included in the report of Devine et al. 2002. Twenty patients were transplanted after TBI/flu-darabine conditioning with or without in vivo T-cell depletion using antithymocyte globulin (ATG) or antilymphocyte globulin (ALG). The authors reported a TRM at 1 year of 37% and OS of 54%. Notably, within the study cohort, 25% of patients had almost leukemic transformation prior to AHSCT.

In 2005, two larger studies were published, both with 21 patients (Rondelli et al. 2005; Kröger et al. 2005). The first retrospective study of the Myeloproliferative Disease-Research Consortium included 21 patients with a median age of 54 years, mainly transplanted from matched sibling donor with peripheral blood stem cells. Multiple conditioning regimens were used (TBI/fludarabine, fludarabine/melphalan, thiothepa/cyclophosphamide, and thio-thepa/fludarabine). All patients had intermediate or high risk according to Lille score at the time of AHSCT, and most had advanced marrow fibrosis. Only one engraftment failure occurred, and after a median follow-up of 31 months, 18 patients were alive and 17 were still in remission. Three patients died during follow-up due to transplant-related causes ($n=2$) or due to relapse ($n=1$) (Rondelli et al. 2005).

Similar results were reported by the German prospective pilot study including 21 patients with a median age of 53 years. The conditioning regimen consisted of busulfan/fludarabine 10 mg/kg, and in vivo T-cell depletion with ATG was followed by AHSCT from related ($n=8$) and unrelated ($n=13$) donors. All patients achieved stable engraftment and were full chimera at day 100 post-AHSCT. Graft-versus-host disease (GvHD) rates were acceptable, and TRM was 16% at 1 year. OS at 3 years after a median follow-up of 22 months was 84%. Hematological response and complete histopathological remission were seen in 100% and 75% of patients respectively. Twenty-five percent showed partial histopathological remission with a continuing decline in fibrosis grade (Kröger et al. 2005). In 2007, a single Italian center reported on 39 patients with a median age of 51 years who received reduced-intensity conditioning with thiothepa/cyclophosphamide. Most of patients received bone marrow from matched-related ($n=22$) or alternative donor ($n=17$). After a median follow-up of 28 months, the overall actuarial survival was 50%. In univariate analysis, a Karnowsky score of 100%, an interval from diagnosis to transplant of <1 year, an HLA-identical sibling donor, and splenectomy pretransplant were significant predictors of favorable outcome (Bacigalupo et al. 2007). Recently, the same group reported on a total of 46 patients with PMF transplanted after the same conditioning regimen. After a median follow-up of 3.8 years, the multivariate analysis showed RBC transfusions >20 units, spleen size >22 cm pre-AHSCT, and alternative donor as independent risk factors for unfavorable outcome post-AHSCT. Patients who had two or more from the previous factors had an extremely poor 5-year survival (8% vs. 77% in those who had ≤1 risk factors, $p=0.0001$) due to increased TRM (HR 6.0, $p=0.006$) and relapse incidence (HR 7.69, $p=0.001$) (Bacigalupo et al. 2010).

Excellent results were shown in a small report of six patients who underwent AHSCT after reduced-intensity busulfan/fludarabine–based conditioning with no TRM after a median follow-up of 16 months post-AHSCT (George et al. 2008).

More recently, the results of the prospective multicenter study of the Chronic Leukemia Working Party of the European Group for Blood and Marrow Transplantation (EBMT) were updated and published after the first presentation in 2007 in abstract form (Kröger et al. 2007b, 2009b). Seventeen transplant centers from three nations participated and enrolled 103 patients with PMF ($n=63$), post-PV and post-ET MF ($n=40$), and a median age of 55 (range, 32–68). Most of the patients were at intermediate or high risk according to Lille score. Conditioning regimen was busulfan (10 mg/kg)/fludarabine with in vivo T-cell depletion with ATG. All but two patients showed leukocyte and platelet engraftment, and the cumulative incidence of TRM at 1 year was 16% which was significantly higher with HLA-mismatched donors. At 3 years, the cumulative incidence of relapse was 22% and significantly influenced by the risk status according to Lille. After a median follow-up of 33 months (range, 12–76), 5-year estimated OS and DFS were 67% and 51%, respectively. In the multivariate analysis, allografting from HLA-mismatched donor and advanced Lille score were independent risk factors for decreased DFS, whereas age >55 years and HLA-mismatched transplantation significantly predicted inferior overall survival (Kröger et al. 2009a, b).

Stewart et al. reported on behalf of the British Society for Blood and Marrow Transplantation of 24 patients who received various dose-reduced conditioning regimens. Four patients (17%) experienced primary graft failure, and the nonrelapse mortality at 3 years was 32%, resulting in overall survival of 31% (Stewart et al. 2010). Lissandre et al. (2011) reported on 24 patients who received various dose-reduced conditioning regimens for myelofibrosis. The nonrelapse mortality at 3 years was 36%, and the 3-year relapse-free survival was 60%.

These data show that AHSCT after dose-reduced conditioning is feasible and results in a substantial reduction of procedure-related mortality. Through

Table 16.2 Dose-reduced conditioning regimen followed by allogeneic stem cell transplantation for myelofibrosis

Author	No. of patients	Conditioning regimen	Median age	Nonrelapse mortality	Overall survival
Hertenstein et al. (2002)	$n=20$	Various fludarabine-based	50 years	37% at 1 year	54% at 1 year
Rondelli et al. (2005)	$n=21$	Various fludarabine-based	54 years	10% at 1 year	85% at 2.5 years
Kröger et al. (2005)	$n=21$	Busulfan 10 mg/kg Fludarabine + ATG	53 years	16% at 1 year	84% at 3 years
Bacigalupo et al. (2010)	$n=46$	Thiothepa-based	51 years	24% at 5 years	45% at 5 years
Kröger et al. (2009b)	$n=103$	Busulfan (10 mg/kg) Fludarabine + ATG	55 years	16% at 1 year	67% at 5 years
Stewart et al. (2010)	$n=24$	Various fludarabine-based	54 years	32% at 3 years	31% at 3 years
Lissandre et al. (2011)	$n=24$	Various fludarabine-based	49 years	36% at 3 years	60% at 3 years (*RFS*)

this approach, the median age of AHSCT candidates was shifted from about 40–55 years. Results of selected studies are listed in Table 16.2.

16.4 Comparison Between Myeloablative and Reduced-Intensity Conditioning

A matter of concern of reduced-dose conditioning is the potential increase in relapse rates due to the incomplete eradication of tumor cells pre-AHSCT. Up to date, there was no direct comparison between the myeloablative and dose-reduced transplantation for myelofibrosis within a prospective trial. However, the Swedish Group for Myeloproliferative Disorders reported in 2006 a retrospective comparative study of a small series of 27 MF patients transplanted in six Swedish centers between 1982 and 2004. Seventeen patients were transplanted after myeloablative and ten after dose-reduced conditioning. Regardless that patients transplanted after reduced-intensity conditioning were older with more comorbidities, they had less TRM (10% vs. 30% respectively) and tended to survive longer (Merup et al. 2006). In 2008, another retrospective multicenter study from the Gruppo Italiano Trapianto di Midollo Osseo (GITMO) included 100 patients who were transplanted between 1986 and 2006 using myeloablative and reduced-intensity conditioning in

48 and 52 patients respectively. Ninety percent of them had intermediate or high Lille score, and 78% received stem cells from matched sibling donors. The cumulative incidence of engraftment at day 90 after transplant was 87% and the cumulative 1-year and 3-year incidence of TRM were 35% and 43% respectively. The estimated 3-year OS and DFS were 42% and 35%, respectively. In the multivariate analysis, predictors of negative outcome were AHSCT before 1995, unrelated donors, and long interval from diagnosis to transplant. The intensity of conditioning regimen did not significantly influence the outcome (Patriarca et al. 2008). Recently, a report from three Canadian and four European transplant centers examined retrospectively 46 consecutive patients with myelofibrosis treated with AHSCT between 1998 and 2005. Twenty-three patients received myeloablative conditioning from whom all but one were treated with TBI-based regimen. Most of the remaining patients received dose-reduced conditioning with busulfan/fludarabine combination. Patients with reduced-intensity conditioning were significantly older (54 vs. 47 years), had longer disease duration, and tended to have more reduced performance status. Those patients had significantly lower deaths due to treatment-related-causes and a borderline improved OS (68% vs. 48% at 3 years $p=0.08$). Relapse rates at 3 years were not different between myeloablative and reduced-intensity settings (Gupta et al. 2009).

Table 16.3 Retrospective between myeloablative and dose-reduced conditioning followed by allogeneic stem cell transplantation for myelofibrosis

Author	No. of patients		Median age	Treatment-related mortality (TRM)		Relapse		Overall survival	
Gupta et al. (2009)	RIC	n=23	54 years	23% (1 year)	p=0.08	14%	n.s.	68% (3 years)	p=0.08
	MAC	n=23	47 years	39% (1 year)		9%		48% (3 years)	
Stewart et al. (2010)	RIC	n=24	54 years	21% (day 100)		46%	p=0.06	31%	n.s.
	MAC	n=27	38 years	54% (day 100)		15%		44%	
Robin et al. (2010)	RIC	n=101	56 years	21% (day 100)	n.s.	n.d.		HR 1	n.s.
	MAC	n=46	47 years	54% (day 100)				HR 0.98	
Patriarca et al. (2008)	RIC	n=52	n. d.	HR 0.93	n.s.	n.d.		HR 0.78	n.s.
	MAC	n=48	n.d.	HR 1				HR 1	

RIC reduced-intensity conditioning, *MAC* myeloablative conditioning

The British Society for Blood and Marrow Transplantation compared retrospectively the outcome of 7 myeloablative and 24 reduced-intensity conditioning regimen in myelofibrosis patients. The median age was significantly younger in the RIC group (38 vs. 54 years, $p<0.001$). The nonrelapse rate did not differ significantly between the myeloablative and the reduced-intensity group (41% vs. 32%, $p=0.4$), but there was a borderline significant higher risk of relapse for the RIC group (46% vs. 15%, $p=0.06$), resulting in a comparable overall survival at 3 years (31% vs. 44%, $p=0.7$) (Stewart et al. 2010).

The French Society for Blood and Marrow Transplantation (SFGM-TC) reported on 197 myelofibrosis patients who received allogeneic stem cell transplantation. Thirty-one percent of the patients received a myeloablative conditioning. No detailed comparison was given in the paper, but nonrelapse mortality ($p=0.4$) and overall survival ($p=0.8$) did not differ between both groups (Robin et al. 2010). Table 16.3 summarizes the results of the comparative trials.

16.5 Specific Considerations

16.5.1 Splenectomy Prior to AHSCT

The presence of massive splenomegaly in PMF patients is probably a surrogate marker of disease bulk. Based thereon, it could be postulated that removal of the enlarged spleen may serve a debulking purpose as well as prevent sequestration of blood progenitors which can lead to delayed engraftment or even graft failure. However, the spleen is an important immune organ and may play a role in immune reconstitution after AHSCT. Furthermore, there is a high reported surgical risk associated with splenectomy in PMF patients (about 6% mortality) (Tefferi et al. 2000; Li and Deeg 2001).

In the setting of myeloablative conditioning, allografting after splenectomy led to faster engraftment and to lower transfusion support needs without significant impact on the 3-year estimated OS in one study (Li et al. 2001). Data regarding the role of splenectomy in the case of dose-reduced AHSCT are few. More recently, in a large study of 103 patients from which 14 patients were splenectomized, splenectomy was associated with an increased incidence of relapse in the multivariate analysis (51% vs. 20% in patients with intact spleen, HR 3.58, $p=0.006$) (Kröger et al. 2009b).

Indeed, one report analyzed the impact of splenomegaly on transplant outcome in ten patients with PMF and splenomegaly who were treated with AHSCT after reduced-intensity conditioning. All patients fully engrafted donor cells, including five patients with extensive splenomegaly who,

Table 16.4 Impact of splenectomy on transplant outcome: splenectomy prior to allogeneic stem cell transplantation

Author	Engraftment	TRM	Relapse	Survival
Robin et al. (2010)	⇑	Ø	Ø	Only male ⇑
Guardiola et al. (1999)	⇑	Ø	Ø	Ø
Kröger et al. (2009b)	⇑	Ø	⇑	Ø
Patriarca et al. (2008)	No difference in graft failure	Ø	Ø	Ø
Kerbauy et al. (2007)	⇑	Ø	Ø	Ø
Li et al. (2001b)	⇑	Ø	Ø	Ø

Ø = no difference, ⇑ = improvement

however, had prolonged time to neutrophil and platelet recovery. In all, patient regression of spleen size was documented within 12 months posttransplant (Ciurea et al. 2008). In contrast, in an Italian study, spleen size >22 cm was an independent risk factor for worse survival (Bacigalupo et al. 2010). In most studies, splenectomy was associated with faster engraftment, and survival benefit for splenectomized patients was seen only for the subgroup of male patients in the French study (Robin et al. 2010). In conclusion, considering the sufficient evidence available that even in the case of massive splenomegaly, donor cell engraftment and full donor chimerism are achievable, together with the significant risks associated with splenectomy pretransplant such as surgical risk, delayed immune reconstitution after AHSCT, and possibly the reported increased relapse, splenectomy is not generally recommended in transplant-eligible patients. Table 16.4 summarizes the effect of splenectomy in these different studies.

16.5.2 The Impact of Cytogenetics and Molecular Genetics on Outcome

Cytogenetic abnormalities are detected in 30–40% of PMF patients at diagnosis (Hussein et al. 2009). In nontransplant settings, del(20q) or del(13q) as well as normal karyotype are associated with a favorable prognosis, whereas most other cytogenetic abnormalities confer a negative prognostic impact. Particularly abnormalities of chromosomes 5, 7, or 17 display markedly a shortened survival (Hussein et al. 2009; Tam et al. 2009). However, cytogenetic findings are not yet implemented in

any of the risk stratification systems for myelofibrosis currently available. Furthermore, the impact of specific genetic abnormalities on transplant outcome is still controversial. After myeloablative AHSCT, one study reported a significant impact of abnormal karyotype on the outcome after transplant (Guardiola et al. 1999). Recently, after reduced-dose conditioning allografting, one study presented in abstract form with 45 patients found a statistically significant negative impact on the DFS in the presence of unfavorable abnormalities (Baurmann et al. 2009), but another larger study (*n* = 103 patients) did not reveal any significant impact of abnormal karyotype (Kröger et al. 2009b). Based thereon, cytogenetic findings currently do not influence outcome after AHSCT, but its possible contribution to the outcome should be addressed in further trials.

Similarly, the role of novel mutations associated with PMF and other myeloproliferative neoplasms in the transplant setting is not well understood. JAK2V617F is a gain of function mutation which occurs in the pseudokinase domain of JAK2 gene and results in a cytokine-independent proliferation advantage in the affected cells (James et al. 2005). This mutation is detected in about 50–60% of PMF cases (Percy and McMullin 2005). In the nontransplant setting, the presence of JAK2V617F and its underlying allele burden probably plays a role in disease phenotype, but the impact on disease prognosis is rather controversial (Vannucchi et al. 2008). In 2006, a German group conducted a retrospective analysis of 30 AHSCT patients for JAK2 status from whom 16 were JAK2V617F positive and found no influence of JAK2V617F mutation on the outcome posttransplant. In contrast, the

Table 16.5 Risk factor for outcome after allogeneic stem cell transplantation

Author	Age	Donor	Disease status	Others
Kröger et al. EBMT (2009a, b)	>55 years	Mismatched unrelated	Lille high	
Robin et al. SFGM (2010)	Ø	Mismatched unrelated	Lille high sAML	Male without splenectomy
Guardiola et al. (1999)	>45 years			Hb <10 g/l Grade III fibrosis
Deeg et al. (2003)	Increasing age		Lille high	Abnormal cytogenetics Marrow fibrosis
Bacigalupo et al. (2010)		Unrelated		>20 transfusions Spleen size >20 cm
Alchalby et al. (2010b)	Advanced age	Mismatched unrelated	Lille high	JAK2 wild type
Kerbauy et al. (2007)	Advanced age			Low platelets Comorbidity score No Bu-targeted

prospective EBMT trial noted a favorable impact of JAK2V617F mutation on OS and DFS post-transplant (Kröger et al. 2009a). More recently, JAK2 positivity has been found as an independent factor for improved survival in 139 patients who received dose-reduced conditioning followed by allogeneic stem cell transplantation for myelofibrosis (Alchalby et al. 2010b). The major risk factors for transplant outcome within the major trials are listed in Table 16.5.

16.5.2.1 Evaluation of Remission and Residual Disease Posttransplant

Monitoring of remission after ASCT for MF depending only on the criteria established by the International Working Group for Myelofibrosis Research and Treatment (IWG-MRT) is often misleading (Tefferi et al. 2006). A complete remission according to those criteria warrants the resolution of the disease-related clinical signs and symptoms as well as cytopenias. However, persistence of such signs after ASCT may be caused by several coexisting treatment-related conditions such as GvHD, graft dysfunction, or toxic medications. On the other hand, normalization of peripheral blood values and resolution of disease-related symptoms and signs do not exclude residual disease. Using specific molecular markers of malignant cells such as the JAK2V617F detected in >50% of MF patients, close monitoring of the molecular remission state became possible. In one study using a

highly sensitive real-time Taqman PCR assay, 21 JAK2V617F-positive patients were monitored in peripheral blood after reduced-intensity conditioning and AHSCT. Seventeen patients cleared JAK2V617F mutation after a median of 89 days post-AHSCT from whom 15 remained JAK2V617F negative after a median follow-up of 20 months. The results of JAK2V617F monitoring correlated inversely with donor cell chimerism. Four of five patients who never reached JAK2V617F negativity during the follow-up fulfilled otherwise the IWG-MRT criteria for complete remission (Kröger et al. 2007a). Similar findings were reported from another group where three patients from whom 15 tested positive for JAK2V617F prior to AHSCT became once more positive post-AHSCT. All of them developed an overt relapse shortly after redetection of JAK2V617F mutation (Steckel et al. 2007). These data suggest that JAK2V617F mutation monitored with a sensitive method is useful as a minimal residual disease marker post-ASCT. In another study, clearance of JAK2 mutation level in peripheral blood as a time-dependent event after allogeneic stem cell transplantation remained an independent risk factor for relapse. JAK2-positive patients who cleared mutation level within 6 months after allogeneic stem cell transplantation had a significant lower risk for clinical relapse (5% vs. 35%, $p=0.03$) (Alchalby et al. 2010b). The same may probably apply for the presence of other disease-specific mutations such as MPLW515L/K. Two groups reported the disappearance of

MPLW515A mutation (Rumi et al. 2010) in one patient and MPLW515L (Alchalby et al. 2010a) in two patients posttransplant respectively. Therefore and based on the experience with the JAK2V617F, it might well be expected that MPLW515L/K/ become positive in the case of malignant relapse. However, more data are needed to confirm the utility of MPL mutations as residual disease markers post-AHSCT.

At the histomorphological level, resolution or regression of bone marrow fibrosis is documented in ~50% of OMF patients after myeloablative conditioning between 6 and 12 months post-AHSCT (11, 12). In the setting of reduced-intensity conditioning, one study documented the kinetics of marrow fibrosis resolution in 24 PMF patients who underwent AHSCT with different degrees of fibrosis grade (MF-2, $n=13$; MF-3, $n=11$). A complete or near-complete resolution of bone marrow fibrosis was seen in 59% of patients by day 100, 90% by day 180, and 100% by 1 year post-AHSCT (Thiele et al. 2005; Kröger et al. 2007c).

Furthermore, one group showed that monitoring of marrow composition by MRI could accurately assess the pattern and extent of myelofibrosis as well as disease status, and correlated with biopsy findings after AHSCT (Sale et al. 2006).

Overall, due to the risk of relapse after AHSCT, posttransplant survey and management is crucial for improving the outcome. Since morphological criteria are frequently insufficient, it is necessary to closely monitor chimerism status and minimal residual disease whenever a reliable marker is available. Bone biopsy and histopathologic examination is necessary for any remission state estimation according to IWG-MRT criteria.

16.5.2.2 Adoptive Immunotherapy Posttransplant for Residual Disease or Relapse

Posttransplant adoptive immunotherapy with DLIs can be given after AHSCT to treat relapse and often results in a marked regression or disappearance of marrow fibrosis (Byrne et al. 2000; Cervantes et al. 2000; Benjamini et al. 2008). Unfortunately, severe GvHD may complicate DLIs administration and increase the treatment morbidity. Recently, 17 patients with PMF, post-PV/ET MF, and secondary

AML postmyelofibrosis received DLIs from related or unrelated donor either for clinical relapse (salvage DLI, $n=9$) or residual disease after AHSCT (preemptive DLI, $n=8$). The median cell dose of the first DLI was 10^6 CD3$^+$ cells per kilogram of body weight (BW; range, $0.5–9 \times 10^6$ cells/kg BW). Second and subsequent half-log-increased DLI were given if no graft-versus-host disease (GvHD) and no significant response were observed. No TRM was documented, but 18% of patients ($n=3$) developed grade II through IV acute GvHD which happened only in the salvage group probably due to the higher DLI dose escalation required. In this group, 44% of patients responded with complete molecular remission, and remarkably, development of GvHD was associated with increased quality of response. In contrast, all patients in the preemptive group responded at the molecular level with only one case of mild chronic liver GvHD. The difference in remission rates between the two groups was statistically significant ($p=0.04$) (Kröger et al. 2009a). The authors concluded that the application of adoptive immunotherapy in a preemptive approach is more successful and less toxic than treating patients with clinical relapse.

16.5.2.3 Role of Second Allogeneic Transplantation for Relapsed Patients

For patients with good performance status who relapsed after dose-reduced intensity allograft and failed or are not eligible for donor lymphocyte infusion, a second allograft can be considered. The German Transplant Group reported on 17 relapsed patients who did not respond to donor lymphocyte infusion ($n=13$) or did not receive DLI due to graft failure or blastic transformation and received a second allograft. The nonrelapse mortality was only 6% at 1 year, and the cumulative incidence of relapse was 24%, resulting in an overall survival of 82% at 1 year (Klyuchnikov et al. 2011).

16.5.2.4 Decision-Making and Risk Assessment Before AHSCT

Due to the highly variable natural history and treatment outcome of myelofibrosis, accurate and dynamic risk assessment systems which can be applied in different time points after diagnosis are urgently needed. Over the last years, several scoring systems for myelofibrosis were developed. The most widely used model is the Lille (Dupriez) score (Dupriez et al. 1996) which includes two classification variables: hemoglobin (<10 g/dl) and white blood cell count (<4×10⁹/l or >30×10⁹/l). High-risk patients with both factors have an OS of 13 months compared to intermediate risk (one factor, 26 months) and low risk (none, 93 months). Both of the largest trials evaluating AHSCT after myeloablative conditioning (Guardiola et al. 1999; Deeg et al. 2003) and one large study in the reduced-dose allografting setting (Kröger et al. 2009a, b) showed that Lille classification maintains its independent significance for the outcome posttransplant. Cervantes scoring system (Cervantes et al. 1998) includes hemoglobin (<10 g/dl), circulating blasts, and constitutional symptoms as stratification factors. Another model from Mayo Clinic (Elliott et al. 2007) included, in addition to hemoglobin (<10 g/dl) and white blood cell count (<4×10⁹/l or >30×10⁹/l), platelet count (<100×10⁹/l) and monocytes (≥1×10⁹/l). The most recent classification system (IPSS score) is based on a study of the IWG-MRT (Cervantes et al. 2009). The IPSS classification distinguishes between four risk groups, depending on the presence of advanced age >65 years, hemoglobin (<10 g/dl) and white blood cell count (>25×10⁹/l), circulating blast cells ≥1%, and constitutional symptoms. The presence of 0 (low risk), 1 (intermediate-1 risk), 2 (intermediate-2 risk) and ≥3 (high risk) of these variables corresponds to a respective median survival of 135, 95, 48, and 27 months. In this study, abnormal karyotype contributed independently to the outcome only in the intermediate-risk group. Studying a cohort of PMF patients in a reduced-intensity allografting setting, one group developed recently a classification system which depends on the presence of RBC transfusions >20 units, spleen size >22 cm, pre-AHSCT, and alternative donor and thus distinguishes a group of patients with two or more factors who had a very poor transplant outcome (Bacigalupo et al. 2010). Unfavorable cytogenetics and the presence of JAK2V617F mutation are other possible contributors to outcome which are not yet implemented in any available prognostic system. Which scor-

ing system should be used in the transplant setting is a critical question. Notably, due to the heterogeneity of the different models, one given myelofibrosis patient may be classified according to one of them to have a high-risk status and according to another to be at low risk. Since the introduction of reduced-intensity conditioning regimens, allogeneic stem cell transplantation has become a reasonable curative treatment option also for elderly patients. Age which is in general an important prognostic factor is also an important risk factor for outcome after transplantation. Nevertheless, elderly patients with advanced disease and no or only few comorbidities can be cured by allogeneic stem cell transplantation (Samuelson et al. 2011).

The optimal time point to perform AHSCT for myelofibrosis is not clearly defined. Transplanting low-risk disease is very likely to be curative, but the possible associated TRM (about 10%) should be balanced against the individual life expectancy without transplantation. On the other hand, deferring AHSCT until the disease becomes very advanced results in a significantly lower cure chance and an increased TRM. We recommend offering AHSCT to intermediate- and high-risk disease given that the patient is transplant eligible and a suitable donor is available. Close monitoring of disease course in low-risk patients is mandatory, and a sustained change toward more advanced disease should lead to consulting a transplant unit experienced in AHSCT for myelofibrosis.

Whenever possible, HLA-identical siblings are donors of choice for AHSCT; however, similar transplant outcome could be achieved with HLA-identical alternative donors using reduced-intensity conditioning (Kröger et al. 2009a, b). The results of AHSCT after dose-reduced conditioning are very encouraging and seem overall not to be inferior to those with myeloablative conditioning. Particularly due to the low associated TRM, reduced-dose allografting is the recommended procedure in elderly patients. Whether it is the case in young patients, it should be confirmed in future randomized studies. In fact, it could be postulated that reduction of the tumor eradication potential of conditioning pre-ASCT may lead to a lesser degree of disease control;

however, this assumption has never been confirmed in the available literature. Moreover, the increased feasibility of posttransplant strategies through availability of sensitive techniques for MRD detection and application of DLIs may make the prevention and management of relapse more successful.

Conclusion

Many significant advances were achieved in the last decade regarding understanding and management of Philadelphia-negative myeloproliferative neoplasms. Much work is still needed at different levels to offer more options to myelofibrosis patients. An important aim is to further reduce AHSCT toxicity and to widen its applicability to older or comorbid patients as well as to improve posttransplant strategies preferably the prophylactic or preemptive approaches to reduce relapse.

References

Alchalby H, Badbaran A, Bock O et al (2010a) Screening and monitoring of MPL W515L mutation with real-time PCR in patients with myelofibrosis undergoing allogeneic stem cell transplantation. Bone Marrow Transplant 45:1404–1407

Alchalby H, Badbaran A, Zabelina T et al (2010b) Impact of JAK2V617F mutation status, allele burden, and clearance after allogeneic stem cell transplantation for myelofibrosis. Blood 116:3572–3581

Bacigalupo A, Dominetto A, Pozzi S et al (2007) Allogeneic hematopoietic stem transplant for patients with idiopathic myelofibrosis using a reduced intensity thiotepa based conditioning regimen. Blood 110: Abstract no. 684

Bacigalupo A, Soraru M, Dominietto A et al (2010) Allogeneic hematopoietic SCT for patients with primary myelofibrosis: a predictive transplant score based on transfusion requirement, spleen size and donor type. Bone Marrow Transplant 45:458–463

Ballen K, Zhang M, Arora M, the Chronic Leukemia Working Committee of the Center for International Blood Marrow Transplant Research (2005) Outcome of bone marrow transplantation for myelofibrosis. Blood 106: Abstract no. 170

Ballen KK, Shrestha S, Sobocinski KA et al (2010) Outcome of transplantation for myelofibrosis. Biol Blood Marrow Transplant 16(3):358–367. Epub 2009 Oct 30

Baurmann H, Burlakova I, Jedlickova Z et al (2009) Allogeneic haematopoietic cell transplantation for myelofibrosis – close post-transplant surveillance is mandatory [abstract no. V59]. Presented the Corporate Annual Conference '09 of the German, Austrian and Swiss Haematology and Oncology Societies. Mannheim/Heidelberg, Germany; 2–6 Oct 2009

Benjamini O, Koren-Michowitz M, Amariglio N et al (2008) Relapse of postpolycythemia myelofibrosis after allogeneic stem cell transplantation in a polycythemic phase: successful treatment with donor lymphocyte infusion directed by quantitative PCR test for V617F-JAK2 mutation. Leukemia 22:1961–1963

Byrne JL, Beshti H, Clark D et al (2000) Induction of remission after donor leucocyte infusion for the treatment of relapsed chronic idiopathic myelofibrosis following allogeneic transplantation: evidence for a 'graft vs. myelofibrosis' effect. Br J Haematol 108: 430–433

Cervantes F, Barosi G, Demory JL et al (1998) Myelofibrosis with myeloid metaplasia in young individuals: disease characteristics, prognostic factors and identification of risk groups. Br J Haematol 102:684–690

Cervantes F, Rovira M, Urbano-Ispizua A (2000) Complete remission of idiopathic myelofibrosis following donor lymphocyte infusion after failure of allogeneic transplantation: demonstration of a graft-versus-myelofibrosis effect. Bone Marrow Transplant 26:697–699

Cervantes F, Passamonti F, Barosi G (2008) Life expectancy and prognostic factors in the classic BCR/ABL-negative myeloproliferative disorders. Leukemia 22: 905–914

Cervantes F, Dupriez B, Pereira A et al (2009) New prognostic scoring system for primary myelofibrosis based on a study of the International Working Group for Myelofibrosis Research and Treatment. Blood 113: 2895–2901

Ciurea SO, Sadegi B, Wilbur A et al (2008) Effects of extensive splenomegaly in patients with myelofibrosis undergoing a reduced intensity allogeneic stem cell transplantation. Br J Haematol 141:80–83

Creemers GJ, Lowenberg B, Hagenbeek A (1992) Allogeneic bone marrow transplantation for primary myelofibrosis. Br J Haematol 82:772–773

Deeg HJ, Gooley TA, Flowers ME et al (2003) Allogeneic hematopoietic stem cell transplantation for myelofibrosis. Blood 102:3912–3918

Devine SM, Hoffman R, Verma A et al (2002) Allogeneic blood cell transplantation following reduced-intensity conditioning is effective therapy for older patients with myelofibrosis with myeloid metaplasia. Blood 99:2255–2258

Dokal I, Jones L, Deenmamode M et al (1989) Allogeneic bone marrow transplantation for primary myelofibrosis. Br J Haematol 71:158–160

Dupriez B, Morel P, Demory JL et al (1996) Prognostic factors in agnogenic myeloid metaplasia: a report on 195 cases with a new scoring system. Blood 88:1013–1018

Elliott MA, Verstovsek S, Dingli D et al (2007) Monocytosis is an adverse prognostic factor for survival in younger patients with primary myelofibrosis. Leuk Res 31:1503–1509

George B, Kerridge I, Gottlieb D et al (2008) A reduced intensity conditioning protocol associated with excellent survival in patients with myelofibrosis. Bone Marrow Transplant 42:567–568

Guardiola P, Anderson JE, Bandini GW et al (1999) Allogeneic stem cell transplantation for agnogenic myeloid metaplasia: a European Group for Blood and Marrow Transplantation, Societe Francaise de Greffe de Moelle, Gruppo Italiano per il Trapianto del Midollo Osseo, and Fred Hutchinson Cancer Research Center Collaborative Study. Blood 93:2831–2838

Gupta V, Kröger N, Aschan J et al (2009) A retrospective comparison of conventional intensity conditioning and reduced-intensity conditioning for allogeneic hematopoietic cell transplantation in myelofibrosis. Bone Marrow Transplant 44:317–320

Hertenstein B, Guardiola P, Finke J et al (2002) Non-myeloablative (NMA) stem cell transplantation (SCT) for myeloid metaplasia with myelofibrosis (MMM): a survey from the Chronic Leukemia Working Party of the EBMT. Blood 100:Abstract no. 70

Hessling J, Kroger N, Werner M et al (2002) Dose-reduced conditioning regimen followed by allogeneic stem cell transplantation in patients with myelofibrosis with myeloid metaplasia. Br J Haematol 119:769–772

Hussein K, Huang J, Lasho T et al (2009) Karyotype complements the International Prognostic Scoring System for primary myelofibrosis. Eur J Haematol 82:255–259

James C, Ugo V, Le Couedic JP et al (2005) A unique clonal JAK2 mutation leading to constitutive signalling causes polycythaemia vera. Nature 434:1144–1148

Kerbauy DM, Gooley TA et al (2007) Hematopoietic cell transplantation as curative therapy for idiopathic myelofibrosis, advanced polycythemia vera, and essential thrombocythemia. Biol Blood Marrow Transplant 13:355–365

Klyuchnikov E, Holler E, Bornhäuser M et al (2011) Donor lymphocyte infusions and/or second allogeneic stem cell transplantation as salvage treatment for relapsed myelofibrosis after reduced-intensity allografting. (manuscript submitted)

Kröger N, Mesa RA (2008) Choosing between stem cell therapy and drugs in myelofibrosis. Leukemia 22:474–486

Kröger N, Zabelina T, Schieder H et al (2005) Pilot study of reduced-intensity conditioning followed by allogeneic stem cell transplantation from related and unrelated donors in patients with myelofibrosis. Br J Haematol 128:690–697

Kröger N, Badbaran A, Holler E et al (2007a) Monitoring of the JAK2-V617F mutation by highly sensitive quantitative real-time PCR after allogeneic stem cell transplantation in patients with myelofibrosis. Blood 109:1316–1321

Kröger N, Holler E, Kobbe G et al (2007b) Dose-reduced conditioning followed by allogeneic stem cell transplantation in patients with myelofibrosis. Results from

a Multicenter Prospective Trial of the Chronic Leukemia Working Party of the European Group for Blood and Marrow Transplantation (EBMT). Blood 110:Abstract no. 683

Kröger N, Thiele J, Zander A et al (2007c) Rapid regression of bone marrow fibrosis after dose-reduced allogeneic stem cell transplantation in patients with primary myelofibrosis. Exp Hematol 35:1719–1722

Kröger N, Alchalby H, Klyuchnikov E et al (2009a) JAK2-V617F-triggered preemptive and salvage adoptive immunotherapy with donor-lymphocyte infusion in patients with myelofibrosis after allogeneic stem cell transplantation. Blood 113:1866–1868

Kröger N, Holler E, Kobbe G et al (2009b) Allogeneic stem cell transplantation after reduced-intensity conditioning in patients with myelofibrosis: a prospective, multicenter study of the Chronic Leukemia Working Party of the European Group for Blood and Marrow Transplantation (EBMT). Blood 114: 5264–5270

Li Z, Deeg HJ (2001) Pros and cons of splenectomy in patients with myelofibrosis undergoing stem cell transplantation. Leukemia 15:465–467

Li Z, Gooley T, Applebaum FR (2001) Splenectomy and hemopoietic stem cell transplantation for myelofibrosis. Blood 97:2180–2181

Lissandre A, Bay J-O, Cahn J-Y et al (2011) Retrospective study of allogeneic haematopoietic stem-cell transplantation for myelofibrosis. Bone Marrow Transplant 46:557–561

Merup M, Lazarevic V, Nahi H, Andreasson B, Malm C, Nilsson L et al (2006) Different outcome of allogeneic transplantation in myelofibrosis using conventional or reduced-intensity conditioning regimens. Br J Haematol 135:367–373

Mesa RA, Verstovsek S, Cervantes F et al (2007) Primary myelofibrosis (PMF), post polycythemia vera myelofibrosis (post-PV MF), post essential thrombocythemia myelofibrosis (post-ET MF), blast phase PMF (PMF-BP): Consensus on terminology by the international working group for myelofibrosis research and treatment (IWG-MRT). Leuk Res 31:737–740

Patriarca F, Bacigalupo A, Sperotto A et al (2008) Allogeneic hematopoietic stem cell transplantation in myelofibrosis: the 20-year experience of the Gruppo Italiano Trapianto di Midollo Osseo (GITMO). Haematologica 93:1514–1522

Percy MJ, McMullin MF (2005) The V617F JAK2 mutation and the myeloproliferative disorders. Hematol Oncol 23:91–93

Rajantie J, Sale GE, Deeg HJ et al (1986) Adverse effect of severe marrow fibrosis on hematologic recovery after chemoradiotherapy and allogeneic bone marrow transplantation. Blood 67:1693–1697

Robin M, Tabrizi R, Mohty M et al (2010) Allogeneic haematopoietic stem cell transplantation for myelofibrosis: a report of the Société Française de Greffe de Moelle et de Thérapie Cellulaire (SFGM-TC). Br J Haematol 152:331–339

Rondelli D, Barosi G, Bacigalupo A et al (2005) Allogeneic hematopoietic stem-cell transplantation with reduced-intensity conditioning in intermediate- or high-risk patients with myelofibrosis with myeloid metaplasia. Blood 105:4115–4119

Rumi E, Passamonti F, Arcaini L et al (2010) Molecular remission after allo-SCT in a patient with post-essential thrombocythemia myelofibrosis carrying the MPL (W515A) mutation. Bone Marrow Transplant 45:798–800

Sale GE, Deeg HJ, Porter BA (2006) Regression of myelofibrosis and osteosclerosis following hematopoietic cell transplantation assessed by magnetic resonance imaging and histologic grading. Biol Blood Marrow Transplant 12:1285–1294

Samuelson S, Sandmaier BM, Heslop HE et al (2011) Allogeneic haematopoietic cell transplantation for myelofibrosis in 30 patients 60–78 years of age. Br J Haematol 153:76–82

Smith RE, Chelmowski MK, Szabo EJ (1990) Myelofibrosis: a review of clinical and pathologic features and treatment. Crit Rev Oncol Hematol 10:305–314

Soll E, Massumoto C, Clift RA et al (1995) Relevance of marrow fibrosis in bone marrow transplantation: a retrospective analysis of engraftment. Blood 86:4667–4673

Steckel NK, Koldehoff M, Ditschkowski M (2007) Use of the activating gene mutation of the tyrosine kinase (VAL617Phe) JAK2 as a minimal residual disease marker in patients with myelofibrosis and myeloid metaplasia after allogeneic stem cell transplantation. Transplantation 83:1518–1520

Stewart WA, Pearce R, Kirkland KE et al on behalf of the British Society for Blood and Marrow Transplantation (2010) The role of allogeneic SCT in primary myelofibrosis: a British Society for Blood and Marrow Transplantation study. Bone Marrow Transplant 45:1587–1593

Tam CS, Abruzzo LV, Lin KI et al (2009) The role of cytogenetic abnormalities as a prognostic marker in primary myelofibrosis: applicability at the time of diagnosis and later during disease course. Blood 113:4171–4178

Tefferi A (2005) Pathogenesis of myelofibrosis with myeloid metaplasia. J Clin Oncol 23:8520–8530

Tefferi A, Mesa RA, Nagorney DM (2000) Splenectomy in myelofibrosis with myeloid metaplasia: a single-institution experience with 223 patients. Blood 95:2226–2233

Tefferi A, Barosi G, Mesa RA et al (2006) International Working Group (IWG) consensus criteria for treatment response in myelofibrosis with myeloid metaplasia, for the IWG for MYelofibrosis Research and Treatment (IWG-MRT). Blood 108:1497–1503

Thiele J, Kvasnicka HM, Dietrich H et al (2005) Dynamics of bone marrow changes in patients with chronic idiopathic myelofibrosis following allogeneic stem cell transplantation. Histol Histopathol 20:879–889

Vannucchi AM, Antonioli E, Guglielmelli P (2008) Clinical correlates of JAK2V617F presence or allele burden in myeloproliferative neoplasms: a critical reappraisal. Leukemia 22:1299–1307

Part V
Research Issues and Perspectives

A Critical Review of the Role and Limitations of JAK Inhibitors in Myelofibrosis Therapy

17

Animesh Pardanani

Contents

A. Pardanani
Division of Hematology, Department of Medicine,
Mayo Clinic, Rochester, MN, USA
e-mail: pardanani.animesh@mayo.edu

17.1 Myeloproliferative Neoplasms: Pathogenesis, Prognosis, and Survival

Myeloproliferative neoplasms (MPN) are stem cell-derived clonal or oligoclonal hemopathies and are phenotypically characterized by the abnormal accumulation of mature-appearing myeloid cells. The shared predilection of MPN for transformation into acute myeloid leukemia (AML) has led to their reclassification – from "myeloproliferative disorders" to "MPN" – per the 2008 World Health Organization classification system for myeloid neoplasms (Vardiman et al. 2009). While *BCR-ABL1* is the disease-causing mutation in chronic myelogenous leukemia (CML) and kinase inhibitors (e.g., imatinib, nilotinib, and dasatinib) that target the mutant oncoprotein have been shown to be therapeutically effective (Druker 2008), the genetic underpinnings of *BCR-ABL1*-negative MPN, which include polycythemia vera (PV), essential thrombocythemia (ET), and primary myelofibrosis (PMF), remain poorly understood and their treatment suboptimal.

While multiple mutations that arise at the stem/progenitor cell level have recently been identified, it is unclear which mutation, if any, represents the primary pathogenetic event. Furthermore, in contrast to chronic myeloid leukemia (CML), the clonal architecture and hierarchy of *BCR-ABL1*-negative MPN appears to be remarkably complex; multiple subclones with overlapping mutations are frequently identified, and dominance of a particular subclone may vary with time in a given patient. The seminal discovery of *JAK2*V617F in 2004 (James et al. 2005) has opened a new era in the science and practice of MPN. The subsequent focus on JAK-STAT-relevant molecules has led to the discovery of *JAK2* exon 12 (Scott et al. 2007), *MPL* (Pikman et al. 2006), and *LNK* (Oh et al. 2010) mutations (Table 17.1). In addition, many other somatic mutations involving a growing list of genes have been described in the last 3 years: *TET2* (Delhommeau et al. 2009), *ASXL1* (Carbuccia et al. 2009), *CBL* (Grand et al. 2009), *IDH1* (Green and Beer 2010; Abdel-Wahab et al. 2010), *IDH2* (Jones et al. 2009; Kilpivaara et al. 2009), *IKZF1* (Jager et al. 2010), *EZH2* (Ernst et al. 2010), and *DNMT3A* (Abdel-Wahab et al. 2011) (Table 17.1). Additional mutations involving *TP53* (Harutyunyan et al. 2011) and *CUX1* (Klampfl et al. 2011; Thoennissen et al. 2011) have been described mostly in blast-phase MPN (Table 17.1). Most of these mutations can be classified as being JAK-STAT relevant (*JAK2, MPL, LNK* and *CBL*) or epigenetically relevant (*TET2, EZH2, DNMT3A, ASXL1*, and possibly *IDH*).

Currently known MPN relevant mutations that activate the JAK-STAT pathway include:

(i) JAK2**V617F**: represents the most prevalent mutation; it occurs in approximately 96% of patients with PV, 55% in ET, and 65% in PMF (James et al. 2005; Kralovics et al. 2005; Levine et al. 2005; Baxter et al. 2005). *JAK2*V617F cooperates with inherited disease susceptibility alleles, such as the JAK2 46/1 haplotype, and other somatic mutations and generally biases towards a PV-like phenotype (Jones et al. 2009; Kilpivaara et al. 2009; Olcaydu et al. 2009). *JAK2*V617F presence or increased allele burden does not appear to affect thrombosis risk or survival in MPN; (Vannucchi et al. 2008a; Passamonti et al. 2010) whereas low allele burden has been associated with inferior survival (Tefferi et al. 2008; Guglielmelli et al. 2009).

(ii) JAK2 **exon 12 mutations**: are relatively specific to *JAK2*V617F-negative PV (3% of all PV cases) and target a hot spot from residues 536–547 with point mutations, deletions, or insertions (Scott et al. 2007; Pardanani et al. 2007; Pietra et al. 2008; Passamonti et al. 2009). Mutation presence is characterized by predominantly erythroid myelopoiesis, subnormal serum erythropoietin level, and younger age at diagnosis.

(iii) **MPL exon 10 mutations**: including *MPL*W515L, *MPL*W515K, and others occur in approximately 3% and 10% of ET and PMF patients, respectively (Pikman et al. 2006; Pardanani et al. 2006; Vannucchi et al. 2008b; Beer et al. 2008; Guglielmelli et al. 2007). *MPL*-mutated ET has been associated with older age, lower hemoglobin level, higher platelet count, microvascular symptoms, and a higher risk of postdiagnosis arterial thrombosis. Similar to *JAK2*V617F, presence of *MPL* mutation does not appear to affect survival, fibrotic, or leukemic transformation (Pardanani et al. 2011a).

(iv) **LNK (SH2B3)**: is an adaptor protein that negatively regulates thrombopoietin-MPL-mediated JAK-STAT pathway activation, including signaling downstream of *MPL*W515L and *JAK2*V617F (Gery et al. 2007, 2009). *LNK* exon 2 mutations are infrequently encountered in chronic-phase MPN and *JAK2*V617F-negative erythrocytosis, but a higher (13%) incidence has been demonstrated in blast-phase MPN (Oh et al. 2010; Pardanani et al. 2010a). Most currently described *LNK* mutations target an exon 2 "hot spot" in the Pleckstrin homology (PH) domain, spanning residues E208-D234. MPN cases harboring *LNK* mutations exhibit a phenotype that is indistinguishable from those harboring *JAK2*V617F or *MPL* exon 10 mutations.

(v) **CBL mutations**: are most frequently associated with juvenile or chronic myelomonocytic leukemia (JMML 17%; CMML 11%) (Loh et al. 2009), usually within the context of 11q acquired uniparental disomy, which suggests a tumor suppressor role for wild-type CBL. In a recent study of MPN patients, *CBL* mutations were identified in 6% of PMF patients (Grand et al. 2009).

Table 17.1 Mutations in *BCR-ABL1*-negative myeloproliferative neoplasms (see text for references)

Mutations	Chromosome location	Mutational frequency	Pathogenetic relevance
JAK2 (Janus kinase 2) *JAK2V617F exon 14 mutation*	9p24	PV ~ 96% ET ~ 55% PMF ~ 65% BP-MPN ~ 50%	Contributes to abnormal myeloproliferation and progenitor cell growth factor hypersensitivity
JAK2 exon 12 mutation	9p24	PV ~ 3%	Contributes to primarily erythroid myeloproliferation
MPL (myeloproliferative leukemia virus oncogene) *MPN-associated MPL mutations involve exon 10*	1p34	ET ~ 3% PMF ~ 10% BP-MPN ~ 5%	Contributes to primarily megakaryocytic myeloproliferation
LNK (as in Links) *a.k.a. SH2B3* (a membrane-bound adaptor protein) *MPN-associated mutations were monoallelic and involved exon 2*	12q24.12	PV ~ rare ET ~ rare PMF ~ rare BP-MPN ~ 10%	Wild-type LNK is a negative regulator of JAK2 signaling
TET2 (TET oncogene family member 2) *Mutations involve several exons*	4q24	PV ~ 16% ET ~ 5% PMF ~ 17% BP-MPN ~ 17% AML ~ 20% MDS ~ 26% CMML ~ 51% SM ~ 29% RARS-T ~ 26%	TET proteins catalyze conversion of 5-methylcytosine (5mC) to 5-hydroxymethylcytosine (5hmC), which favors demethylated DNA. Both TET1 and TET2 display this catalytic activity *IDH* and *TET2* mutations might share a common pathogenetic effect, which might include abnormal DNA hypermethylation and impaired myelopoiesis
ASXL1 (additional sex combs-like 1) *Exon 12 mutations*	20q11.1	ET ~ 3% PMF ~ 13% BP-MPN ~ 18% AML ~ 11% MDS ~ 11% CMML ~ 43%	Wild-type ASXL1 is needed for normal hematopoiesis and might be involved in co-activation of transcription factors and transcriptional repression

(continued)

Table 17.1 (continued)

Mutations	Chromosome location	Mutational frequency	Pathogenetic relevance
IDH1/IDH2 (isocitrate dehydrogenase) *Exon 4 mutations*	2q33.3/15q26.1	PV ~ 2% ET ~ 1% PMF ~ 4% BP-MPN ~ 20% AML ~ 14% MDS ~ 5%	*IDH* mutations induce loss of activity for the conversion of isocitrate to 2-ketoglutarate (2-KG) and gain of function in the conversion of 2-KG to 2-hydroxyglutarate (2-HG). 2-HG might be the mediator of impaired TET2 function in cells with mutant *IDH* expression
EZH2 (enhancer of zeste homolog 2) *Mutations involve several exons*	7q36.1	PV ~ 3% PMF ~ 7% MDS ~ 6% CMML ~ 13% aCML ~ 13% HES/CEL ~ 3%	Wild-type EZH2 is part of a histone methyltransferase (polycomb repressive complex 2 associated with H3 Lys-27 trimethylation). MPN-associated *EZH2* mutations might have a tumor suppressor activity, which contrasts with the gain-of-function activity for lymphoma-associated *EZH2* mutations
DNMT3A (DNA cytosine methyltransferase 3a) *Most frequent mutations affect amino acid R882*	2p23	PV ~ 7% PMF ~ 7% BP-MPN ~ 14% AML ~ 22% MDS ~ 8%	DNA methyl transferases are essential In establishing and maintaining DNA methylation patterns in mammals
CBL (Casitas B-lineage lymphoma proto-oncogene) *Exon 8/9 mutations*	11q23.3	PV ~ rare ET ~ rare MF ~ 6%	CBL is an E3 ubiquitin ligase that marks mutant kinases for degradation. Transforming activity requires loss of this function
IKZF1 (IKAROS family zinc finger 1) (*mostly deletions including intragenic*)	7p12	CP-MPN ~ rare BP-MPN ~ 19%	IKZF1 is a transcription regulator and putative tumor suppressor

MPN myeloproliferative neoplasms, *ET* essential thrombocythemia, *PV* polycythemia vera, *PMF* primary myelofibrosis, *MF* includes both PMF and post-ET/PV myelofibrosis, *BP-MPN* blast-phase MPN, *CP-MPN* chronic-phase MPN, *SM* systemic mastocytosis, *CMML* chronic myelomonocytic leukemia, *AML* acute myeloid leukemia, *MDS* myelodysplastic syndromes, *RARS-T* refractory anemia with ring sideroblasts, *aCML* atypical chronic myeloid leukemia, *BCR-ABL1*-negative, *HES/CEL* hypereosinophilic syndrome/chronic eosinophilic leukemia

Survival in WHO-defined ET is near normal, and the risk of leukemic or fibrotic transformation is less than 1% (Barbui et al. 2011). The incidence of thrombosis is substantially higher in "high risk for thrombosis" patients (age >60 years or history of thrombosis), but not necessarily in those with "low risk for thrombosis" (absence of both risk factors). Survival in PV exceeds 22 years in "low risk for survival" patients (age <65 years and without leukocytosis) and is approximately 9 years in "high risk for survival" patients (presence of both adverse factors) (Gangat et al. 2007). In one representative PV study (Gangat et al. 2007), after a median follow-up of approximately 5 years, the cumulative incidences of leukemic or fibrotic transformation were approximately 7% and 12%, respectively. The risk factors for thrombosis in PV are similar to those in ET. Prognosis in PMF is based on the Dynamic International Prognostic Scoring System-plus (*DIPSS*-plus) model, and median survivals range from >15 years in low-risk to 1.3 years in high-risk patients (Gangat et al. 2011). The risk of leukemic transformation in PMF is significantly higher than that seen in either PV or ET, and the 10-year risk was reported at 12% for "low risk for leukemia" patients (absence of both thrombocytopenia and unfavorable karyotype) and 31% for "high risk for leukemia" patients (presence of either thrombocytopenia or unfavorable karyotype) (Gangat et al. 2011).

17.2 Myeloproliferative Neoplasms: Scope of the Unmet Therapeutic Need

17.2.1 Myelofibrosis

Myelofibrosis presents either de novo (PMF) or post-PV or ET. Current drug therapy for PMF is not curative, and there is little evidence to suggest a favorable effect on the risk of leukemic transformation or survival. Consequently, palliative therapies, particularly those targeting anemia, hepatosplenomegaly, and/or constitutional symptoms, have considerable clinical value in this population. Palpable splenomegaly and hepatomegaly are present in 90% and 50% of PMF patients, respectively

(Gangat et al. 2011; Cervantes et al. 2009). The resulting intra-abdominal mass effect causes significant morbidity, including abdominal pain, early satiety, cough, diarrhea, and leg edema. Hydroxyurea is the commonest first-line treatment for symptomatic splenomegaly; however, its efficacy in the presence of massive splenomegaly appears to be modest and may exacerbate preexisting cytopenias (Martinez-Trillos et al. 2010; Siragusa et al. 2009). The use of splenectomy and splenic/hepatic radiation in the setting of hydroxyurea-refractory organomegaly is limited by postoperative thrombosis/bleeding or infection and occurrence of severe cytopenias, respectively (Mishchenko and Tefferi 2010). Anemia is a common problem with 35–54% of PMF cases presenting with a hemoglobin <10 g/dL (Gangat et al. 2011; Cervantes et al. 2009). Patients with symptomatic anemia can be treated with androgens (e.g., oral fluoxymesterone 10 mg BID), prednisone (0.5–1.0 mg/kg/day), or danazol (600 mg/day) (Cervantes et al. 2007), thalidomide (Elliott et al. 2002; Thomas et al. 2006), or lenalidomide (Tefferi et al. 2006). Response rates are approximately 20%, and response durations average 1–2 years. Thalidomide and lenalidomide are limited by peripheral neuropathy and myelosuppression, respectively; the latter is particularly effective in the presence of del (5q31) (Tefferi et al. 2007). Use of erythropoiesis-stimulating agents is limited by their relative ineffectiveness in transfusion-dependent patients and their propensity to exacerbate splenomegaly. The presence of constitutional symptoms has a profoundly adverse impact on the functional ability and quality of life of myelofibrosis patients. The frequency of self-reported symptoms is as follows: fatigue 84%, bone pain 47%, night sweats 56%, pruritus 50%, and fever 18% (Mesa et al. 2007, 2009). Current treatments for myelofibrosis are inadequate for alleviating disease-associated constitutional symptoms.

17.2.2 Polycythemia Vera/Essential Thrombocythemia

In general, these patients have a relatively good prognosis, with median survival exceeding 15–20 years (Gangat et al. 2007; Passamonti et al.

2008). Controlled studies have confirmed the antithrombotic value of low-dose aspirin in PV (all-risk categories) (Landolfi et al. 2004) and hydroxyurea in ET (high-risk disease) (Cortelazzo et al. 1995; Harrison et al. 2005). In addition, phlebotomy is indicated in all patients with PV with a generally advocated hematocrit target of <45%. Use of hydroxyurea in high-risk PV and low-dose aspirin in ET is also recommended based on currently available data. PV or ET patients who are either intolerant or resistant to hydroxyurea can be treated with interferon-alpha (INF-α) (younger patients) (Quintas-Cardama et al. 2009; Kiladjian et al. 2008) or busulfan (older patients) (Shvidel et al. 2007; "Leukemia and Hematosarcoma" Cooperative Group, EORTC 1981). Use of IFN-α is limited by its significant adverse event profile (including for pegylated INF-α) and its uncertain effects on disease-related complications and survival. Wider use of busulfan has been limited by the fear, real or otherwise, of leukemogenicity. Based on the above, it is hard to argue that there is a truly unmet need in the treatment of ET or PV, including hydroxyurea-refractory disease. Furthermore, because of the indolent natural history of ET, it would be very difficult to demonstrate a therapeutic advantage for a new drug over the *status quo*; previous attempts in that regard have met with failure (Harrison et al. 2005). The matter is further complicated by the recent revelation that extreme thrombocytosis in ET was associated with a lower risk of arterial thrombosis (Carobbio et al. 2011), an observation that does not necessarily support the need to lower platelet count in ET. A similar argument can be made for PV, although it is associated with more severe symptoms such as pruritus.

17.3 Myeloproliferative Neoplasms: Therapeutic Use of JAK Inhibitor ATP Mimetics

JAK-STAT can be inhibited by several classes of drugs including (1) ATP-mimetic small molecule kinase inhibitors, such as ruxolitinib (INCB018424), SAR302503 (TG101348), CYT387, lestaurtinib (CEP-701), SB1518, AZD1480, BMS911543,

LY2784544, and XL019 and (2) histone deacetylase inhibitors, such as panobinostat (LBH589), vorinostat (MK0683), givinostat (ITF2357), and SB939 (*clinicalTrials.gov*). For the purposes of the current review, we will focus on the ATP-mimetic JAK inhibitors (Table 17.2) and discuss their role and limitations in MPN therapy.

17.3.1 Myelofibrosis

Data from clinical trials (phases 1, 2, and/or 3) where at least 50 patients have been treated are available for INCB018424, SAR302503, and CYT387 (see Table 17.2 for references). All three drugs appear to have substantial activity against hydroxyurea-refractory splenomegaly; the response is evident within the first cycle of treatment, with peak response being observed within the first 3 months. The spleen responses are dose dependent and durable through 12 cycles of treatment in those remaining on therapy. Not infrequently, dose maximization for splenomegaly control is limited by dose-dependent myelosuppression. In our experience, markedly enlarged spleens ($\geq$15–20 cm below the costal margin) were less likely to achieve complete resolution. Interruption of JAK inhibitor treatment is associated with relapse of splenomegaly; relapse can be within days (INCB018424) or weeks (SAR302503), which likely relates to the dissimilar half-lives of the two drugs (2–3 h vs. 16–34 h, respectively) and possibly differences in the mode of action (predominant anticytokine versus anticlonal activity, respectively). Treatment-emergent anemia appears to be associated with some (INCB018424, SAR302503) but not other (CYT387) JAK inhibitors; the significant anemia (and splenomegaly) improvement seen with CYT387, if confirmed, indicates the possibility of an optimal inhibitor profile that balances JAK-1 and JAK-2 inhibitory activities, for myelofibrosis treatment. INCB018424, SAR302503, and CYT387 have all been shown to produce a significant improvement in myelofibrosis-associated constitutional symptoms; responses were seen within the first few weeks, and unlike the response

Table 17.2 JAK2 inhibitors that have reached phase 2 clinical trials in myeloproliferative neoplasms

Anti-JAK2 ATP-mimetic	Targets other than JAK2	Disease features shown to be favorably affected	Side effects
Ruxolitinib (phase 1/2/3 study) (Verstovsek et al. 2010a, c, 2011; Harrison et al. 2011)	JAK1	Splenomegaly Constitutional symptoms Pruritus Cachexia	Thrombocytopenia (DLT) Anemia "Acute relapse of symptoms and re-enlargement of spleen upon drug discontinuation" "Systemic inflammatory response syndrome (SIRS) upon drug discontinuation"
SAR302503 (phase 1/2 study) (Pardanani et al. 2011b)	FLT3 RET	Splenomegaly Constitutional symptoms Pruritus Leukocytosis Thrombocytosis $JAK2$V617F burden	Increased amylase/lipase (DLT) Anemia Thrombocytopenia Nausea/vomiting Diarrhea Increased transaminases
CEP-701 (lestaurtinib) (phase 2 study) (Moliterno et al. 2009; Santos et al. 2010)	FLT3 TrkA	Splenomegaly Anemia Pruritus	Diarrhea Nausea/vomiting Anemia Thrombocytopenia
CYT387 (phase 1/2 study) (Pardanani et al. 2011c)	JAK1 TYK2 JNK1 CDK2	Anemia Splenomegaly Constitutional symptoms Pruritus	Increased amylase/lipase (DLT) Headache (DLT) Thrombocytopenia Increased transaminases Peripheral neuropathy "First dose" effect characterized by transient hypotension and light-headedness
SB1518 (phase 1/2 study) (Deeg et al. 2011)	FLT3	Splenomegaly	(DLT=GI symptoms) Diarrhea Nausea Thrombocytopenia

DLT dose-limiting toxicity, *GI* gastrointestinal

in splenomegaly, there was not a clear dose dependency. These improvements were durable for at least a year (INCB018424 and SAR302503) and were associated with a significant weight gain (INCB018424). The toxicity profile of JAK inhibitors is dissimilar; frequent gastrointestinal toxicities (CEP-701, SAR302503) may reflect the off-target FLT3 inhibitory activity. In contrast, abrupt discontinuation of INCB018424 may be associated with acute relapse of disease-related features including splenomegaly, likely reflecting a "cytokine flare" that can be associated with serious complications such as systemic inflammatory response syndrome (SIRS)-like picture with respiratory and hemodynamic compromise, splenic infarction, etc.; a gradual taper over a 2–4-week period is recommended to decrease the possibility of its occurrence. CYT387 is associated with transient hypotension, flushing, and light-headedness after administration of the first dose.

Outstanding issues include identification of an optimal starting dose/schedule; given the patient heterogeneity, we favor a predefined dynamic schedule that triggers dose changes based on specific response and toxicity criteria. Treatment can be commenced with an "induction" dose to maximize response (particularly splenomegaly) followed by a lower "maintenance" dose; we have seen alleviation of treatment-emergent anemia with SAR302503 using this approach. It may be also possible to avert/attenuate treatment-related myelosuppression, particularly anemia, by combining

JAK inhibitors with other agents such as pomalido-mide, androgens, or erythropoietin. Finally, the identification of primary end points for clinical trials with JAK inhibitors in myelofibrosis that will support labeling claims remains challenging; short of improvement in survival, we favor anemia response as a physiologic end point (as compared to spleen response) given prognostic implications of anemia-/transfusion-dependence in this disease. Patient reported outcome (PRO) instruments in myelofibrosis (e.g., MFSAF) await validation within the context of a clinical trial (Mesa et al. 2009); thus far, data from such instruments have been relegated as secondary end points in clinical trial design.

17.3.2 Polycythemia Vera/Essential Thrombocythemia

Widespread use of JAK inhibitors in PV or ET will have to wait until long-term safety of these agents is demonstrated. JAK-2 selective inhibitors (SAR302503) may be particularly useful, given their potent activity in normalizing leuko-cytosis/thrombocytosis (Pardanani et al. 2011b). In contrast, JAK-1/2 inhibitors (INCB018424, CYT387) may be somewhat less effective, as evidenced by the modest activity of INCB018424 at normalizing the platelet count in ET (Verstovsek et al. 2010a; Pardanani et al. 2011c).

Conclusions

Eradication or suppression of clonal myeloproliferation is essential for modifying disease natural history in MPN. Effective targeting of the primary clonal process will also abrogate the paraneoplastic effects of the disease including constitutional symptoms, cachexia, and extramedullary hematopoiesis. Unfortunately, our current understanding of the molecular pathogenesis of *BCR-ABL1*-negative MPN is incomplete despite the description of a multitude of somatic mutations that are neither disease specific nor necessarily clonally predominant. Consequently, a better understanding of oncogenic pathways rather than an accumulation of secondary mutations is more

likely to lead to identification of a suitable drug target in *BCR-ABL1*-negative MPN. In this regard, we need to query further the precise pathogenetic contribution of JAK-STAT and other aberrant pathways and consider the potential need for multitargeted therapy.

In general, it may not be rational to use a non-specific JAK inhibitor, such as INCB018424 (Verstovsek et al. 2010a) or CYT387 (Pardanani et al. 2011c), for the treatment of ET or PV, including hydroxyurea-refractory cases. The evidence so far suggests that such drugs are inferior to conventional second-line drug therapy (e.g., INF-α (Quintas-Cardama et al. 2009; Kiladjian et al. 2008), busulfan (Shvidel et al. 2007; "Leukemia and Hematosarcoma" Cooperative Group, EORTC 1981), and pipobroman (Passamonti et al. 2000, 2004; Petti et al. 1998; De Sanctis et al. 2003)) for PV or ET in controlling either thrombocytosis or leukocytosis. All three aforementioned second-line drugs induce phlebotomy independence in almost all patients with PV, and response rates for thrombocytosis or leukocytosis often exceed 80% for both PV and ET, which is superior to what has been seen so far with current JAK inhibitors (Verstovsek et al. 2010a). On the other hand, considering the fact that virtually all patients with PV carry a *JAK2* mutation and that such patients may sometimes suffer from drug-refractory pruritus, it is reasonable to investigate the therapeutic value of more selective anti-JAK2 drugs such as SAR302503 (Pardanani et al. 2010b) or SB1518 (Verstovsek et al. 2010b). In this regard, we underscore the fact that induction of phlebotomy-independence or control of other cytosis does not necessarily imply meaningful health outcome in these patients, and one has to demonstrate either selective anticlonal activity or reduction of thrombosis, fibrotic/leukemic transformation, or premature death in a controlled setting.

As for MF, cytokine modulation rather than direct cytotoxicity may underlie the predominant mechanism of action for some of the currently available JAK inhibitors (Pardanani et al.

2011b; Verstovsek et al. 2010c). This is not to undermine the potential antiproliferative value of new and improved JAK2 inhibitors but to underscore the suboptimal activity of currently available drugs in this regard. Current information suggests that more selective JAK2 inhibitors, such as SAR302503 (Pardanani et al. 2011b), might be superior in controlling myeloproliferation without losing activity against constitutional symptoms. Selective targeting of JAK2 also spares patients from the pathogenetically unnecessary and potentially harmful cotargeting of JAK1. However, because physiologic erythropoiesis heavily depends on JAK2 signaling, anemia is an expected and problematic side effect of such drugs (Pardanani et al. 2011b), and it is currently not known if combining these drugs with other erythropoietic agents or increasing their mutant JAK2 selectivity would overcome the particular problem.

There is now evidence for pathogenetic contribution of immune response from the host and abnormal cytokine expression in MPN (Tefferi et al. 2011). Therefore, one could argue for the value of drugs with broad anticytokine activity, such as JAK1/JAK2 inhibitors. The counterargument is uncomplicated; the primary disease process in MPN is clonal myeloproliferation, and targeting its paraneoplastic effects can only provide an incomplete and transient benefit. We do recognize and appreciate the palliative value of JAK1/JAK2 inhibitors in MF patients with symptomatic splenomegaly or severe constitutional symptoms. However, such patients might be served better if they were to participate in clinical trials with newer JAK inhibitors or other novel agents.

Acknowledgments I have received a research grant from the Henry J Predolin Foundation.

Conflict of Interest Statement I am principal investigator or co-investigator on clinical trials that are supported by TargeGen, Sanofi-Aventis, Incyte, BMS, Cytopia, YM BioSciences, Celgene, and Novartis. No payments outside of clinical trial support were paid to either myself or my institution. Support for laboratory investigations relevant to the clinical trials or preclinical laboratory research has been provided by TargeGen and Cytopia.

References

Abdel-Wahab O, Manshouri T, Patel J, Harris K, Yao J, Hedvat C et al (2010) Genetic analysis of transforming events that convert chronic myeloproliferative neoplasms to leukemias. Cancer Res 70:447–452

Abdel-Wahab O, Pardanani A, Rampal R, Lasho TL, Levine RL, Tefferi A (2011) DNMT3A mutational analysis in primary myelofibrosis, chronic myelomonocytic leukemia and advanced phases of myeloproliferative neoplasms. Leukemia 25:1219–1220

Barbui T, Thiele J, Passamonti F, Rumi E, Boveri E, Ruggeri M et al (2011) Survival and disease progression in essential thrombocythemia are significantly influenced by accurate morphologic diagnosis: an international study. J Clin Oncol 29:3179–3184

Baxter EJ, Scott LM, Campbell PJ, East C, Fourouclas N, Swanton S et al (2005) Acquired mutation of the tyrosine kinase JAK2 in human myeloproliferative disorders. Lancet 365:1054–1061

Beer PA, Campbell PJ, Scott LM, Bench AJ, Erber WN, Bareford D et al (2008) MPL mutations in myeloproliferative disorders: analysis of the PT-1 cohort. Blood 112:141–149

Carbuccia N, Murati A, Trouplin V, Brecqueville M, Adelaide J, Rey J et al (2009) Mutations of ASXL1 gene in myeloproliferative neoplasms. Leukemia 23:2183–2186

Carobbio A, Thiele J, Passamonti F, Rumi E, Ruggeri M, Rodeghiero F et al (2011) Risk factors for arterial and venous thrombosis in WHO-defined essential thrombocythemia: an international study of 891 patients. Blood 117:5857–5859

Cervantes F, Mesa R, Barosi G (2007) New and old treatment modalities in primary myelofibrosis. Cancer J 13:377–383

Cervantes F, Dupriez B, Pereira A, Passamonti F, Reilly JT, Morra E et al (2009) New prognostic scoring system for primary myelofibrosis based on a study of the International Working Group for Myelofibrosis Research and Treatment. Blood 113:2895–2901

Cortelazzo S, Finazzi G, Ruggeri M, Vestri O, Galli M, Rodeghiero F et al (1995) Hydroxyurea for patients with essential thrombocythemia and a high risk of thrombosis. N Engl J Med 332:1132–1136

De Sanctis V, Mazzucconi MG, Spadea A, Alfo M, Mancini M, Bizzoni L et al (2003) Long-term evaluation of 164 patients with essential thrombocythaemia treated with pipobroman: occurrence of leukaemic evolution. Br J Haematol 123:517–521

Deeg HJ, Odenike O, Scott BL, Estrov Z, Cortes JE, Thomas DA et al (2011) Phase II study of SB1518, an orally available novel JAK2 inhibitor, in patients with myelofibrosis. J Clin Oncol, ASCO Annual Meeting Proceedings (Post-Meeting Edition) 29(15_Suppl.):6515

Delhommeau F, Dupont S, Della Valle V, James C, Trannoy S, Masse A et al (2009) Mutation in TET2 in myeloid cancers. N Engl J Med 360:2289–2301

Druker BJ (2008) Translation of the Philadelphia chromosome into therapy for CML. Blood 112:4808–4817

Elliott MA, Mesa RA, Li CY, Hook CC, Ansell SM, Levitt RM et al (2002) Thalidomide treatment in myelofibrosis with myeloid metaplasia. Br J Haematol 117:288–296

Ernst T, Chase AJ, Score J, Hidalgo-Curtis CE, Bryant C, Jones AV et al (2010) Inactivating mutations of the histone methyltransferase gene EZH2 in myeloid disorders. Nat Genet 42:722–726

Gangat N, Strand J, Li CY, Wu W, Pardanani A, Tefferi A (2007) Leucocytosis in polycythaemia vera predicts both inferior survival and leukaemic transformation. Br J Haematol 138:354–358

Gangat N, Caramazza D, Vaidya R, George G, Begna K, Schwager S et al (2011) DIPSS plus: a refined Dynamic International Prognostic Scoring System for primary myelofibrosis that incorporates prognostic information from karyotype, platelet count, and transfusion status. J Clin Oncol 29:392–397

Gery S, Gueller S, Chumakova K, Kawamata N, Liu L, Koeffler HP (2007) Adaptor protein Lnk negatively regulates the mutant MPL, MPLW515L associated with myeloproliferative disorders. Blood 110:3360–3364

Gery S, Cao Q, Gueller S, Xing H, Tefferi A, Koeffler HP (2009) Lnk inhibits myeloproliferative disorder-associated JAK2 mutant, JAK2V617F. J Leukoc Biol 85:957–965

Grand FH, Hidalgo-Curtis CE, Ernst T, Zoi K, Zoi C, McGuire C et al (2009) Frequent CBL mutations associated with 11q acquired uniparental disomy in myeloproliferative neoplasms. Blood 113:6182–6192

Green A, Beer P (2010) Somatic mutations of IDH1 and IDH2 in the leukemic transformation of myeloproliferative neoplasms. N Engl J Med 362:369–370

Guglielmelli P, Pancrazzi A, Bergamaschi G, Rosti V, Villani L, Antonioli E et al (2007) Anaemia characterises patients with myelofibrosis harbouring Mpl mutation. Br J Haematol 137:244–247

Guglielmelli P, Barosi G, Specchia G, Rambaldi A, Lo Coco F, Antonioli E et al (2009) Identification of patients with poorer survival in primary myelofibrosis based on the burden of JAK2V617F mutated allele. Blood 114:1477–1483

Harrison CN, Campbell PJ, Buck G, Wheatley K, East CL, Bareford D et al (2005) Hydroxyurea compared with anagrelide in high-risk essential thrombocythemia. N Engl J Med 353:33–45

Harrison CN, Kiladjian JJ, Al-Ali HK, Gisslinger H, Waltzman RJ, Stalbovskaya V et al (2011) Results of a randomized study of the JAK inhibitor ruxolitinib (INC424) versus best available therapy (BAT) in primary myelofibrosis (PMF), post-polycythemia vera-myelofibrosis (PPV-MF) or post-essential thrombocythemia-myelofibrosis (PET-MF). J Clin Oncol, ASCO Annual Meeting Proceedings (Post-Meeting Edition) 29(18_Suppl.):LBA6501

Harutyunyan A, Klampfl T, Cazzola M, Kralovics R (2011) p53 lesions in leukemic transformation. N Engl J Med 364:488–490

Jager R, Gisslinger H, Passamonti F, Rumi E, Berg T, Gisslinger B et al (2010) Deletions of the transcription factor Ikaros in myeloproliferative neoplasms. Leukemia 24:1290–1298

James C, Ugo V, Le Couedic JP, Staerk J, Delhommeau F, Lacout C et al (2005) A unique clonal JAK2 mutation leading to constitutive signalling causes polycythaemia vera. Nature 434:1144–1148

Jones AV, Chase A, Silver RT, Oscier D, Zoi K, Wang YL et al (2009) JAK2 haplotype is a major risk factor for the development of myeloproliferative neoplasms. Nat Genet 41:446–449

Kiladjian JJ, Cassinat B, Chevret S, Turlure P, Cambier N, Roussel M et al (2008) Pegylated interferon-alfa-2a induces complete hematologic and molecular responses with low toxicity in polycythemia vera. Blood 112: 3065–3072

Kilpivaara O, Mukherjee S, Schram AM, Wadleigh M, Mullally A, Ebert BL et al (2009) A germline JAK2 SNP is associated with predisposition to the development of JAK2(V617F)-positive myeloproliferative neoplasms. Nat Genet 41:455–459

Klampfl T, Harutyunyan A, Berg T, Gisslinger B, Schalling M, Bagienski K et al (2011) Genome integrity of myeloproliferative neoplasms in chronic phase and during disease progression. Blood 118:167–176

Kralovics R, Passamonti F, Buser AS, Teo SS, Tiedt R, Passweg JR et al (2005) A gain-of-function mutation of JAK2 in myeloproliferative disorders. N Engl J Med 352:1779–1790

Landolfi R, Marchioli R, Kutti J, Gisslinger H, Tognoni G, Patrono C et al (2004) Efficacy and safety of low-dose aspirin in polycythemia vera. N Engl J Med 350:114–124

"Leukemia and Hematosarcoma" Cooperative Group, European Organization for Research on Treatment of Cancer (EORTC) (1981) Treatment of polycythaemia vera by radiophosphorus or busulphan: a randomized trial. Br J Cancer 44:75–80

Levine RL, Wadleigh M, Cools J, Ebert BL, Wernig G, Huntly BJ et al (2005) Activating mutation in the tyrosine kinase JAK2 in polycythemia vera, essential thrombocythemia, and myeloid metaplasia with myelofibrosis. Cancer Cell 7:387–397

Loh ML, Sakai DS, Flotho C, Kang M, Fliegauf M, Archambeault S et al (2009) Mutations in CBL occur frequently in juvenile myelomonocytic leukemia. Blood 114:1859–1863

Martinez-Trillos A, Gaya A, Maffioli M, Arellano-Rodrigo E, Calvo X, Diaz-Beya M et al (2010) Efficacy and tolerability of hydroxyurea in the treatment of the hyperproliferative manifestations of myelofibrosis: results in 40 patients. Ann Hematol 89:1233–1237

Mesa RA, Niblack J, Wadleigh M, Verstovsek S, Camoriano J, Barnes S et al (2007) The burden of fatigue and quality of life in myeloproliferative disorders (MPDs): an international Internet-based survey of 1179 MPD patients. Cancer 109:68–76

Mesa RA, Schwager S, Radia D, Cheville A, Hussein K, Niblack J et al (2009) The Myelofibrosis Symptom Assessment Form (MFSAF): an evidence-based brief inventory to measure quality of life and symptomatic response to treatment in myelofibrosis. Leuk Res 33:1199–1203

Mishchenko E, Tefferi A (2010) Treatment options for hydroxyurea-refractory disease complications in myeloproliferative neoplasms: JAK2 inhibitors, radiotherapy, splenectomy and transjugular intrahepatic portosystemic shunt. Eur J Haematol 85:192–199

Moliterno AR, Hexner E, Roboz GJ, Carroll M, Luger S, Mascarenhas J et al (2009) An open-label study of CEP-701 in patients with JAK2 V617F-positive PV and ET: update of 39 enrolled patients. Blood 114:Abstract 753

Oh ST, Simonds EF, Jones C, Hale MB, Goltsev Y, Gibbs KD Jr et al (2010) Novel mutations in the inhibitory adaptor protein LNK drive JAK-STAT signaling in patients with myeloproliferative neoplasms. Blood 116:988–992

Olcaydu D, Harutyunyan A, Jager R, Berg T, Gisslinger B, Pabinger I et al (2009) A common JAK2 haplotype confers susceptibility to myeloproliferative neoplasms. Nat Genet 41:450–454

Pardanani AD, Levine RL, Lasho T, Pikman Y, Mesa RA, Wadleigh M et al (2006) MPL515 mutations in myeloproliferative and other myeloid disorders: a study of 1182 patients. Blood 108:3472–3476

Pardanani A, Lasho TL, Finke C, Hanson CA, Tefferi A (2007) Prevalence and clinicopathologic correlates of JAK2 exon 12 mutations in JAK2V617F-negative polycythemia vera. Leukemia 21:1960–1963

Pardanani A, Lasho T, Finke C, Oh ST, Gotlib J, Tefferi A (2010a) LNK mutation studies in blast-phase myeloproliferative neoplasms, and in chronic-phase disease with TET2, IDH, JAK2 or MPL mutations. Leukemia 24:1713–1718

Pardanani A, Gotlib JR, Jamieson C, Cortes JE, Talpaz M, Stone RM et al (2010b) Longer-term follow up with TG101348 therapy in myelofibrosis confirms sustained improvement in splenomegaly, disease-related symptoms, and JAK2V617F allele burden. ASH Annual Meeting Abstracts 116:459

Pardanani A, Guglielmelli P, Lasho TL, Pancrazzi A, Finke CM, Vannucchi AM et al (2011a) Primary myelofibrosis with or without mutant MPL: comparison of survival and clinical features involving 603 patients. Leukemia. doi:101038/leu2011161

Pardanani A, Gotlib JR, Jamieson C, Cortes JE, Talpaz M, Stone RM et al (2011b) Safety and efficacy of TG101348, a selective JAK2 inhibitor, in myelofibrosis. J Clin Oncol 29:789–796

Pardanani A, Caramazza D, George G, Lasho TL, Hogan WJ, Litzow MR et al (2011c) Safety and efficacy of CYT387, a JAK-1/2 inhibitor, for the treatment of myelofibrosis. J Clin Oncol, ASCO Annual Meeting Proceedings (Post-Meeting Edition) 29(15_Suppl.):6514

Passamonti F, Brusamolino E, Lazzarino M, Barate C, Klersy C, Orlandi E et al (2000) Efficacy of pipobroman in the treatment of polycythemia vera: long-term results in 163 patients. Haematologica 85:1011–1018

Passamonti F, Rumi E, Malabarba L, Arcaini L, Orlandi E, Brusamolino E et al (2004) Long-term follow-up of young patients with essential thrombocythemia treated with pipobroman. Ann Hematol 83:495–497

Passamonti F, Rumi E, Arcaini L, Boveri E, Elena C, Pietra D et al (2008) Prognostic factors for thrombosis, myelofibrosis, and leukemia in essential thrombocythemia: a study of 605 patients. Haematologica 93:1645–1651

Passamonti F, Schnittger S, Girodon F, Kiladjian J-J, McMullin MF, Ruggeri M et al (2009) Molecular and clinical features of the myeloproliferative neoplasm associated with JAK2 exon 12 mutations: a European Multicenter Study. ASH Annual Meeting Abstracts 114:3904

Passamonti F, Rumi E, Pietra D, Elena C, Boveri E, Arcaini L et al (2010) A prospective study of 338 patients with polycythemia vera: the impact of JAK2 (V617F) allele burden and leukocytosis on fibrotic or leukemic disease transformation and vascular complications. Leukemia 24:1574–1579

Petti MC, Spadea A, Avvisati G, Spadea T, Latagliata R, Montefusco E et al (1998) Polycythemia vera treated with pipobroman as single agent: low incidence of secondary leukemia in a cohort of patients observed during 20 years (1971–1991). Leukemia 12:869–874

Pietra D, Li S, Brisci A, Passamonti F, Rumi E, Theocharides A et al (2008) Somatic mutations of JAK2 exon 12 in patients with JAK2 (V617F)-negative myeloproliferative disorders. Blood 111:1686–1689

Pikman Y, Lee BH, Mercher T, McDowell E, Ebert BL, Gozo M et al (2006) MPLW515L is a novel somatic activating mutation in myelofibrosis with myeloid metaplasia. PLoS Med 3:e270

Quintas-Cardama A, Kantarjian H, Manshouri T, Luthra R, Estrov Z, Pierce S et al (2009) Pegylated interferon alfa-2a yields high rates of hematologic and molecular response in patients with advanced essential thrombocythemia and polycythemia vera. J Clin Oncol 27:5418–5424

Santos FP, Kantarjian HM, Jain N, Manshouri T, Thomas DA, Garcia-Manero G et al (2010) Phase 2 study of CEP-701, an orally available JAK2 inhibitor, in patients with primary or post-polycythemia vera/essential thrombocythemia myelofibrosis. Blood 115:1131–1136

Scott LM, Tong W, Levine RL, Scott MA, Beer PA, Stratton MR et al (2007) JAK2 exon 12 mutations in polycythemia vera and idiopathic erythrocytosis. N Engl J Med 356:459–468

Shvidel L, Sigler E, Haran M, Klepfish A, Duek A, Berrebi A et al (2007) Busulphan is safe and efficient treatment in elderly patients with essential thrombocythemia. Leukemia 21:2071–2072

Siragusa S, Vaidya R, Tefferi A (2009) Hydroxyurea effect on marked splenomegaly associated with primary myelofibrosis: response rates and correlation with JAK2V617F allele burden. Blood (ASH Annual Meeting Abstracts) 114:Abstract 4971

Tefferi A, Cortes J, Verstovsek S, Mesa RA, Thomas D, Lasho TL et al (2006) Lenalidomide therapy in myelofibrosis with myeloid metaplasia. Blood 108:1158–1164

Tefferi A, Lasho TL, Mesa RA, Pardanani A, Ketterling RP, Hanson CA (2007) Lenalidomide therapy in del(5) (q31)-associated myelofibrosis: cytogenetic and JAK2V617F molecular remissions. Leukemia 21: 1827–1828

Tefferi A, Lasho TL, Huang J, Finke C, Mesa RA, Li CY et al (2008) Low JAK2V617F allele burden in primary myelofibrosis, compared to either a higher allele burden or unmutated status, is associated with inferior overall and leukemia-free survival. Leukemia 22:756–761

Tefferi A, Vaidya R, Caramazza D, Finke C, Lasho T, Pardanani A (2011) Circulating interleukin (IL)-8, IL-2R, IL-12, and IL-15 levels are independently prognostic in primary myelofibrosis: a comprehensive cytokine profiling study. J Clin Oncol 29:1356–1363

Thoennissen NH, Lasho T, Thoennissen GB, Ogawa S, Tefferi A, Koeffler HP (2011) Novel CUX1 missense mutation in association with 7q- at leukemic transformation of MPN. Am J Hematol 86:703–705

Thomas DA, Giles FJ, Albitar M, Cortes JE, Verstovsek S, Faderl S et al (2006) Thalidomide therapy for myelofibrosis with myeloid metaplasia. Cancer 106:1974–1984

Vannucchi AM, Antonioli E, Guglielmelli P, Pardanani A, Tefferi A (2008a) Clinical correlates of JAK2V617F presence or allele burden in myeloproliferative neoplasms: a critical reappraisal. Leukemia 22:1299–1307

Vannucchi AM, Antonioli E, Guglielmelli P, Pancrazzi A, Guerini V, Barosi G et al (2008b) Characteristics and clinical correlates of MPL 515W>L/K mutation in essential thrombocythemia. Blood 112:844–847

Vardiman JW, Thiele J, Arber DA, Brunning RD, Borowitz MJ, Porwit A et al (2009) The 2008 revision of the World Health Organization (WHO) classification of myeloid neoplasms and acute leukemia: rationale and important changes. Blood 114:937–951

Verstovsek S, Passamonti F, Rambaldi A, Barosi G, Rosen PJ, Levine R et al (2010a) Durable responses with the JAK1/ JAK2 inhibitor, INCB018424, in patients with polycythemia vera (PV) and essential thrombocythemia (ET) refractory or intolerant to hydroxyurea (HU). Blood (ASH Annual Meeting Abstracts) 116:Abstract 313

Verstovsek S, Deeg HJ, Odenike O, Zhu J, Kantarjian H, Estrov Z et al (2010b) Phase 1/2 study of SB1518, a novel JAK2/FLT3 inhibitor, in the treatment of primary myelofibrosis. ASH Annual Meeting Abstracts 116:3082

Verstovsek S, Kantarjian H, Mesa RA, Pardanani AD, Cortes-Franco J, Thomas DA et al (2010c) Safety and efficacy of INCB018424, a JAK1 and JAK2 inhibitor, in myelofibrosis. N Engl J Med 363:1117–1127

Verstovsek S, Mesa RA, Gotlib JR, Levy RS, Gupta V, DiPersio JF et al (2011) Results of COMFORT-I, a randomized double-blind phase III trial of JAK 1/2 inhibitor INCB18424 (424) versus placebo (PB) for patients with myelofibrosis (MF). J Clin Oncol, ASCO Annual Meeting Proceedings (Post-Meeting Edition) 29(15_Suppl.):6500

Ongoing Clinical Trials in Myeloproliferative Neoplasms

18

Fabio P.S. Santos and Srdan Verstovsek

Contents

F.P.S. Santos
Hematology and Oncology Department,
Hospital Israelita Albert Einstein,
São Paulo, SP, Brazil

S. Verstovsek (✉)
Department of Leukemia,
The University of Texas M. D. Anderson Cancer Center,
Houston, TX, USA
e-mail: sverstov@mdanderson.org

18.1 Introduction

The classic Philadelphia-negative (Ph-negative) myeloproliferative neoplasms (MPNs) are a group of neoplastic disorders characterized by variable degrees of peripheral blood (PB) cell proliferation (i.e., erythrocytosis, and/or leukocytosis, and/or thrombocytosis), splenomegaly, bone marrow (BM) fibrosis, and an increased risk of thrombotic episodes and transformation to acute myeloid leukemia (AML) (Swerdlow et al. 2008). Classic Ph-negative MPNs include polycythemia vera (PV), essential thrombocythemia (ET), and primary myelofibrosis (PMF) (Swerdlow et al. 2008). MF can also develop secondary to disease transformation from PV and ET. The prognosis of these Ph-negative MPNs is quite heterogeneous, as some patients can have a disease with indolent course and median survival of 15–20+ years (PV, ET), while in other cases, the disease can follow a very aggressive course, as in MF where the median survival ranges from 5 to 7 years only (Cervantes et al. 2009).

Currently, treatment options for patients with Ph-negative MPNs are few and far between (Tefferi 2011). Patients with PV and ET are usually managed with anti-platelet agents and cytoreductive drugs (e.g., hydroxyurea) when their risk of thrombosis is deemed to be elevated (e.g., older age, previous thrombotic episodes). Treatment of MF is palliative and directed to alleviation of symptoms caused by cytopenias and massive splenomegaly. Allogeneic stem cell transplantation (SCT) is potentially curative, but only a minority of patients with MF can benefit from the procedure due to

T. Barbui and A. Tefferi (eds.), *Myeloproliferative Neoplasms*, Hematologic Malignancies,
DOI 10.1007/978-3-642-24989-1_18, © Springer-Verlag Berlin Heidelberg 2012

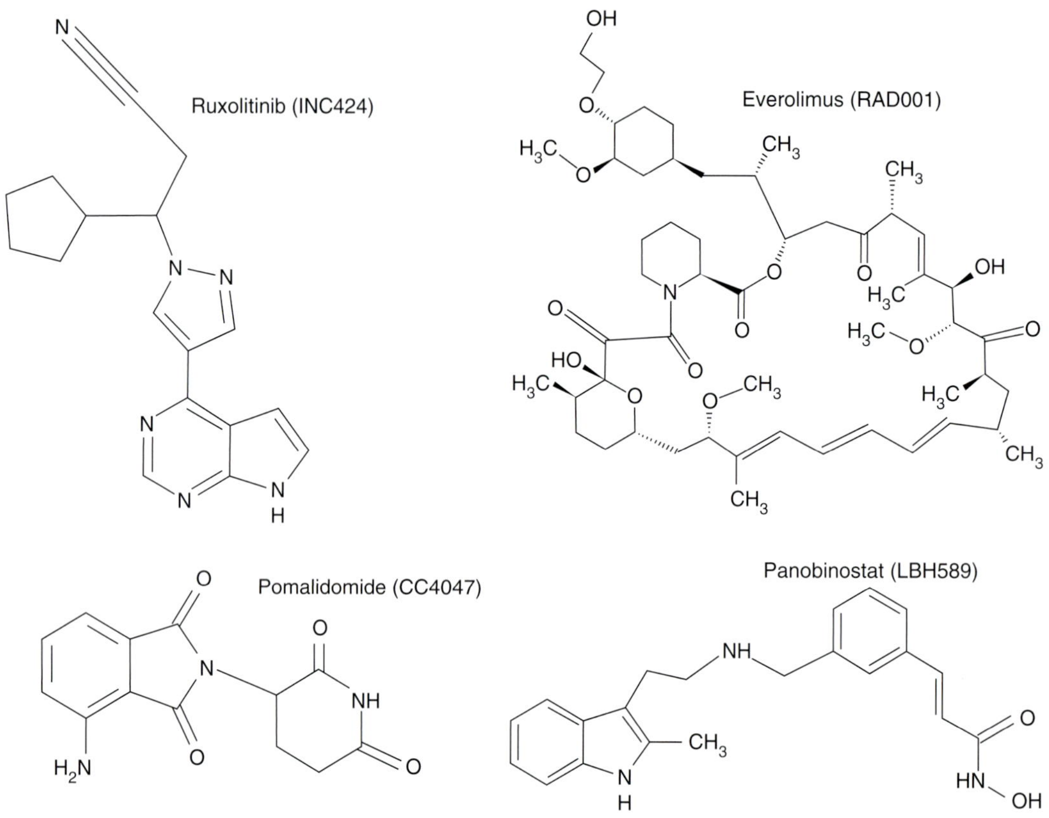

Fig. 18.1 Chemical structures of selected drugs in current development for classic Ph-negative MPNs. Ruxolitinib (JAK2 inhibitor), everolimus (mTOR inhibitor), pomali- domide (immunomodulatory drug), panobinostat (HDAC inhibitor)

issues with age and comorbidities (Kroger et al. 2009). Fortunately, the scenario for patients with Ph-negative MPNs seems to be changing. Over the past 5 years, many new drugs have been in devel- opment for treatment of patients with Ph-negative MPNs. This surge in new drugs is mainly due to a greater understanding of the pathophysiology of Ph-negative MPNs. It is now known that most patients with Ph-negative MPNs harbor activating mutations in the hematopoietic cytokines signal- ing pathways, such as *JAK2* V617F (PV ~90%, MF ~50%, ET ~50%), *JAK2* exon 12 mutations (PV ~5%) and *MPL* W515K/L (ET ~5%, MF ~10%) (Baxter et al. 2005; James et al. 2005; Kralovics et al. 2005; Levine et al. 2005; Pikman et al. 2006; Scott et al. 2007). Mutations in other genes have also been described, including *TET2*, *ASXL1*, *EZH2*, *LNK*, *IDH*, and *IZKF1*, and their role in pathogenesis is currently being investigated

(Tefferi 2010). There are several different classes of compounds in clinical trials for patients with Ph-negative MPNs at present (Fig. 18.1). In this chapter, we will review current clinical results in studies of JAK2 inhibitors (Table 18.1) and the most important other drugs (Table 18.2).

18.2 JAK2 Inhibitors

18.2.1 Rationale

Since the discovery of the JAK2 V617F mutation by four independent groups in 2005, the prospect of using enzyme inhibitors to target this mutated kinase, similar to imatinib in CML, has been allur- ing investigators (Baxter et al. 2005; James et al. 2005; Kralovics et al. 2005; Levine et al. 2005). JAK2 tyrosine kinases (TKs) are part of the JAK

Table 18.1 Complete and ongoing clinical trials with JAK2 inhibitors for patients with classic Ph-negative MPNs

Study	Compound	Disease	Phase	N	Results
Verstovsek et al. 2010b	Ruxolitinib	MF	I/II	153	CI: 44% (spleen response); improvement in exercise ability and systemic symptoms; cytopenias (thrombocytopenia, anemia)
NCT00952289	Ruxolitinib versus placebo	MF	III	309	NA
NCT00934544	Ruxolitinib versus best medical therapy	MF	III	219	NA
NCT01340651	Ruxolitinib sustained release	MF	II	NA	NA
NCT01317875	Ruxolitinib low dose	MF	I/II	NA	NA
Verstovsek et al. 2010c	Ruxolitinib	PV/ET	I/II	73	PV: 100% response; ET: 62% response; improvement systemic symptoms; cytopenias (thrombocytopenia, anemia)
NCT01243944	Ruxolitinib versus best medical therapy	PV	III	NA	NA
Pardanani et al. 2011	TG101348	MF	I/II	59	CI: 39% (spleen response); improvement in systemic symptoms; leukocytosis; thrombocytosis; cytopenias; GI toxicity
Pardanani et al. 2010	CYT387	MF	I/II	60	CI (spleen response): 47%; CI (anemia): 50%; thrombocytopenia; nausea; vomiting
Santos et al. 2010	CEP-701	MF	II	22	CI: 27% (spleen response and cytopenias); GI toxicity; cytopenias
Hexner et al. 2009	CEP-701	MF	I/II	26	Reduction in splenomegaly; GI toxicity; cytopenias
Moliterno et al. 2009	CEP-701	PV/ET	I/II	39	Reduction in spleen size: 83%; reduction in phlebotomy requirements: 3/5 (60%); GI toxicity; five thrombotic episodes
Verstovsek et al. 2010a	SB1518	MF	I/II	33	Reduction in splenomegaly; GI toxicity
Seymour et al. 2010	SB1518	MF	I/II	20	Reduction in splenomegaly; improvement in transfusion dependency; GI toxicity
NCT01243944	AZD1480	MF	I	NA	NA
NCT01134120	LY2784544	MF	I	NA	NA

CI clinical improvement, *ET* essential thrombocythemia, *GI* gastrointestinal, *MF* myelofibrosis, *NA* not available, *PV* polycythemia vera

Table 18.2 Clinical trials with drugs other than JAK2 inhibitors for patients with classic Ph-negative MPNs

Study	Compound	Disease	Phase	N	Results
Rambaldi et al. 2010	Givinostat	PV/ET/MF	II	29	PV/ET: response 54%; MF: response 3/16 patients; diarrhea; cytopenias; QT prolongation
NCT00928707	Givinostat+hydroxyurea	PV	II	NA	NA
DeAngelo et al. 2009	Panobinostat	MF	I	13	Responses in four patients (spleen and transfusion independency); thrombocytopenia
DeAngelo et al. 2010	Panobinostat	MF	II	31	Depletion of JAK2 V617F phosphorylation and phospho STAT3/5
Mascarenhas et al. 2009	Panobinostat	MF	I/II	15	Responses in four patients (spleen response); thrombocytopenia
Vannucchi et al. 2010	Everolimus	MF	I/II	30	CI: 23% (spleen response); improvement in pruritus; mouth ulcers; hypertriglicerydemia
Tefferi et al. 2009	Pomalidomide±prednisone	MF	II	84	CI: 16–36% (anemia); thrombocytopenia; anemia
Begna et al. 2011	Pomalidomide	MF	II	58	CI: 17% (anemia); 58% increase platelet; better response in JAK2 V617F–positive patients
NCT00946270	Pomalidomide	MF	II	NA	NA
NCT00949364	Pomalidomide	MF	II	NA	NA
NCT01178281	Pomalidomide versus placebo	MF	III	NA	NA
NCT01291784	GC1008	MF	I	NA	NA
NCT00287261	Zoledronic acid	MF	II	NA	NA

CI clinical improvement, *ET* essential thrombocythemia, *MF* myelofibrosis, *NA* not available, *PV* polycythemia vera family of TKs that associate with the intracellular portion of cytokine receptors that do not possess intrinsic TK activity (e.g., erythropoietin receptor [EPOR], granulocyte colony-stimulating factor [G-CSF] receptor [GCSFR], thrombopoietin receptor [MPL]) (Leonard and O'Shea 1998). When the putative ligand binds to the receptor, JAK TKs are activated and cross-phosphorylate each other and the receptor, increasing their activity and permitting binding of secondary messengers to the cytokine receptor, such as STATs (signal transducers and activators of transcriptions) (Leonard and O'Shea 1998). STATs are latent cytoplasmic transcription factors which bind to phosphorylated tyrosine residues on the intracellular portion of cytokine receptors. This is followed by phosphorylation and activation of the STAT molecule by activated JAK kinases, STAT homodimerization, translocation to the nucleus, and activation of transcription of target genes (Yu and Jove 2004). STAT3 and STAT5a/b are the STAT family members most commonly implicated in neoplastic disorders, including Ph-negative MPNs, and some of their target genes are *CCND1* (cellular proliferation), *VEGF* (angiogenesis) and *BCL2L1*, and *MCL1* (resistance to apoptosis) (Yu and Jove 2004). Other pathways activated by JAK2 TKs include the Ras-Raf-MAPK (mitogen-activated protein kinase) pathway (Winston and Hunter 1995; Mizuguchi et al. 2000) and the phosphatidylinositol-3-kinase (PI3K) of the PI3K-Akt-mTOR pathway (Al-Shami and Naccache 1999; Bouscary et al. 2003).

The JAK2 V617F mutation leads to constitutive signaling of the JAK2 TK (James et al. 2005). The V617F mutation is located in the pseudokinase domain (JAK homology 2 [JH2] domain). The JH2 domain interacts with and inhibits activity of the true TK domain (JH1) since aberrant JAK enzymes lacking the JH2 domain possess an increased TK activity (Saharinen and Silvennoinen 2002). The V617F mutation disrupts this important interaction between the JH2 domain and the JH1 domain, and it is believed that this is the molecular mechanism through which the V617F mutation leads to constitutive JAK2 activation (Lindauer et al. 2001; Dusa et al. 2010). When JAK2 V617F is expressed in EPOR-positive BaF/3 cells, it confers EPO-hypersensitivity and EPO-independent growth and survival (Levine et al. 2005). Intracellularly, there is increased phosphorylation and activation of STAT5 and other downstream targets, such as Akt (James et al. 2005). In mice expressing JAK2 V617F in hematopoietic stem cells (HSC), there is development of a disease clinically similar to human PV, with increased red cell mass, splenomegaly, and hypercellularity of the BM (Lacout et al. 2006; Wernig et al. 2006; Mullally et al. 2010). Some mice later develop fibrosis in the BM, akin to human MF (Lacout et al. 2006; Wernig et al. 2006). More recently, laboratory studies have revealed a non-canonical role for JAK2 besides activating intracellular signaling pathways related to cell proliferation and survival. Dawson et al. demonstrated that JAK2 is present in the nucleus of HSCs and that it phosphorylates histone H3 at residue Y41 (H3Y41), preventing binding of the Heterochromatin Protein 1-α (HP1α) (Dawson et al. 2009). HP1α is responsible for mediating gene silencing through epigenetic mechanisms (Bannister et al. 2001; Lachner et al. 2001), and indeed, increased expression of the oncogene *LMO2* was detected in JAK2 V617F–positive cells. Inhibition of JAK2 was associated with reduced phosphorylation of H3Y41 and reduced expression of *LMO2* (Dawson et al. 2009). In a similar manner, another report demonstrated that JAK2 phosphorylation of the histone arginine methyltransferase enzyme PRMT5 was associated with decreased enzyme activity, decreased arginine methylation at histone targets, increased erythroid colony formation and proliferation (Liu et al. 2011). Thus, it is becoming clearer that JAK2 V617F exerts its effects on hematopoietic cells both through canonical targets (e.g., JAK-STAT pathway) and non-canonical targets (e.g., epigenetic modulation through histone modifications), making JAK2 a central component of targeted therapy for classic Ph-negative MPNs.

18.2.2 Current Clinical Trials

18.2.2.1 Ruxolitinib in Myelofibrosis

Ruxolitinib (formerly known as INCB018424/ INC424; Incyte, Wilmington, DE) is a dual JAK1/ JAK2 inhibitor currently in clinical trials for both MF and PV. It is the JAK2 inhibitor which is most advanced in clinical development. Pre-clinical studies demonstrated that ruxolitinib inhibited both JAK1 (half-maximal inhibitory concentration [IC50] 3.3 nM) and JAK2 (IC50 2.8 nM) and had decreased activity versus JAK3 (IC50 322 nM) (Quintas-Cardama et al. 2010). Ruxolitinib inhibited phosphorylation of JAK2 downstream target STAT3 and reduced viability of cells expressing EPOR and JAK2 V617F. In an animal model of MPN, mice who received ruxolitinib had a decrease in splenomegaly and pro-inflammatory cytokines levels (Quintas-Cardama et al. 2010). Ruxolitinib also inhibited proliferation of erythroid progenitors from patients with PV to a greater degree than cells from normal donors (Quintas-Cardama et al. 2010).

The results of a phase I/II clinical trial with ruxolitinib for patients with MF (PMF or post-PV/ET) were recently published (Verstovsek et al. 2010b). In this study, 153 patients received ruxolitinib at different dose schedules. An individualized dose schedule of 15 mg twice daily (10 mg twice daily if platelets $<100 \times 10^9$/L) with further escalation to 20–25 mg twice daily if no response was observed represented the best balance between efficacy and safety. Dose-limiting toxicity (DLT) was thrombocytopenia. According to the International Working Group on Myelofibrosis Research and Treatment (IWG-MRT) response criteria, 44% of patients with splenomegaly had a clinical improvement (CI) with a decrease $\geq$50% in spleen size. Response rate in the cohort receiving the optimized dose schedule was 52%. At 12 months, 73% of patients in the 15 mg twice daily cohort maintained response. Importantly, response rate was seen in patients with both wild-type and mutated JAK2 and also in patients with post-PV/ET MF, showing that ruxolitinib is effective in all subgroups of MF. Other observed significant beneficial effects included an improvement in systemic symptoms, exercise capacity, and quality of life in the majority of patients. At 1 month, the majority of patients reported a greater than 50% improvement in their Myelofibrosis Symptom Assessment Form (MFSAF) score. Improvement in cytokine profile (decrease in pro-inflammatory cytokines and increase in EPO and leptin) accompanied the improvement in systemic symptoms. There was no decrease in BM fibrosis, and patients with JAK2 V617F had a mean decrease in allele burden of only 13%. Hematological toxicity was the most common reported side effect seen with ruxolitinib and consisted mainly of new-onset anemia and thrombocytopenia. However, the rate of grade 3–4 myelosuppression was substantially improved in the cohort which started with the dose-adjusted schedule of 15 mg twice daily rather than at maximum dose of 25 mg twice daily (2.9% versus 23.4% [grade 3–4 thrombocytopenia]; 8.3% versus 26.7% [grade 3–4 anemia]). Other side effects included diarrhea (all grades, 5.9%; grade 3–4, 0%), fatigue (all grades, 4.3%; grade 3–4, 1.3%) and headache (all grades, 3.3%; grade 3–4, 0%). Even though the study was not randomized to detect an improvement in survival or disease transformation, only three patients transformed to AML (rate of 0.016 patients/year), less than expected based on historical cohorts (Barosi et al. 2007). Interestingly, a recent publication showed that patients with MF who present with increased levels of pro-inflammatory cytokines (e.g., interleukin-8 [IL-8], IL-2R) have a worse survival compared to other patients (median survival 17 versus 80 months; $p < 0.0001$) (Tefferi et al. 2011). Since ruxolitinib normalizes the cytokine profile of patients with MF, it would be interesting to see with longer follow-up if that translates into improved survival for these patients.

The results of the phase I/II trial with ruxolitinib were exciting and led to the launching of two phase III trials with ruxolitinib in the USA and Europe. Both clinical trials (**CO**ntrolled **M**yelo**F**ibrosis study with **OR**al JAK inhibitor **T**reatment I and II [COMFORT-I/II]) enrolled patients with PMF or post-PV/ET MF who required therapy and had a high or intermediate-2 risk score by the MF International Prognostic Score System (IPSS). In COMFORT-I (www.clinicaltrials.gov register number NCT00952289), 309 patients were randomized (1:1) in a double-blind fashion between ruxolitinib (initial doses 15–20 mg twice daily) and placebo. Primary endpoint was the rate of patients with $\geq$35% decrease in spleen volume, as assessed by magnetic resonance imaging (MRI) or computed tomography (CT) at 24 weeks (corresponds roughly to a 50% decrease in spleen size by physical examination). Secondary endpoint was the duration of maintenance of a ≥35% reduction from baseline in spleen volume among subjects initially randomized to receive ruxolitinib. A recent press release from Incyte revealed that the study primary endpoint was achieved (Incyte 2010), with 42% of patients receiving ruxolitinib having achieved the endpoint, versus <1% of placebo patients ($p < 0.0001$). The COMFORT-II trial (NCT00934544) is a phase III controlled, open-label, randomized (2:1) study comparing ruxolitinib (initial doses 15–20 mg twice daily) versus best available therapy for patients with MF requiring therapy and with an IPSS risk of intermediate-2 or high. Primary endpoint was the rate of patients with ≥35% decrease in spleen volume, as assessed by MRI/CT at 48 weeks. Secondary endpoint was the duration of maintenance of a ≥35% reduction from baseline in spleen volume. A total of 219 patients have been randomized in nine countries. Preliminary data in a press release from Incyte have stated that ruxolitinib provided a statistically significant reduction in spleen size compared to best available therapy (Incyte 2011). Full data from these studies are expected in an upcoming medical meeting.

Two other ongoing clinical trials with ruxolitinib deserve mention. The first trial (NCT01317875) is a phase IB study which will determine the maximum safe starting dose (MSSD) for patients with MF (PMF and post-PV/ET) who have baseline platelet counts $<100 \times 10^9/L$. This is important since as many as 30% of patients with MF may develop platelet counts below these levels at some point during disease course (Gangat et al. 2010). Patients will receive ruxolitinib at initial dose of 5 mg twice daily, with escalation in increments of 5 mg in successive cohorts until the MSSD is determined. Then additional patients will be treated with ruxolitinib at the MSSD to confirm activity and safety. The other clinical trial (NCT01340651) will explore the activity and toxicity of a sustained release formulation of ruxolitinib administered to 40 patients with PMF or post-PV/ET MF. After 16 weeks of therapy with the sustained release formulation, patients will transition to an equivalent regimen of immediate release, twice daily ruxolitinib.

18.2.2.2 Ruxolitinib for PV and ET

A phase II trial is also evaluating ruxolitinib for patients with hydroxyurea-refractory or intolerant PV and ET (NCT00726232). Additional inclusion criteria included hematocrit (Hct) >45% or dependence on phlebotomies (for patients with PV) and platelet count $>650 \times 10^9/L$ (for patients with ET). Results were presented recently in an abstract form (Verstovsek et al. 2010c). A total of 73 patients were enrolled (PV = 34; ET = 39). Best clinically active dose was determined to be 10 mg twice daily for PV and 25 mg twice daily for ET.

In PV, therapy with ruxolitinib led to a hematocrit <45% in the absence of phlebotomies in 97% of patients, and all continued to maintain response at last follow-up. There was also improvement (≥50%) in splenomegaly (59% of those evaluable), normalization of leukocytosis ($\geq 15 \times 10^9/L$) and thrombocytosis ($\geq 650 \times 10^9/L$) in 63% and 69%, respectively. Complete remission (CR) rate was 62%, and 38% had a partial response (PR), for an overall response rate (ORR) of 100%. Patients also reported improvement in pruritus, night sweats, and bone pain. Side effects included anemia (all grades, 74%; grade 3–4, 0%), thrombocytopenia (all grades, 29%; grade 3–4, 6%), leukopenia (grade 1–2, only 15%) and weight gain (grade 1–2, only 15%).

For patients with ET, therapy with ruxolitinib normalized platelet counts to ≤ upper limit of normal after a median of 0.5 months in 49% of patients. Among four patients with palpable splenomegaly, all experienced ≥50% reduction or normalization in spleen size. ORR was 62% (CR: 41%; PR 21%). More common side effects were anemia (grade 1–2, only 74%) and weight gain (grade 1–2, only 23%). Grade 3 adverse events were leukopenia ($N = 2$), peripheral neuropathy ($N = 1$) and GI disturbances ($N = 1$).

A decrease in the JAK2 V617F allele burden of at least 20% was obtained in 42% of PV patients and 56% of ET patients. However, similar to MF, clinical responses were unrelated to the presence of the JAK2 V617F mutation and/or reduction in JAK2 V617F mutated allele burden.

Currently, there is a randomized, open-label phase III trial for patients with PV underway. The RESPONSE trial (study of efficacy and safety in polycythemia vera subjects who are resistant to or intolerant of hydroxyurea: JAK Inhibitor INC424 (INCB018424) tablets versus best available care) (NCT01243944) compares ruxolitinib (initial dose 10 mg twice daily) to best available therapy in patients with hydroxyurea-refractory or hydroxyurea-intolerant PV. Primary endpoint is the proportion of patients who achieve a response (absence of phlebotomy requirement and ≥35% reduction from baseline in spleen volume as determined by MRI/CT) at 32 weeks of therapy. Secondary endpoints include the percentage of patients who achieve CR at 32 weeks and the percentage of all randomized patients who both achieve response at 32 weeks and maintain that response for ≥48 weeks from the time response was initially documented. The study has recently started, with an estimated enrolment of 300 patients. Results are expected in 2013.

18.2.2.3 TG101348

TG101348 is an orally available, selective JAK2 inhibitor. TG101348 has selective activity against JAK2 (IC50=3 nM) when compared to JAK1 (IC50=105 nM) and JAK3 (IC50=996 nM) (Geron et al. 2008; Wernig et al. 2008). In preclinical studies, TG101348 inhibited JAK2 activity and phosphorylation of downstream targets, induced apoptosis of JAK2 V617F–positive cells and had activity in a murine model of PV (Geron et al. 2008; Wernig et al. 2008).

Results of a phase I/II trial with TG101348 were recently published (Pardanani et al. 2011). In this study, 59 patients with high- or intermediate-risk MF (PMF or post-PV/ET) received treatment with TG101348 in successive dose escalation cohorts ranging from 30 to 800 mg once daily, in a classic 3 + 3 design, with expansion at MTD. JAK2 V617F mutation was positive in 86% of cases, splenomegaly ≥10 cm could be found in 83% of patients, and 36% were transfusion dependent. The MTD was 680 mg once daily, and DLTs included asymptomatic grade 3–4 hyperamylasemia and

hyperlipasemia. Most frequent non-hematological side effects included nausea (all grades, 69.5%; grade 3–4, 3.4%), vomiting (all grades, 57.6%; grade 3–4, 3.4%), diarrhea (all grades, 64.4%; grade 3–4, 10.2%) and abdominal pain (grade 1–2, only 10.2%). Myelosuppressive complications included new-onset transfusion-dependent anemia (grade 3–4, 35.1%) and thrombocytopenia (grade 3–4, 23.7%). Among patients treated at the MTD cohort, incidence of grade 3–4 anemia and thrombocytopenia was 54.2% and 27%, respectively. Similar to other compounds, responses consisted of improvement in spleen size, systemic symptoms, and decreased PB cell counts. After six cycles of therapy, a CI in splenomegaly by IWG-MRT criteria was observed in 39% of patients, and 45% of those in the MTD cohort. There was significant improvement in systemic symptoms after 2–6 cycles of therapy: early satiety (56% complete resolution), fatigue (63% improvement), night sweats (64% complete resolution), cough (67% complete resolution), and pruritus (50% complete resolution). Normalization of WBC count and platelet count was observed in 56% and 90% of patients who presented with leukocytosis and thrombocytosis. No improvement in transfusion-dependent anemia was observed. Median JAK2 V617F allele burden at beginning of therapy was 20% (range 3–100%), with 45% of patients having an allele burden greater than 20% (median 60%; range 23–100%). There was a decrease in JAK2 V617F allele burden after six cycles, with a median value of 17% (p=0.04). Results were more dramatic for the subgroup with high JAK2 V617F allele burden, who had a median allele burden of 31% (p=0.002) after six cycles of therapy. Currently, patients enrolled in the phase I/II trial have been transferred to an extension study (NCT00724334) to evaluate long-term effects of TG101348. Future clinical trials with this drug will evaluate different dose schedules in order to decrease side effects and maintain the efficacy, followed by a phase III study for patients with MF.

18.2.2.4 CYT387

The compound CYT387 (YM Biosciences Inc., Mississauga, Canada) is a novel dual JAK1/JAK2 inhibitor in clinical trials for patients with MF. In vitro CYT387 inhibits JAK1, JAK2, and TYK2 with IC50 values of 11, 18, and 17 nM, respectively (Tyner et al. 2010), while having no activity against JAK3 (IC50 = 155 nM). CYT387 inhibited cell lines dependent on JAK2, such as EPOR-JAK2 V617F transduced Ba/F3 cells (IC50 = 500 nM), Ba/F3 cells transduced with MPLW515L (IC50 = 200 nM) and endogenous erythroid colonies from patients with JAK2 V617F–positive PV (Pardanani et al. 2009; Tyner et al. 2010). Inhibition of proliferation was associated with apoptosis and decreased phosphorylation of JAK2, ERK1/2, and STAT5, consistent with on target activity (Tyner et al. 2010). In an animal model of PV-like MPN, treatment with CYT387 normalized leukocytosis, erythrocytosis, and spleen size (Tyner et al. 2010). Normalization of pro-inflammatory cytokines was also observed.

Initial results of a phase I/II clinical trial with CYT387 (NCT00935987) have been presented in abstract form (Pardanani et al. 2010). Sixty patients were recruited; 80% had a spleen size ≥10 cm, and 55% were transfusion dependent. Twenty-three percent of patients had failed a previous JAK2 inhibitor (either TG101348 or ruxolitinib). MTD was determined to be 300 mg/day, and DLT included grade 3 headache and grade 3 hyperlipasemia at 400 mg/day. Currently, the study is being expanded at the MTD, aiming for a total of 140 patients recruited. Improvement in pruritus was documented in 92% of patients, alongside improvements in night sweats, bone pain, and fever. A reduction in splenomegaly ≥50% to qualify as a CI by IWG-MRT criteria occurred in 47% of patients. More strikingly was the response observed in anemia. Fifty percent of evaluable patients had an anemia CI by IWG-MRT criteria. Among 19 evaluable patients who received the MTD of 300 mg/day, 56% had a response. The response rate was 69% in 16 transfusion-dependent patients treated at the MTD. Grade 3–4 myelosuppressive complications included anemia (7%), thrombocytopenia (26%), and neutropenia (5%). Other common side effects were nausea (grade 1, only 15%), diarrhea (grade 1, only 12%), increased transaminases (all grades, 23%; grade 3, 3%) and increased bilirubin (grade 1, 16%). The beneficial effect of CYT387 in Hb level in patients with MF has not been observed with other JAK2 inhibitors in clinical trials. Further maturation of data and results of this study are awaited in the near future.

18.2.2.5 Other JAK2 Inhibitors in Clinical Development

CEP-701 (lestaurtinib) is an indolocarbazole alkaloid that has activity as a FLT3 and JAK2 (IC50 = 1 nM) inhibitor (Hexner et al. 2008). One single centre phase II trial treated 22 patients with JAK2 V617F–positive MF with CEP-701, and responses were seen in six patients only (27%), consisting of reduction in splenomegaly ($N=3$), reduction in splenomegaly with improvement in cytopenias ($N=2$) and transfusion independency ($N=1$) (Santos et al. 2010). Main toxicities were cytopenias and gastrointestinal disturbances. Another phase I/II clinical trial (NCT00668421) is exploring the possibility that different preparation of CEP-701 might have increased efficacy in treating patients with MF. However, preliminary results have demonstrated at best modest efficacy (Hexner et al. 2009), and final results are awaited. Pharmacological issues may hamper the efficacy of CEP-701 by limiting its ability to inhibit target kinases. In a clinical trial of patients with relapsed FLT3-mutated AML who were randomized between salvage chemotherapy and salvage chemotherapy plus CEP-701, there was a strong correlation between achieving FLT3 inhibition and CR rate (39% [FLT3 inhibition] versus 9% [no FLT3 inhibition]; $p=0.004$) (Levis et al. 2011). Lack of FLT3 inhibition was associated with variable levels of CEP-701, due to binding to plasma proteins such as alpha1-glycoprotein acid.

The JAK2 inhibitor SB1518 has selective activity against JAK2 (IC50 = 19 nM), and inhibits proliferation of JAK2 V617F–positive cells in association with decreased JAK2 and STAT5 phosphorylation. Two phase I clinical trials (NCT00719836 and NCT00745550) are evaluating SB1518 for therapy of MF, and preliminary results have been reported for both (Seymour et al. 2010; Verstovsek et al. 2010a). MTD was 500 mg/day in both trials, but the dose of 400 mg/day was chosen for phase II evaluation since there is no increase in plasma drug levels above this dosage. In one study, there was significant reduction in spleen size and systemic symptoms (Verstovsek et al. 2010a). Toxicities included diarrhea (81%; grade 3, 6%), nausea (grade 1–2, only 41%) and vomiting (grade 1–2, 22%). One advantage of SB1518 over other JAK2 inhibitors is that it appears not to be myelosuppressive, and the drug can be safely used in patients with platelet count $<100 \times 10^9$/L (Seymour et al. 2010; Verstovsek et al. 2010a). Phase 3 study of this agent in MF is planned.

The selective JAK2 inhibitor AZD1480 was shown to inhibit JAK2 activity and phosphorylation of STAT5 in Ba/F3 cells transduced with the chimeric protein TEL-JAK2 (Hedvat et al. 2009). No activity against TEL-JAK1, TEL-JAK3, and TEL-TYK2 was seen, confirming the selectivity of AZD1480 against JAK2 (Hedvat et al. 2009). AZD1480 reduced tumor growth in xenograft models of solid tumor cell lines, and the compound is currently being evaluated in a phase I/II clinical trial in patients with PMF and post-PV/ET MF (NCT00910728).

Most JAK2 inhibitors in clinical development affect both mutated and wild-type JAK2. That would be expected since the mutation is located in the pseudokinase domain, and these drugs compete with adenosine triphosphate (ATP) for the ATP binding site on the tyrosine kinase domain. Recently, results of pre-clinical studies with the JAK2 inhibitor LY2784544 were presented (Ma et al. 2010). In vitro, LY2784544 has selective activity against the mutated JAK2 V617F. LY2784544 inhibited JAK2 V617F signaling at a concentration 41-fold lower than JAK2 wild type (IC50 = 55 nM [V617F] versus 2.260 nM [wild type]) (Ma et al. 2010). LY2784544 preferentially inhibited proliferation on JAK2 V617F–positive cells as compared with wild-type JAK2 cells (IC50 = 113 nM versus 1,356 nM). In a mouse model of MPN, LY2784544 decreased the burden of mutated JAK2 V617F cells but had no effect on unmutated erythroid cells. Currently, a phase I/II trial (NCT01134120) is underway to confirm the selectivity of LY2784544 for JAK2 V617F and determine whether this would reflect in the side effect profile of the drug.

18.3 Histone Deacetylase Inhibitors

18.3.1 Rationale

Epigenetics are biochemical modifications of chromatin that regulate gene expression without affecting DNA sequencing (Herman and Baylin 2003). Main epigenetic mechanisms are DNA methylation and post-transcriptional histone modifications (e.g., acetylation, methylation). Epigenetic abnormalities in cancer cells can lead to silencing of tumor suppressor genes (Herman and Baylin 2003). Several post-transcriptional histone modifications can occur which modulate gene expression. Histone acetylation of lysine residues is typically associated with increased gene expression (Marks et al. 2001). Histone acetylation is modulated through acetylases (HATs, histone acetyltransferases) and deacetylases (HDACs, histone deacetylases). Besides histones, HDACs can deacetylate several other target proteins, including transcription factors (e.g., p53, STAT1, STAT3), signaling mediators, steroid receptors, chaperone proteins (heat shock protein 90 [Hsp90]) and DNA repair enzymes (Ku70) (Xu et al. 2007). Acetylation of the chaperone protein Hsp90 prevents its association with client proteins, such as BCR-ABL and JAK2 (Bali et al. 2005; Wang et al. 2009). Inhibition of Hsp90 leads to client protein degradation by the proteasome (Bali et al. 2005).

A series of epigenetic abnormalities has been described in Ph-negative MPNs. We have already mentioned the effect of JAK2 V617F on histone H3Y41 phosphorylation status and its implication for gene expression regulation (Dawson et al. 2009). Wang et al. described increased activity of several histone deacetylases, particularly those of class I (HDACs 1, 2, 8) and class III, in MF cells (Wang et al. 2008). In another study, increased expression of genes for HDACs 6, 9, and 11 were found in samples from patients with MPNs compared to controls (Skov et al. 2010). More recently, mutations of genes involved in epigenetic regulation of gene expression have been described in patients with Ph-negative MPNs, including *EZH2* (Ernst et al. 2010), *TET2* (Ko et al. 2010) and *DNMT3A* (Abdel-Wahab et al. 2011).

HDAC inhibitors (HDACIs) are compounds which inhibit activity of HDACs and can lead to increased histone acetylation and gene expression. In pre-clinical studies, several HDAC inhibitors have demonstrated activity against JAK2 V617F–positive cells. Some of HDACIs in clinical trials for MPNs include givinostat (formerly known as ITF2357; Italfarmaco, Milan, Italy) and panobinostat (formerly known as LBH589; Novartis, Basel, Switzerland). Givinostat is a synthetic class I HDACI (Guerini et al. 2008; Rambaldi et al. 2010). In vitro, givinostat preferentially inhibited proliferation of JAK2 V617F cells compared to JAK2 wild-type cells (Guerini et al. 2008). This was associated with decreased intracellular levels of total and phosphorylated JAK2 V617F and phosphorylated STAT3 and STAT5. There was no change in JAK2 V617F mRNA, indicating that down-modulation of JAK2 V617F occurred most probably at the protein level (Guerini et al. 2008). The HDACI panobinostat induced JAK2 V617F degradation by the proteasome and was synergic with the JAK2 inhibitor TG101209 in inducing apoptosis of BM mononuclear CD34+ cell from patients with MF (Wang et al. 2009). Wang et al. also demonstrated that panobinostat inhibited JAK2 V617F phosphorylation and phosphorylation of downstream messengers, including STAT3, STAT5, Akt, and ERK1/2 (Wang et al. 2009).

18.3.2 Current Clinical Trials

A pilot study with givinostat in MF was recently published (Rambaldi et al. 2010). Twenty-nine patients with JAK2 V617F–positive MPNs (PV = 12, ET = 1, MF = 16) received treatment with givinostat 50 mg twice daily. Responses were seen in 54% of PV/ET patients (CR = 1, PR = 6) according to European LeukemiaNet criteria (Barosi et al. 2009). Responses in MF were more modest, only three of 16 patients had a major response. Side effects included diarrhea (62%, mostly grade 1–2), anemia (21%, mostly grade 1–2), thrombocytopenia (10%), fatigue (17%), and QTc elongation (17%) (Rambaldi et al. 2010). There is a phase II clinical trial with

givinostat ongoing for patients with PV who did not respond to hydroxyurea (NCT00928707). Patients will be randomized between two doses of givinostat (50 mg once or twice daily) to be used in combination with the maximum tolerated dose of hydroxyurea already in use before study beginning. Endpoints include the response rate at 12 weeks of therapy, safety, and molecular responses at 24 weeks of treatment.

Panobinostat was evaluated in a phase I trial for patients with hematological malignancies, including 13 patients with MF (DeAngelo et al. 2009). Most patients received panobinostat thrice weekly, and the MTD was 60 mg/dose. Grade 3–4 side effects included thrombocytopenia (33%), fatigue (28%, DLT), neutropenia (28%), and anemia (12%). Among the 13 patients with MF, four had CI by IWG-MRT criteria, including one patient who became transfusion independent. These results were followed by two studies evaluating panobinostat solely in patients with MF (Mascarenhas et al. 2009; DeAngelo et al. 2010). Mascarenhas et al. reported on a phase I study in 15 MF patients (NCT01298934); the drug was given at doses ranging from 20 to 30 mg thrice weekly, and MTD had not been determined. Thrombocytopenia was the DLT. Responses were seen in four patients, all CI with reduction in splenomegaly (Mascarenhas et al. 2009). In another trial presented last year (NCT00931762), 31 patients with MF were treated with panobinostat (initial dose: 60 mg thrice weekly) (DeAngelo et al. 2010). Treatment with panobinostat led to depletion of phosphorylated JAK2 V617F, STAT3, STAT5, Akt, and ERK1/2. Interestingly, there was a decrease in the allele burden ranging from 10% to 90%. Clinical response data is still not mature but will be presented in the near future.

18.4 Mammalian Target of Rapamycin Inhibitors

18.4.1 Rationale

The PI3K-Akt-mTOR pathway is abnormally activated in several types of cancer (Panwalkar et al. 2004). In erythroid cells, activation of the

PI3K pathway occurs in response to EPO stimulation and leads to resistance to apoptosis and increased proliferation by downregulation of the cyclin-dependent kinase inhibitor p27 (Bouscary et al. 2003). PI3K can be activated directly by JAK2, and this leads to downstream activation of the serine/threonine kinase Akt and subsequently mTOR (Al-Shami and Naccache 1999). Activated mTOR is a serine/threonine kinase which regulates cell growth, proliferation, and metabolism (Panwalkar et al. 2004). Disruption of the PI3K-Akt-mTOR pathway can be demonstrated in JAK2 V617F–positive MPNs, which show increased phosphorylation and activity of Akt (James et al. 2005; Grimwade et al. 2009).

18.4.2 Current Clinical Trials

Rapamycin (sirolimus) is the first mTOR inhibitor to be discovered; it is currently used mostly as an immunosuppressant in solid organ transplantation. More recently, new mTOR inhibitors were developed, such as everolimus (RAD001; Novartis), which is a 40-O-(2-hydroxyethyl) derivative of sirolimus. Everolimus was tested in 30 patients with MF in a phase I/II clinical trial (Vannucchi et al. 2010). The MTD was determined to be 10 mg/daily. Most common side effects included mouth ulcers, hypertriglicerydemia, and anemia. Fifty-two percent of evaluable patients reported disappearance of systemic symptoms, and pruritus improved in 74% of cases. According to IWG-MRT criteria, the CI rate was 23%, with reduction in splenomegaly. Correlative studies demonstrated a reduction in levels of cyclin D1 (an mTOR target gene) but no changes in JAK2 V617F allele burden (Vannucchi et al. 2010).

18.5 Immunomodulatory Drugs

18.5.1 Rationale

Immunomodulatory drugs (IMiDs) are medications which modulate immune responses and have diverse anti-cytokine and anti-angiogenic activities (Corral et al. 1999). In Ph-negative MPNs, particularly MF, there is a systemic deregulation of the immunologic milieu, with increased levels of pro-inflammatory and fibrogenic cytokines such as IL-2R, IL-8, IL-12, IL-15, transforming growth factor-beta1 (TGF-β1), bone morphogenetic protein 1 (BMP1), tumor necrosis factor-α (TNF-α), and vascular endothelial growth factor (VEGF) (Lundberg et al. 2000; Schmitt et al. 2000; Ciurea et al. 2007; Bock et al. 2008; Tefferi et al. 2011). Pro-inflammatory cytokines are related to development of systemic symptoms and are associated with worse survival in MF (Tefferi et al. 2011). There are three available IMiDs: thalidomide, lenalidomide, and pomalidomide. Thalidomide was the first IMiD to be evaluated in MF (Barosi et al. 2001). Response rates, by IWG-MRT criteria, are in the range of 28–32%, either alone or in combination with prednisone (Jabbour et al. 2009; Thapaliya et al. 2011). Lenalidomide is a much more potent thalidomide derivative. Three clinical trials with lenalidomide have been published in MF (one single agent; two in combination with prednisone) (Tefferi et al. 2006; Quintas-Cardama et al. 2009; Mesa et al. 2010). Response rate is 23–30%, with improvements seen in anemia (19–30%) and splenomegaly (10–42%) (Quintas-Cardama et al. 2009; Mesa et al. 2010).

18.5.2 Current Clinical Trials

Pomalidomide (formerly CC-4047; Celgene) is a thalidomide analog which has 10,000-fold greater anti-TNF-α activity (Galustian et al. 2009). The first published study of pomalidomide evaluated 84 patients with MF who were randomized among four arms: pomalidomide 2 mg daily plus placebo ($N=22$), pomalidomide 2 mg daily plus prednisone ($N=19$), pomalidomide 0.5 mg daily plus prednisone ($N=22$) and prednisone alone ($N=21$) (Tefferi et al. 2009). Observed benefit was limited to improvement in Hb, and response rates were 23% (pomalidomide 2 mg + placebo), 16% (pomalidomide 2 mg + prednisone), 36% (pomalidomide 0.5 mg + prednisone) and 19% (prednisone alone). Thrombocytopenia (11%) and anemia (10%) were the most common side effects, but overall, the drug was very well tolerated. In a phase I/II trial, the MTD of pomalidomide was determined to be 3.0 mg/day, and DLT was myelosuppression (Mesa et al. 2009). In accordance with the results of the randomized study, better response rates were observed in patients who received low-dose pomalidomide (63% CI in anemia).

Currently, there are four ongoing studies with pomalidomide for MF. Begna et al. reported in abstract form the results of a phase II study of low-dose pomalidomide alone (0.5 mg/day) in 58 patients with MF (NCT00669578) (Begna et al. 2010). The main eligibility criterion was transfusion dependence or Hb < 10 g/dL. The rate of CI in anemia was 17% by IWG-MRT criteria. An increase in platelet count in thrombocytopenic patients was observed in 58% of cases. No patient had an improvement in splenomegaly. Interestingly, the JAK2 V617F mutation was a positive predictive marker of response (RR 24% [positive] versus 0% [negative]; $p = 0.03$). Responders developed basophilia in the first month of therapy (RR 38% [present] versus 6% [absent]; $p = 0.02$) and did not have marked splenomegaly (38% versus 11%; $p = 0.05$). Two other phase II studies of similar design are currently being conducted (NCT00946270 and NCT00949364), but no results are available at the time of this writing. A phase III randomized study of pomalidomide versus placebo in patients with MF who are transfusion dependent (NCT01178281) is also underway. Patients will be randomized to either pomalidomide (0.5 mg/day) or placebo; primary endpoint is rate of transfusion independence after 6 months of therapy.

18.6 Anti-fibrotic Drugs

18.6.1 Rationale

As mentioned, in MF, there is an increased production of cytokines associated with BM fibrosis and osteosclerosis, such as TGF-β and BMP-1 (Castro-Malaspina et al. 1981; Kimura et al. 1989; Martyre et al. 1994; Rameshwar et al. 1994; Ciurea et al. 2007). In mouse models of thrombopoietin-induced MF, transplantation of TGF-β-null murine hematopoietic cells retrovirally transduced with murine TPO does not elicit BM fibrosis into recipient mice, despite eliciting other features of the disease including leukocytosis and thrombocytosis (Chagraoui et al. 2002). This suggests that TGF-β has a central role in the pathogenesis of fibrotic BM seen in this disorder.

18.6.2 Current Clinical Trials

GC1008 (Genzyme, Cambridge, MA) is a monoclonal antibody (IgG4) that targets and binds TGF-β proteins. Results of a phase I study in patients with metastatic, advanced melanoma and renal cell cancer were presented (Morris et al. 2008). The MTD was 15 mg/kg/dose. No DLT was observed. Side effects included rash, fatigue, headache, epistaxis, and diarrhea (Morris et al. 2008). Currently, a phase I trial (NCT01291784) in patients with MF is being conducted. Patients will receive a starting dose of 1 mg/kg/dose every 4 weeks for six applications.

18.7 Bisphosphonates

18.7.1 Rationale

In MF, increased bone formation with osteosclerosis can be observed in BM biopsies (Thiele and Kvasnicka 2005), and patients frequently complain of bone pain (Mesa et al. 2007). Histomorphometric studies in MF have revealed an uncoupling between bone formation and reabsorption, with a resultant increase in osteoblasts' activity and a decreased number of osteoclasts (Schmidt et al. 2007). The dysplastic megakaryocytes of MF probably play a role in the abnormal bone metabolism observed, as megakaryocytes can increase osteoblasts activity and inhibit osteoclasts (Kacena et al. 2006). In two mouse models of MF, the GATA-1 low and the TPO-high mice, there is an increased number of megakaryocytes, accompanied by an increased bone mass and osteosclerosis (Yan et al. 1996; Vannucchi et al. 2002; Kacena et al. 2004). Increased levels of TGF-β and osteoprotegerin are probably related to the increased in bone formation seen in MF (Chagraoui et al. 2002, 2003; Kakumitsu et al. 2005).

Bisphosphonates (BPPs) are organic analogs of the pyrophosphate molecule, with a carbon atom substituting the central oxygen atom. BPPs inhibit bone absorption by osteoclasts, re-establishing the equilibrium between bone re-absorption and bone formation (Rodan and Fleisch 1996). BPPs are used for treating several non-malignant and malignant conditions, such as osteoporosis, Paget's disease of the bone, solid tumors bone metastasis, and multiple myeloma. Even though there is increased bone formation in MF, BPPs indirectly diminish bone formation by decreasing bone absorption and bone turnover (Chavassieux et al. 1997). In this regard, BPPs have been successfully used for treatment of predominantly osteoblastic (with increased bone formation) metastatic lesions of prostate cancer. Thus, BPPs could potentially have a role in MF by reverting the increased bone turnover seen in this disorder (Diamond et al. 2002).

18.7.2   Current Clinical Trials

At the present time, activity of BPPs in patients with MF is limited to case reports. Sivera et al. reported on a patient with MF who was treated with oral etidronate (6 mg/kg/day on alternate months) due to severe bone pain (Sivera et al. 1994). After 3 months of therapy, there was complete disappearance of pain and fever, and this was associated with a significant improvement in Hb and WBC. In another report, therapy with clodronate (30 mg/kg/day) led to transfusion independence and reversal of BM fibrosis in a single patient with MF (Froom et al. 2002). In other reports, there was efficacy of BPPs for treating bone pain associated with MF (Perkins et al. 2004; Assous et al. 2005). Currently, there is one clinical trial with BPPs ongoing in MF (NCT00287261). In this international, multi-center phase II trial, patients with MF requiring therapy will receive zoledronic acid (4 mg/dose) infusions every 3 weeks for a total of 12 infusions. Primary endpoint is the effect of zoledronic

acid on Hb level and spleen size. Other endpoints include measures of safety and toxicity in this patient population, effect on transfusion needs, LDH, WBC count, platelets, constitutional symptoms, performance status, and BM histology. Trial has been completed, but no results have been presented so far.

Conclusions

In recent years, the outlook for patients with chronic Ph-negative MPNs has changed with new discoveries on molecular biology of these diseases and the subsequent development of new compounds directed against those molecular defects. With standardization of diagnostic and response criteria, the reporting of clinical trials will be more uniform and will facilitate analysis of results obtained with different agents. JAK2 inhibitors and other compounds, such as pomalidomide, are on the verge of making the transition from clinical trials to routine clinical use. There is still much room for improvement though. We need to better understand how these drugs work, and through which mechanism(s) they are producing benefits for individual patients. We need biomarkers to determine which patients will respond to a specific agent. And, similarly to conventional chemotherapy used for treating solid tumors and other hematological malignancies, we need to study combination therapy, to see if there is any improvement in the response rate when the medications are combined. With coordinated efforts and appropriate design of clinical trials, we can hope to overcome these challenges and improve outcomes for patients with these diseases, not just in controlling disease signs and symptoms but potentially in eliminating it.

References

Abdel-Wahab O, Pardanani A, Rampal R et al (2011) DNMT3A mutational analysis in primary myelofibrosis, chronic myelomonocytic leukemia and advanced phases of myeloproliferative neoplasms. Leukemia. doi:10.1038/leu.2011.82

Al-Shami A, Naccache PH (1999) Granulocyte-macrophage colony-stimulating factor-activated signaling pathways in human neutrophils. Involvement of Jak2 in the stimulation of phosphatidylinositol 3-kinase. J Biol Chem 274:5333–5338

Assous N, Foltz V, Fautrel B et al (2005) Bone involvement in myelofibrosis: effectiveness of bisphosphonates. Joint Bone Spine 72:591–592

Bali P, Pranpat M, Bradner J et al (2005) Inhibition of histone deacetylase 6 acetylates and disrupts the chaperone function of heat shock protein 90: a novel basis for antileukemia activity of histone deacetylase inhibitors. J Biol Chem 280:26729–26734

Bannister AJ, Zegerman P, Partridge JF et al (2001) Selective recognition of methylated lysine 9 on histone H3 by the HP1 chromo domain. Nature 410:120–124

Barosi G, Grossi A, Comotti B et al (2001) Safety and efficacy of thalidomide in patients with myelofibrosis with myeloid metaplasia. Br J Haematol 114:78–83

Barosi G, Bergamaschi G, Marchetti M et al (2007) JAK2 V617F mutational status predicts progression to large splenomegaly and leukemic transformation in primary myelofibrosis. Blood 110:4030–4036

Barosi G, Birgegard G, Finazzi G et al (2009) Response criteria for essential thrombocythemia and polycythemia vera: result of a European LeukemiaNet consensus conference. Blood 113:4829–4833

Baxter EJ, Scott LM, Campbell PJ et al (2005) Acquired mutation of the tyrosine kinase JAK2 in human myeloproliferative disorders. Lancet 365:1054–1061

Begna K, Mesa RA, Pardanani A et al (2010) A phase-2 trial of low-dose pomalidomide in myelofibrosis with anemia [abstract]. Blood 116: Abstract 4109

Begna KH, Mesa RA, Pardanani A et al (2011) A phase-2 trial of low-dose pomalidomide in myelofibrosis. Leukemia 25:301–304

Bock O, Hoftmann J, Theophile K et al (2008) Bone morphogenetic proteins are overexpressed in the bone marrow of primary myelofibrosis and are apparently induced by fibrogenic cytokines. Am J Pathol 172: 951–960

Bouscary D, Pene F, Claessens YE et al (2003) Critical role for PI 3-kinase in the control of erythropoietin-induced erythroid progenitor proliferation. Blood 101:3436–3443

Castro-Malaspina H, Rabellino EM, Yen A et al (1981) Human megakaryocyte stimulation of proliferation of bone marrow fibroblasts. Blood 57:781–787

Cervantes F, Dupriez B, Pereira A et al (2009) New prognostic scoring system for primary myelofibrosis based on a study of the International Working Group for Myelofibrosis Research and Treatment. Blood 113:2895–2901

Chagraoui H, Komura E, Tulliez M et al (2002) Prominent role of TGF-beta 1 in thrombopoietin-induced myelofibrosis in mice. Blood 100:3495–3503

Chagraoui H, Tulliez M, Smayra T et al (2003) Stimulation of osteoprotegerin production is responsible for osteosclerosis in mice overexpressing TPO. Blood 101: 2983–2989

Chavassieux PM, Arlot ME, Reda C et al (1997) Histomorphometric assessment of the long-term effects of alendronate on bone quality and remodeling in patients with osteoporosis. J Clin Invest 100: 1475–1480

Ciurea SO, Merchant D, Mahmud N et al (2007) Pivotal contributions of megakaryocytes to the biology of idiopathic myelofibrosis. Blood 110:986–993

Corral LG, Haslett PA, Muller GW et al (1999) Differential cytokine modulation and T cell activation by two distinct classes of thalidomide analogues that are potent inhibitors of TNF-alpha. J Immunol 163:380–386

Dawson MA, Bannister AJ, Gottgens B et al (2009) JAK2 phosphorylates histone H3Y41 and excludes HP1alpha from chromatin. Nature 461:819–822

DeAngelo DJ, Spencer A, Fischer T et al (2009) Activity of oral Panobinostat (LBH589) in patients with myelofibrosis [abstract]. Blood 114:Abstract 2898

DeAngelo DJ, Tefferi A, Fiskus W et al (2010) A phase II trial of Panobinostat, an orally available deacetylase inhibitor (DACi), in patients with primary myelofibrosis (PMF), post essential thrombocythemia (ET), and post polycythemia vera (PV) myelofibrosis [abstract]. Blood 116:Abstract 630

Diamond T, Smith A, Schnier R et al (2002) Syndrome of myelofibrosis and osteosclerosis: a series of case reports and review of the literature. Bone 30:498–501

Dusa A, Mouton C, Pecquet C et al (2010) JAK2 V617F constitutive activation requires JH2 residue F595: a pseudokinase domain target for specific inhibitors. PLoS One 5:e11157

Ernst T, Chase AJ, Score J et al (2010) Inactivating mutations of the histone methyltransferase gene EZH2 in myeloid disorders. Nat Genet 42:722–726

Froom P, Elmalah I, Braester A et al (2002) Clodronate in myelofibrosis: a case report. Am J Med Sci 323: 115–116

Galustian C, Meyer B, Labarthe MC et al (2009) The anti-cancer agents lenalidomide and pomalidomide inhibit the proliferation and function of T regulatory cells. Cancer Immunol Immunother 58:1033–1045

Gangat N, Caramazza D, Vaidya R et al (2010) DIPSS plus: a refined dynamic international prognostic scoring system for primary myelofibrosis that incorporates prognostic information from karyotype, platelet count, and transfusion status. J Clin Oncol. doi:10.1200/JCO.2010.32.2446

Geron I, Abrahamsson AE, Barroga CF et al (2008) Selective inhibition of JAK2-driven erythroid differentiation of polycythemia vera progenitors. Cancer Cell 13:321–330

Grimwade LF, Happerfield L, Tristram C et al (2009) Phospho-STAT5 and phospho-Akt expression in chronic myeloproliferative neoplasms. Br J Haematol 147:495–506

Guerini V, Barbui V, Spinelli O et al (2008) The histone deacetylase inhibitor ITF2357 selectively targets cells bearing mutated JAK2(V617F). Leukemia 22:740–747

Hedvat M, Huszar D, Herrmann A et al (2009) The JAK2 inhibitor AZD1480 potently blocks Stat3 signaling and oncogenesis in solid tumors. Cancer Cell 16: 487–497

Herman JG, Baylin SB (2003) Gene silencing in cancer in association with promoter hypermethylation. N Engl J Med 349:2042–2054

Hexner EO, Serdikoff C, Jan M et al (2008) Lestaurtinib (CEP701) is a JAK2 inhibitor that suppresses JAK2/STAT5 signaling and the proliferation of primary erythroid cells from patients with myeloproliferative disorders. Blood 111:5663–5671

Hexner E, Goldberg JD, Prchal JT et al (2009) A multicenter, open label phase I/II study of CEP701 (Lestaurtinib) in adults with myelofibrosis; a report on phase I: a study of the myeloproliferative disorders research consortium (MPD-RC) [abstract]. Blood 114:Abstract 754

Incyte (2010) Incyte announces positive top-line results from COMFORT-I pivotal phase III trial of INCB18424 in myelofibrosis, a debilitating, life-threatening blood cancer. Press Release http://investor.incyte.com/phoenix.zhtml?c=69764&p=irol-newsArticle&ID=150951 7&highlight=20December2010

Incyte (2011) Incyte's ruxolitinib (INCB18424) meets primary endpoint in second phase III study. Press release http://investor.incyte.com/phoenix.zhtml?c=69764&p=irol-newsArticle&ID=1539173&highlight=15March2011

Jabbour E, Kantarjian H, Parikh SA et al (2009) Comparison of thalidomide and lenalidomide for the treatment of patients (pts) with myelofibrosis (MF) [abstract]. Blood 114:Abstract 2901

James C, Ugo V, Le Couedic JP et al (2005) A unique clonal JAK2 mutation leading to constitutive signalling causes polycythaemia vera. Nature 434:1144–1148

Kacena MA, Shivdasani RA, Wilson K et al (2004) Megakaryocyte-osteoblast interaction revealed in mice deficient in transcription factors GATA-1 and NF-E2. J Bone Miner Res 19:652–660

Kacena MA, Gundberg CM, Horowitz MC (2006) A reciprocal regulatory interaction between megakaryocytes, bone cells, and hematopoietic stem cells. Bone 39:978–984

Kakumitsu H, Kamezaki K, Shimoda K et al (2005) Transgenic mice overexpressing murine thrombopoietin develop myelofibrosis and osteosclerosis. Leuk Res 29:761–769

Kimura A, Katoh O, Hyodo H et al (1989) Transforming growth factor-beta regulates growth as well as collagen and fibronectin synthesis of human marrow fibroblasts. Br J Haematol 72:486–491

Ko M, Huang Y, Jankowska AM et al (2010) Impaired hydroxylation of 5-methylcytosine in myeloid cancers with mutant TET2. Nature 468:839–843

Kralovics R, Passamonti F, Buser AS et al (2005) A gain-of-function mutation of JAK2 in myeloproliferative disorders. N Engl J Med 352:1779–1790

Kroger N, Holler E, Kobbe G et al (2009) Allogeneic stem cell transplantation after reduced-intensity conditioning in patients with myelofibrosis: a prospective, multicenter study of the Chronic Leukemia Working Party of the European Group for Blood and Marrow Transplantation. Blood 114:5264–5270

Lachner M, O'Carroll D, Rea S et al (2001) Methylation of histone H3 lysine 9 creates a binding site for HP1 proteins. Nature 410:116–120

Lacout C, Pisani DF, Tulliez M et al (2006) JAK2V617F expression in murine hematopoietic cells leads to MPD mimicking human PV with secondary myelofibrosis. Blood 108:1652–1660

Leonard WJ, O'Shea JJ (1998) Jaks and STATs: biological implications. Annu Rev Immunol 16:293–322

Levine RL, Wadleigh M, Cools J et al (2005) Activating mutation in the tyrosine kinase JAK2 in polycythemia vera, essential thrombocythemia, and myeloid metaplasia with myelofibrosis. Cancer Cell 7:387–397

Levis M, Ravandi F, Wang ES et al (2011) Results from a randomized trial of salvage chemotherapy followed by lestaurtinib for patients with FLT3 mutant AML in first relapse. Blood 117:3294–3301

Lindauer K, Loerting T, Liedl KR et al (2001) Prediction of the structure of human Janus kinase 2 (JAK2) comprising the two carboxy-terminal domains reveals a mechanism for autoregulation. Protein Eng 14:27–37

Liu F, Zhao X, Perna F et al (2011) JAK2V617F-mediated phosphorylation of PRMT5 downregulates its methyltransferase activity and promotes myeloproliferation. Cancer Cell 19:283–294

Lundberg LG, Lerner R, Sundelin P et al (2000) Bone marrow in polycythemia vera, chronic myelocytic leukemia, and myelofibrosis has an increased vascularity. Am J Pathol 157:15–19

Ma L, Zhao B, Walgren R et al (2010) Efficacy of LY2784544, a small molecule inhibitor selective for mutant JAK2 kinase, in JAK2 V617F-induced hematologic malignancy models [abstract]. Blood 116:Abstract 4087

Marks P, Rifkind RA, Richon VM et al (2001) Histone deacetylases and cancer: causes and therapies. Nat Rev Cancer 1:194–202

Martyre MC, Romquin N, Le Bousse-Kerdiles MC et al (1994) Transforming growth factor-beta and megakaryocytes in the pathogenesis of idiopathic myelofibrosis. Br J Haematol 88:9–16

Mascarenhas J, Wang X, Rodriguez A et al (2009) A phase I study of LBH589, a novel histone deacetylase inhibitor in patients with primary myelofibrosis (PMF) and post-polycythemia/essential thrombocythemia myelofibrosis (post-PV/ET MF) [abstract]. Blood 114:Abstract 308

Mesa RA, Niblack J, Wadleigh M et al (2007) The burden of fatigue and quality of life in myeloproliferative disorders (MPDs): an international Internet-based survey of 1179 MPD patients. Cancer 109:68–76

Mesa RA, Pardanani AD, Hussein K et al (2009) Phase1/-2 study of Pomalidomide in myelofibrosis. Am J Hematol 85:129–130

Mesa RA, Yao X, Cripe LD et al (2010) Lenalidomide and prednisone for myelofibrosis: Eastern Cooperative

Oncology Group (ECOG) phase 2 trial E4903. Blood 116:4436–4438

Mizuguchi R, Noto S, Yamada M et al (2000) Ras and signal transducer and activator of transcription (STAT) are essential and sufficient downstream components of Janus kinases in cell proliferation. Jpn J Cancer Res 91:527–533

Moliterno AR, Hexner E, Roboz GJ et al (2009) An open-label study of CEP-701 in patients with JAK2 V617F-positive PV and ET: update of 39 enrolled patients [abstract]. Blood 114:Abstract 753

Morris JC, Shapiro GI, Tan AR et al (2008) Phase I/II study of GC1008: a human anti-transforming growth factor-beta (TGFβ) monoclonal antibody (MAb) in patients with advanced malignant melanoma (MM) or renal cell carcinoma (RCC) [abstract]. J Clin Oncol 26:Abstract 9028

Mullally A, Lane SW, Ball B et al (2010) Physiological Jak2V617F expression causes a lethal myeloproliferative neoplasm with differential effects on hematopoietic stem and progenitor cells. Cancer Cell 17:584–596

Panwalkar A, Verstovsek S, Giles FJ (2004) Mammalian target of rapamycin inhibition as therapy for hematologic malignancies. Cancer 100:657–666

Pardanani A, Lasho T, Smith G et al (2009) CYT387, a selective JAK1/JAK2 inhibitor: in vitro assessment of kinase selectivity and preclinical studies using cell lines and primary cells from polycythemia vera patients. Leukemia 23:1441–1445

Pardanani A, George G, Lasho T et al (2010) A phase I/II study of CYT387, an oral JAK-1/2 inhibitor, in myelofibrosis: significant response rates in anemia, splenomegaly, and constitutional symptoms [abstract]. Blood 116:Abstract 460

Pardanani A, Gotlib JR, Jamieson C et al (2011) Safety and efficacy of TG101348, a selective JAK2 inhibitor, in myelofibrosis. J Clin Oncol 29:789–796

Perkins P, Curtin NJ, Green AR et al (2004) Pain from myelofibrosis treated with regular pamidronate. Br J Haematol 127:366–367

Pikman Y, Lee BH, Mercher T et al (2006) MPLW515L is a novel somatic activating mutation in myelofibrosis with myeloid metaplasia. PLoS Med 3:e270

Quintas-Cardama A, Kantarjian HM, Manshouri T et al (2009) Lenalidomide plus prednisone results in durable clinical, histopathologic, and molecular responses in patients with myelofibrosis. J Clin Oncol 27:4760–4766

Quintas-Cardama A, Vaddi K, Liu P et al (2010) Preclinical characterization of the selective JAK1/2 inhibitor INCB018424: implications for the treatment of myeloproliferative neoplasms. Blood 115:3109–3117

Rambaldi A, Dellacasa CM, Finazzi G et al (2010) A pilot study of the histone-deacetylase inhibitor givinostat in patients with JAK2V617F positive chronic myeloproliferative neoplasms. Br J Haematol 150:446–455

Rameshwar P, Denny TN, Stein D et al (1994) Monocyte adhesion in patients with bone marrow fibrosis is required for the production of fibrogenic cytokines.

Potential role for interleukin-1 and TGF-beta. J Immunol 153:2819–2830

Rodan GA, Fleisch HA (1996) Bisphosphonates: mechanisms of action. J Clin Invest 97:2692–2696

Saharinen P, Silvennoinen O (2002) The pseudokinase domain is required for suppression of basal activity of Jak2 and Jak3 tyrosine kinases and for cytokine-inducible activation of signal transduction. J Biol Chem 277:47954–47963

Santos FP, Kantarjian HM, Jain N et al (2010) Phase 2 study of CEP-701, an orally available JAK2 inhibitor, in patients with primary or post-polycythemia vera/essential thrombocythemia myelofibrosis. Blood 115:1131–1136

Schmidt A, Blanchet O, Dib M et al (2007) Bone changes in myelofibrosis with myeloid metaplasia: a histomorphometric and microcomputed tomographic study. Eur J Haematol 78:500–509

Schmitt A, Jouault H, Guichard J et al (2000) Pathologic interaction between megakaryocytes and polymorphonuclear leukocytes in myelofibrosis. Blood 96:1342–1347

Scott LM, Tong W, Levine RL et al (2007) JAK2 exon 12 mutations in polycythemia vera and idiopathic erythrocytosis. N Engl J Med 356:459–468

Seymour JF, To B, Goh A et al (2010) First report of the phase I study of the novel oral JAK2 inhibitor SB1518 in patients with myelofibrosis [abstract]. Haematologica 95 [suppl. 2]:Abstract 1444

Sivera P, Cesano L, Guerrasio A et al (1994) Clinical and haematological improvement induced by etidronate in a patient with idiopathic myelofibrosis and osteosclerosis. Br J Haematol 86:397–398

Skov V, Larsen TS, Thomassen M et al (2010) Increased gene expression of histone deacetylases in patients with Philadelphia-negative chronic myeloproliferative neoplasms [abstract]. Blood 116:Abstract 4119

Swerdlow SH, Campo E, Harris NL et al (2008) World health organization classification of tumours of haematopoietic and lymphoid tissues. IARC Press, Lyon

Tefferi A (2010) Novel mutations and their functional and clinical relevance in myeloproliferative neoplasms: JAK2, MPL, TET2, ASXL1, CBL, IDH and IKZF1. Leukemia 24:1128–1138

Tefferi A (2011) How I treat myelofibrosis. Blood 117:3494–3504

Tefferi A, Cortes J, Verstovsek S et al (2006) Lenalidomide therapy in myelofibrosis with myeloid metaplasia. Blood 108:1158–1164

Tefferi A, Verstovsek S, Barosi G et al (2009) Pomalidomide is active in the treatment of anemia associated with myelofibrosis. J Clin Oncol 27:4563–4569

Tefferi A, Vaidya R, Caramazza D et al (2011) Circulating interleukin (IL)-8, IL-2R, IL-12, and IL-15 levels are independently prognostic in primary myelofibrosis: a comprehensive cytokine profiling study. J Clin Oncol 29:1356–1363

Thapaliya P, Tefferi A, Pardanani A et al (2011) International working group for myelofibrosis research

and treatment response assessment and long-term follow-up of 50 myelofibrosis patients treated with thali-
domide-prednisone based regimens. Am J Hematol
86:96–98

Thiele J, Kvasnicka HM (2005) Hematopathologic findings in chronic idiopathic myelofibrosis. Semin Oncol
32:380–394

Tyner JW, Bumm TG, Deininger J et al (2010) CYT387, a
novel JAK2 inhibitor, induces hematologic responses
and normalizes inflammatory cytokines in murine
myeloproliferative neoplasms. Blood 115:5232–5240

Vannucchi AM, Bianchi L, Cellai C et al (2002)
Development of myelofibrosis in mice genetically
impaired for GATA-1 expression (GATA-1(low)
mice). Blood 100:1123–1132

Vannucchi AM, Guglielmelli P, Lupo L et al (2010) A
phase 1/2 study of RAD001, a mTOR inhibitor, in
patients with myelofibrosis: final results [abstract].
Blood 116:Abstract 314

Verstovsek S, Deeg HJ, Odenike O et al (2010a) Phase 1/2
study of SB1518, a novel JAK2/FLT3 inhibitor, in the
treatment of primary myelofibrosis [abstract]. Blood
116:Abstract 3082

Verstovsek S, Kantarjian H, Mesa RA et al (2010b) Safety
and efficacy of INCB018424, a JAK1 and JAK2 inhibitor, in myelofibrosis. N Engl J Med 363:1117–1127

Verstovsek S, Passamonti F, Rambaldi A et al (2010c)
Durable responses with the JAK1/ JAK2 inhibitor,
INCB018424, in patients with polycythemia vera (PV)
and essential thrombocythemia (ET) refractory or
intolerant to hydroxyurea (HU) [abstract]. Blood
116:Abstract 313

Wang JC, Chen C, Dumlao T et al (2008) Enhanced histone deacetylase enzyme activity in primary myelofibrosis. Leuk Lymphoma 49:2321–2327

Wang Y, Fiskus W, Chong DG et al (2009) Cotreatment
with panobinostat and JAK2 inhibitor TG101209
attenuates JAK2V617F levels and signaling and exerts
synergistic cytotoxic effects against human myeloproliferative neoplastic cells. Blood 114:5024–5033

Wernig G, Mercher T, Okabe R et al (2006) Expression of
Jak2V617F causes a polycythemia vera-like disease
with associated myelofibrosis in a murine bone marrow transplant model. Blood 107:4274–4281

Wernig G, Kharas MG, Okabe R et al (2008) Efficacy of
TG101348, a selective JAK2 inhibitor, in treatment of
a murine model of JAK2V617F-induced polycythemia
vera. Cancer Cell 13:311–320

Winston LA, Hunter T (1995) JAK2, Ras, and Raf are
required for activation of extracellular signal-regulated
kinase/mitogen-activated protein kinase by growth
hormone. J Biol Chem 270:30837–30840

Xu WS, Parmigiani RB, Marks PA (2007) Histone
deacetylase inhibitors: molecular mechanisms of
action. Oncogene 26:5541–5552

Yan XQ, Lacey D, Hill D et al (1996) A model of myelofibrosis and osteosclerosis in mice induced by overexpressing thrombopoietin (mpl ligand): reversal of
disease by bone marrow transplantation. Blood
88:402–409

Yu H, Jove R (2004) The STATs of cancer – new molecular targets come of age. Nat Rev Cancer 4:97–105

Index

T. Barbui and A. Tefferi (eds.), *Myeloproliferative Neoplasms*, Hematologic Malignancies,
DOI 10.1007/978-3-642-24989-1, © Springer-Verlag Berlin Heidelberg 2012